Progress in
Medicine 2021

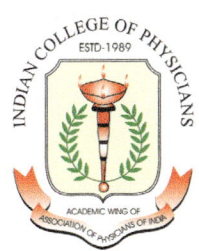

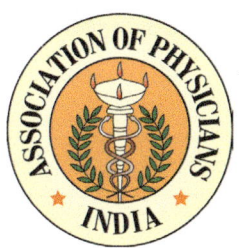

Progress in Medicine 2021

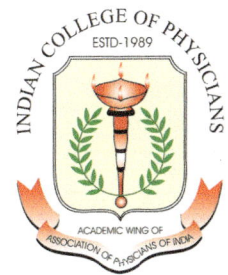 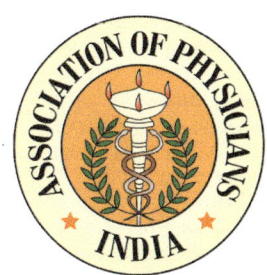

Editor-in-Chief

Shashank R Joshi

MD DM FICP FACP (USA) FACE (USA) FRCP (London, Glasgow and Edinburgh)
(Padma Shri Awardee)
Dean Indian College of Physicians (2020–21)
Past President Association of Physicians of India
Chair, International Diabetes Federation, South East Asia
President Indian Academy of Diabetes
Endocrinologist, Joshi Clinic, Lilavati Hospital, Sir HN Reliance and Bhatia Hospitals
Emeritus Editor JAPI
Past President, Endocrine Society of India, Hypertension Society of India, RSSDI,
International College of Nutrition
Adjunct Faculty, JSS and Jaipur National University
Mumbai, Maharashtra, India

Foreword

YP Munjal

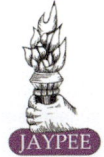

JAYPEE BROTHERS MEDICAL PUBLISHERS
The Health Sciences Publisher
New Delhi | London

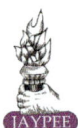 **Jaypee Brothers Medical Publishers (P) Ltd**

Headquarters
EMCA House
23/23-B, Ansari Road, Daryaganj
New Delhi 110 002, India
Landline: +91-11-23272143, +91-11-23272703
+91-11-23282021, +91-11-23245672
E-mail: jaypee@jaypeebrothers.com

Corporate Office
Jaypee Brothers Medical Publishers (P) Ltd.
4838/24, Ansari Road, Daryaganj
New Delhi 110 002, India
Phone: +91-11-43574357
Fax: +91-11-43574314
E-mail: jaypee@jaypeebrothers.com

Overseas Office
JP Medical Ltd.
83, Victoria Street, London
SW1H 0HW (UK)
Phone: +44-20 3170 8910
Fax: +44(0)20 3008 6180
E-mail: info@jpmedpub.com

Website: www.jaypeebrothers.com
Website: www.jaypeedigital.com

© 2022, Jaypee Brothers Medical Publishers

The views and opinions expressed in this book are solely those of the original contributor(s)/author(s) and do not necessarily represent those of editor(s) of the book.

All rights reserved by the author. No part of this publication may be reproduced, stored or transmitted in any form or by any means, electronic, mechanical, photocopying, recording or otherwise, without the prior permission in writing of the publishers.

All brand names and product names used in this book are trade names, service marks, trademarks or registered trademarks of their respective owners. The publisher is not associated with any product or vendor mentioned in this book.

Medical knowledge and practice change constantly. This book is designed to provide accurate, authoritative information about the subject matter in question. However, readers are advised to check the most current information available on procedures included and check information from the manufacturer of each product to be administered, to verify the recommended dose, formula, method and duration of administration, adverse effects and contraindications. It is the responsibility of the practitioner to take all appropriate safety precautions. Neither the publisher nor the author(s)/editor(s) assume any liability for any injury and/or damage to persons or property arising from or related to use of material in this book.

This book is sold on the understanding that the publisher is not engaged in providing professional medical services. If such advice or services are required, the services of a competent medical professional should be sought.

Every effort has been made where necessary to contact holders of copyright to obtain permission to reproduce copyright material. If any have been inadvertently overlooked, the publisher will be pleased to make the necessary arrangements at the first opportunity. The **CD/DVD-ROM** (if any) provided in the sealed envelope with this book is complimentary and free of cost. **It is Not meant for sale.**

Inquiries for bulk sales may be solicited at: jaypee@jaypeebrothers.com

Progress in Medicine 2021 / Shashank R Joshi

First Edition: **2022**

ISBN: 978-93-5465-112-0

Printed at: Replika Press Pvt. Ltd.

Dedication

I dedicate this book to my mentor and my Teacher late Professor Siddarth N Shah and my Father late Professor Rameshchandra D Joshi.

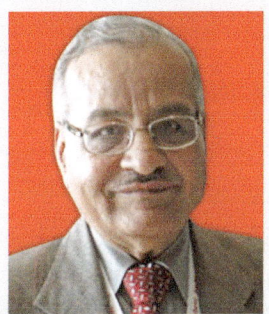
Professor Siddarth N Shah

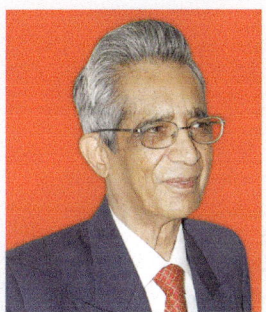
Professor Rameshchandra D Joshi

DISCLAIMER

This book contain views and opinion of group of experts, not policies of Association of Physicians of India or Indian College of Physicians or Editors. The authors/contributors are themselves responsible to get permission to reproduce data/illustrations/figures/tables from other sources. The editors and publishers have accepted manuscripts in good faith and on the condition that all authors have adhered to the highest standards of publication ethics. More and more research publication of original scientific material will change opinion and views of experts of medicine. The editors and publishers have made sincere efforts to ensure information provided in the book is latest. As new data and drugs become available—treatment, concepts and guidelines will change. Readers are thus advised to cross check information provided in this book with the product inserts provided with the drug manufacturers. Readers are advised to cross check any information provided in this book.

CME Committee for eAPICON 2021

Chief Advisor
Dr YP Munjal, Gurugram

Presidents
Dr KK Pareek, Kota   **Dr S Arulrhaj, Tuticorin**   Dr Kamlesh Tewary, Muzaffarpur

Deans
Dr Shashank R Joshi (2020–21)
Dr Amal Kumar Banerjee, Howrah   Dr Rajesh Upadhyay, New Delhi

Members

Dr Mangesh Tiwaskar, Mumbai	**Dr Vikram Londhey, Mumbai**
Dr Charu K Jani, Mumbai	**Dr Shyam Sundar, Varanasi**
Dr Ashit M Bhagwati, Mumbai	**Dr Y Sathyanarayana Raju, Hyderabad**
Dr Narayan G Deogaonkar, Nashik	**Dr Shibendu Ghosh, Hooghli**
Dr Girish Mathur, Kota	**Dr D Selvaraj, Tuticorin**
Dr Liyakhat Ali Gauri, Bikaner	**Dr CL Nawal, Jaipur**
Dr Jyotirmoy Pal, Talbukur	**Dr Nihar Mehta, Mumbai**
Dr Prakash Keswani, Jaipur	**Dr RM Chhabra, New Delhi**
Dr K Mugundhan, Salem	**Dr RN Sarkar, Kolkata**
Dr Narinder Pal Singh, New Delhi	**Dr Devi Ram, Purnea**
Dr Udai Lal, Hyderabad	**Dr Naval Chandra, Hyderabad**
Dr BB Rewari, New Delhi	**Dr Anupam Prakash, New Delhi**
Dr Jai Bhagwan, Gurugram	**Dr Hem Shanker Sharma, Bhagalpur**
Dr Sudhir Mehta, Jaipur	**Dr Agam C Vora, Mumbai**
Dr PS Karmakar, Kolkata	**Dr MPS Chawla, New Delhi**
Dr Aditya P Misra, New Delhi	**Dr V Palaniappan, Guziliamparai**
Dr Sanjiv Maheshwari, Ajmer	**Dr Sekhar Chakraborty, Siliguri**
Dr Soumitra Ghosh, Kolkata	**Dr Munish Prabhakar, Gurugram**
Dr Sandeep Garg, New Delhi	**Dr Devendra Prasad Singh, Bhagalpur**
Dr Shriram V Kulkarni, Khopoli	**Dr Atul Bhasin, New Delhi**
Dr Trupti H Trivedi, Mumbai	**Dr Ashok K Taneja, Gurugram**
Dr AK Mukherjee, Kolkata	**Dr GD Ramchandani, Kota**

CME Committee for eAPICON 2021

Dr M Ravikeerthy, Bangalore
Dr S Chandrasekar, Chennai
Dr Amit Saraf, Mumbai
Dr Jayanta Kumar Panda, Cuttack
Dr Udas C Ghosh, Kolkata
Dr Milind Y Nadkar, Mumbai
Dr Sandhya Kamath, Mumbai

Dr PK Maheshwari, Agra
Dr Puneet Saxena, Jaipur
Dr Gurpreet Singh Wander, Ludhiana
Dr S Sreenivasa Kamath, Kochi
Dr Satya Brata Ganguly, Kolkata
Dr R Rajasekaran, Kumbakonam
Dr Man Mohan Mehndiratta, New Delhi

Editorial Board

Editor-in-Chief
Shashank R Joshi

Executive Editor
Jimit Vadgama
L Srinivas Murthy

Asssociate Editors
Nihar Mehta
Amit Saraf
Agam Vora
Mangesh Tiwaskar

Advisors
BR Bansode
Milind Nadkar
Alaka Deshpande
Amit Ghosh
Trupti Trivedi
Banshi Saboo
A Bhagwati
Vikram Londey
SV Kulkarni

Foreword

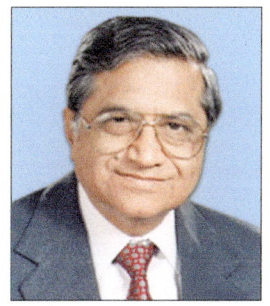

The last 2 years have been dramatically fearful and life changing for many practitioners, teachers, and medical students in the history of medicine. The COVID pandemic has changed the way we interact with each other. It is good we learn the things and how we deliver or distribute the knowledge among us. With the successful completion of the 76th annual virtual conference APICON 2021, we, the members of this scientific committee and the editorial board of the book *Progress in Medicine 2021*, have the pleasure and honor to present this book before you. This book has been a big task as there was an enormous responsibility of making a scientifically excellent book. Although it was very difficult to connect with each other during this pandemic and the editorial process became lengthy and difficult, we had the support of the wonderful editorial team and the prestigious authors.

Various national and international experts have contributed chapters in this book and they have applied science and principal of best of their field. Each and every chapter has been composed thoroughly and has undergone rigorous editorial process. All the chapters reflect the cutting-edge nature of the updates in medicine combined with the clinical knowledge and practical guidance by experienced authors.

This "Progress in Medicine 2021" book contains chapters based on all major specialties, which include a mix of state-of-the-art updated knowledge with clinical skills and practical knowledge in easy-to-learn language that all the consultant physician teachers and medical students in medical colleges, including undergraduate students, can benefit from.

Both knowledge and education are achieved by incorporating the information from multiple sources and channelizing it through a medium like this book. I hope that physicians and readers of this wonderful book will have their knowledge updated and their whole learning experience can be complete by transforming this updated knowledge into their clinical practice day by day. I congratulate Dr Shashank Joshi and his team for this nice educational book which is the need of the hour.

YP Munjal
Director, Physicians Research Foundation (PRF)

Preface

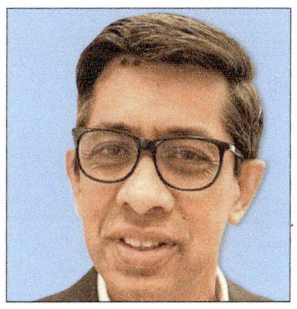

Medicine is ever-changing and no one even remotely dreamt in 2019 that in 2020, the world will be disrupted by a tiny RNA virus which will lead to COVID-19. APICON 2021 in Jaipur had to be converted into a virtual event in March and this year, the CME program of ICP was also a virtual meeting. This Postgraduate Medicine book got interrupted by the second COVID-19 wave, which hit us in April, and is now ready for its final outcome. It has encompassed various aspects of clinical medicine which were covered in the CME and I am grateful to all the authors who contributed to the same despite their extraordinary busy schedules. My virtual tenure as a Dean was predominately spent in public health, shaping COVID policies for the state of Maharashtra as well as a virtual clinical care which has now moved into a hybrid mode.

In the last 2 years, we saw a paradigm shift in the way clinical medicine and academic medicine evolved. Medical professions across all sectors all over the world rose to the call of the rampaging waves of COVID with newer variants such as the Delta which we saw in India. I am grateful to the faculty council which supported me throughout this tenure and our incoming Dean, Dr Rajesh Upadhya, as well as the outgoing Dean, Dr Amal Kumar Banerjee. We had a tragedy at API when our Guru Professor Siddharth N Shah suffered an untimely demise and we all pray he attains *moksha and sadgati*. The loss was a blow, but we all live and cherish his vision for API, ICP, and PRF. Our mentor Professor, YP Munjal, guided us in the time of crisis with his wisdom and action and we were ably supported by Presidents Drs Arul Raj, Kamlesh Tewari, and Shyam Sunder. I am thankful to Drs Pritam Gupta, BB Thakur, KK Parekh, Girish Mathur, and J Pal. I would also like to thank my own Mumbai API colleagues Drs Mangesh Tiwaskar, Agam Vora, Milind Nadkar, Ashsit Bhagwati, Alaka Deshpande, Amit Saraf, Nihar Mehta, Charu Jani, Trupti Trivedi, BR Bansode, and SV Kulkarni, among many. This book would not have been possible without the support of Dr Jimit Vagdama, who helped me with the final edits, and my small editorial team of Drs L Srinivas Murthy, Nihar Mehta, Amit Saraf, and Agam Vora.

I would also like to thank Mrs Sunita Shukla from the API office, Mr Harshnandan Trivedi from Urvi Compugraphics, and Mr Aniruddh Sapatnekar from One MD as well as all the industry which made academic contributions to e-APICON, namely Abbott, USV, and Novo Nordisk, among many others. I have to specially thank Microlabs for their generous participation to ensure that the knowledge of this book spreads to all. I would like to especially thank Mr Jitendar P Vij (Group Chairman), and Mr MS Mani (Group President) from Jaypee Brothers Medical Publishers. I would also like to extend my thanks to the team of Mr Shashikumar Sambhoo (Pharma Head), Dr Richa Saxena (Associate Director-Professional Publishing), Ms Pooja Bhandari (Production Head), and Ms Upasana Kak (Development Editor). I wish all of you a happy reading and a COVID-safe time. Long live ICP!! Long live API!! Long live PRF!!

Jai Hind!

Shashank R Joshi

Contributors

EDITOR-IN-CHIEF

Shashank R Joshi MD DM FICP FACP (USA) FACE (USA) FRCP (London, Glasgow and Edinburgh)
(Padma Shri Awardee)
Dean Indian College of Physicians (2020–21)
Past President Association of Physicians of India
Chair, International Diabetes Federation, South East Asia
President Indian Academy of Diabetes
Endocrinologist, Joshi Clinic, Lilavati Hospital, Sir HN Reliance and Bhatia Hospitals
Emeritus Editor JAPI
Past President, Endocrine Society of India, Hypertension Society of India, RSSDI, International College of Nutrition
Adjunct Faculty, JSS and Jaipur National University
Mumbai, Maharashtra, India

CONTRIBUTING AUTHORS

Aarathy Kannan MD Dip Diab
Consultant Physician and Diabetologist
Department of Medicine
Sundaram Arulrhaj Hospitals
Thoothukudi, Tamil Nadu, India

Aditi S Patankar MD (General Medicine)
Assistant Professor
Department of Medicine
Lokmanya Tilak Municipal Medical College and General Hospital, Sion
Mumbai, Maharashtra, India

Alan F Almeida MD (Internal Medicine) MNAMS (Nephrology) FISN
Consulting Nephrologist and Transplant Physician
Section Coordinator Nephrology Director of Clinical Research
PD Hinduja Hospital and Medical Research Center
Mumbai, Maharashtra, India

Amit A Saraf MD FICP FRCP (London, Edinburgh and Glasgow) FACP (Philadelphia) FCPS
Director, Department of Internal Medicine, Jupiter Hospital
Mumbai, Maharashtra, India

Amit K Ghosh MD FACP FRCP
Consultant, General Internal Medicine
Professor of Medicine – Mayo Clinic College of Medicine and Science
Section of Executive and Development, Division of General Internal Medicine
Mayo Clinic, Rochester, Minnesota, USA

Aniket Hase MBBS DNB (General Medicine) DNB (Nephrology)
Consultant Nephrologist
Jupiter Hospital
Thane, Maharashtra, India

Anil Modak MD (General Medicine)
Associate Professor
Department of Medicine
NKP Salve Institute of Medicine and Research Center and
Lata Mangeshkar Hospital
Nagpur, Maharashtra, India

Arijit Kayal MBBS (WBUHS)
MD (Pharmacology)
DM Resident
Calcutta School of Tropical Medicine
Kolkata, West Bengal, India

Contributors

Asha N Shah MD
Professor of Medicine
GCS Medical College Ahmedabad
Ex Professor and HOD Medicine
Additional Dean
BJ Medical College
Ahmedabad, Gujarat, India

Ajit Desai MD (Medicine) DM (Cardiology) DNB (Cardiology) AFACC (USA)
Additional Director-Jaslok Cardiology
Breach Candy; HN Reliance; Nanavati
Asian Heart; Holy Family Hosptials
Mumbai, Maharashtra, India

Ayan Kumar Dey DNB (Nephrology) [Gold Medal] Fellowship in Nephrology (Toronto) DNB (Internal Medicine)
Junior Consultant
Department of Nephrology
PD Hinduja Hospital
Mumbai, Maharashtra, India

Bitukaur Sodhi DNB (Medicine)
Resident
Department of Internal Medicine
Jupiter Hospital
Mumbai, Maharashtra, India

Chandra Sekar DNB (Internal Medicine)
PG Resident
Department of Internal Medicine
Sundaram Arulrhaj Hospitals
Thoothukudi, Tamil Nadu, India

Dipanjan Haldar MD DM (Clinical Hematology)
Consultant Hematology and BMT
Jupiter Hospital
Thane, Maharashtra, India

Faizur Rahman DNB (Internal Medicine)
PG Resident
Department of Internal Medicine
Sundaram Arulrhaj Hospitals
Thoothukudi, Tamil Nadu, India

Ganpathi Bantwal MD DM (Endocrinology) DNB (Endocrinology) MNAMS
Professor of Endocrinology
Department of Endocrinology,
St John's Medical College and Hospital
Bengaluru, Karnataka, India

Gauri Pathak-Oak MD (General Medicine)
Professor
Department of Medicine
Lokmanya Tilak Municipal Medical
College and General Hospital, Sion,
Mumbai, Maharashtra, India

Hathur Basavanagowdappa MBBS MD (General Medicine)
Professor of Medicine
JSS Medical College, JSS Academy of
Higher Education and Research
Mysuru, Karnataka, India

Iram Syed MBBS
Senior Resident, Bombay Hospital
Mumbai, Maharashtra, India

Jagdish Hiremath MD DM (Cardiology), DNB (Cardiology), FACC
Director, Cath Lab and Consultant
Cardiologist Ruby Hall Clinic
Pune, Maharashtra, India

Jimit Vadgama MD C Diab
Consultant Endocrine,
Diabetes and Metabolic Physician,
Swaminarayan Diabetes,
Thyroid and Hormone Clinic
Surat, Gujarat, India

Kamal Sharma MD (Medicine) DNB (Medicine) DM (Cardiology) DNB (Cardiology) MNAMS FACC FSCAI FESC
Senior Interventional Cardiologist
Ahmedabad, Gujarat, India

Khusrav Beji Bajan MD EDIC
Consultant – Intensivist and
HOD – Emergency Medicine,
Department of Critical Care and
Emergency Medicine PD Hinduja Hospital
Medical Research Centre
Mumbai, Maharashtra, India

KS Lokesh MBBS DNB (TB and Respiratory Diseases/Pulmonary Medicine)
Assistant Professor
Department of Respiratory Medicine
JSS Medical College, JSS Academy of
Higher Education and Research
Mysuru, Karnataka, India

Contributors xix

Leong Hoe Nam MBBS (S'pore) MRCP (UK)
MMed (Intern Medicine, S'pore)
FAMS (Infectious Disease)
Medical Director
Senior Consultant Infectious Diseases
Physician
Adjunct A/Professor,
Duke-NUS Graduate Medical School
Visiting Consultant
Singapore General Hospital
Visiting Consultant
National Cancer Centre Singapore
Visiting Consultant
Dover Park Hospice, Singapore

L Sreenivasamurthy MD FRCP (Edinburgh)
FICP PDCR
Professor and Head of Unit
Department of General Medicine
Dr BR Ambedkar Medical College
Lifecare Hospital and Research Centre
Bengaluru, Karnataka, India

Manikandan DNB (Internal Medicine)
PG Resident
Department of Internal Medicine
Sundaram Arulrhaj Hospitals
Thoothukudi, Tamil Nadu, India

MA Shekar MD (General Medicine)
FRCP (Edinburgh)
Director
Apoorva Diabetes Foundation, Mysuru
Retired Professor of Medicine and Head
Department of Endocrinology
Mysore Medical College and Research
Institute, Mysuru
Former Director
Karnataka Institute of Endocrinology
and Research
Bengaluru, Karnataka, India

Nihar Mehta MD DNB (Medicine)
DNB (Cardiology)
Consultant Cardiologist
Department of Cardiology
Jaslok Hospital and Research Centre
Mumbai, Maharashtra, India

Nikesh Jain DNB (Medicine)
DNB (Cardiology)
Consultant Cardiologist
Jaslok Hospital and Research Centre
KJ Somaiya Superspeciality Hospital
Mumbai, Maharashtra, India

Niteen D Karnik MD (General Medicine)
FICP PGDMLS
Professor and Head
Department of Medicine
Lokmanya Tilak Municipal Medical
College and General Hospital, Sion
Mumbai, Maharashtra, India

Niwrutti Hase MD (Medicine)
DNB (Nephroogy) FICP
Director Clinical Nephrology and
Kidney Transplant
Jupiter Hospital Thane
Ex Professor and Head Department of
Nephrology, Seth GS Medical College and
KEM Hospital
Mumbai, Maharashtra, India

Om Shrivastav MBBS MD Fellowship in
Infectious Diseases and Immunology (Australia)
Consultant Infectious Diseases and
Immunology, Sir HN Reliance Foundation
Jaslok Hospital
Visiting Professor Infectious Diseases
Dr DY Patil Medical College
Navi Mumbai, Maharashtra, India

Pratibha Singhal MD DNB
Consultant, Interventional Pulmonologist
Bombay Hospital and
Sir HN Reliance Hospital
Mumbai, Maharashtra, India

Santanu K Tripathi MBBS MD
(Pharmacology) DM (Clinical Pharmacology)
Professor and Head
Department of Clinical and Experimental
Pharmacology, Kolkata
School of Tropical Medicine
Kolkata, West Bengal, India

S Arulrhaj MD PhD FRCP (Glasgow)
FRCP (London) MBA
Chief Physician and Intensivist
Sundaram Arulrhaj Hospitals
Thoothukudi, Tamil Nadu, India

SB Gupta MD (Internal Medicine) FACC FCSI
FISE FICP
Ex-Consultant Physician Cardiologist
Asian Heart Institute Mumbai
Former Head
Department of Medicine and Cardiology
Central Railway Headquarters Hospital
Mumbai, Maharashtra, India

Contributors

Shashank R Joshi MD DM FICP FACP (USA) FACE (USA) FRCP (London, Glasgow and Edinburgh)
(*Padma Shri Awardee*)
Dean Indian College of Physicians (2020–21)
Past President Association of Physicians of India
Chair, International Diabetes Federation, South East Asia
President Indian Academy of Diabetes
Endocrinologist, Joshi Clinic, Lilavati Hospital, Sir HN Reliance and Bhatia Hospitals
Emeritus Editor JAPI
Past President, Endocrine Society of India, Hypertension Society of India, RSSDI, International College of Nutrition
Adjunct Faculty, JSS and Jaipur National University
Mumbai, Maharashtra, India

Shambo S Samajdar MBBS MD DM (Clinical Pharmacology) Post Graduate Dip in Endo and Diabetes (RCP, UK) Fellowship in Respiratory and Critical Care (WBUHS)
Clinical Pharmacologist
Department of Clinical Pharmacology,
School of Tropical Medicine,
Kolkata and Consultant at Diabetes and Allergy-Asthma Therapeutics
Specialty Clinic
Kolkata, West Bengal, India

Sudhir Bhandari MD DNB MNAMS FRCP (London) FRCP (Edinburgh) FACE FACP FICP FRSSDI
Senior Professor of Medicine
Consultant of Internal Medicine
Diabetes and Endocrinology
Honourable Physician to HE the Governor of Rajasthan
Principal and Controller
Sawai Man Singh Hospital and Medical College
Jaipur, Rajasthan, India

Suhas Erande MD (Medicine)
G Dip Diabetes (Australia)
Founder and Consultant Diabetologist
Akshay Hospital and Diabetic Speciality Centre and Insulin Pump Centre
Pune, Maharashtra, India

Sunanda Chaoji MD (General Medicine)
Associate Professor in Medicine
NKP Salve Institute of Medicine and Research Center and
Lata Mangeshkar Hospital
Nagpur, Maharashtra, India

Tanuja Manohar MD (General Medicine)
Professor in Medicine
NKP Salve Institute of Medicine and Research Center and
Lata Mangeshkar Hospital
Nagpur, Maharashtra, India

Yogesh Solanki MD (Genereal Medicine)
DNB (Cardiology)
Resident, Department of Cardiology
Jaslok Hospital and Research Centre
Mumbai, Maharashtra, India

Contents

1.	**Combating Physician Burnout** *Amit K Ghosh*	1
2.	**Is Clinical Medicine a Forgotten Art?** *MA Shekar*	7
3.	**Pedagogy in Medicine: How to be an Expert Medical Educator—Evidence-based Review** *Amit K Ghosh*	10
4.	**Acute Rheumatic Fever** *Anil Modak, Sunanda Chaoji, Tanuja Manohar*	15
5.	**Angiotensin Receptor Blocker and Angiotensin-converting Enzyme Inhibitors: Newer Insights** *Nihar Mehta, Yogesh Solanki*	21
6.	**Subclinical Hyperthyroidism** *Jimit Vadgama*	32
7.	**Approach to Sleep Apnea** *Hathur Basavanagowdappa, KS Lokesh*	37
8.	**Jaundice in Pregnancy** *Tanuja Manohar*	42
9.	**Cardiometabolic-based Chronic Disease; Is it Adiposity-based Chronic Disease and Dysglycemic-based Chronic Disease?** *Kamal Sharma*	47
10.	**Endocrine Hypertension** *L Sreenivasamurthy*	56
11.	**GINA 2020: What's New and Why?** *Pratibha Singhal, Iram Syed*	65
12.	**Heart Rate an Independent Risk Factor and the Proficient Study** *Jagdish Hiremath*	74
13.	**Hypertensive Emergencies** *Amit A Saraf, Bitukaur Sodhi*	77

14.	Hyponatremia in the Intensive Care Unit: Step Wise Approach to Diagnosis and Management *Niwrutti Hase, Aniket Hase*	84
15.	Importance of Influenza Vaccination in Adult Population *Leong Hoe Nam*	92
16.	Interpreting the Link Between Hyperuricemia and Cardiometabolic Disorders and Management *Ayan Kumar Dey, Alan F Almeida*	95
17.	Masked Hypertension: How Worrisome? *SB Gupta*	103
18.	Myelodysplastic Syndrome: What a Physician Should Know? *Dipanjan Haldar*	108
19.	Approach to Metabolic Syndrome *L Sreenivasamurthy*	114
20.	Nonalcoholic Fatty Liver Disease: What is in the Name? *Suhas Erande*	128
21.	Vagal Nerve Stimulation and Baroreceptor Activation Therapy: An Emerging Modality for Refractory Heart Failure *Kamal Sharma*	134
22.	A Century of Basal Glucose Regulation: From Longer to Flatter to more Predictable Insulins *Ganpathi Bantwal*	137
23.	Pyrexia of Unknown Origin *Asha N Shah*	141
24.	Evolving Epidemiology of COVID, Clinical Presentation, and Triage *Niteen D Karnik, Aditi S Patankar, Gauri Pathak-Oak*	147
25.	COVID-19 and Diabetes Mellitus *Sudhir Bhandari*	154
26.	Digital Outreach: Reaching the Unreached *S Arulrhaj, Aarathy Kannan, Chandra Sekar, Faizur Rahman, Manikandan*	162
27.	Asthma, Biologics, and Clinical Pharmacology *Shambo S Samajdar, Arijit Kayal, Shashank R Joshi*	174
28.	An Approach to Diabetic Autonomic Neuropathy *Shambo S Samajdar, Santanu K Tripathi, Shashank R Joshi*	188

29.	**Pharmacokinetic Considerations in Prescribing Chronic Kidney Disease Patients** *Shambo S Samajdar, Shashank R Joshi*	196
30.	**Protection of the Healthcare Workers in the Coronavirus Disease Pandemic** *Khusrav Beji Bajan*	215
31.	**The Immunology of Sepsis** *Om Shrivastav*	218
32.	**Coronavirus Disease and Cardiovascular System** *Ajit Desai, Nikesh Jain*	225
33.	**Nutrition in Diabetes: Relevance and Current Evidence** *Shashank R Joshi*	238
	Index	243

1 Combating Physician Burnout

Amit K Ghosh

INTRODUCTION

The term "burnout" was coined by the psychologist Herbert Freudenberger in the 1970s and gained prominence in the research literature after American psychologist Christina Maslach developed the Maslach Burnout Inventory (MBI) in 1981.[1] Burnout is a syndrome of emotional exhaustion, loss of meaning at work, feelings of ineffectiveness, and a tendency to view people as objects rather than as human beings.[2] The three domains of emotional health assessed in the MBI include emotional exhaustion (I feel emotionally drained from my work), depersonalization (I have become more callous toward people since I took this job), and reduced sense of personal accomplishment (lack of feeling that I am positively influencing people's lives through my work).[3] Physician burnout is associated with adverse effects at the personal (relationship difficulties, substance abuse, depression, and suicide) and professional levels (decreased productivity, work and career dissatisfaction, suboptimal patient care, and physician turnover).[4] Owing to these negative spin-offs, physician burnout is considered a public health crisis and also a threat to future medical practice worldwide.[5]

BURDEN OF PHYSICIAN BURNOUT

The prevalence of burnout amount attending physicians in United States (US) is about 55% when all specialties were considered.[2] Burnout is also prevalent among medical trainees (medical students, residents, and fellows) and has been associated with self-reported medical errors and suboptimal patient care. On an International level, burnout was also reported in many countries including India.[3]

At present, most widely used and validated instruments to measure burnout include the MBI, mini-Z survey, and the Copenhagen Burnout Inventory (CBI). The MBI is the reference standard in medical research to measure burnout in various work settings. The full-length MBI is a 22-item questionnaire covering domains of emotional exhaustion, depersonalization, and personal accomplishment. Licenses need to be purchased for use of the MBI for work-related or research use. An abbreviated two-item version developed by the Mayo Clinic has been validated and used in numerous physician surveys.[3]

The mini-Z survey is used by the American College of Physicians is shorter than the MBI and free to use.[6] Additionally, the mini-Z survey is more applicable to physician settings as it includes questions on time constraints for documentation and time spent on electronic medical records at home. The CBI[7] is a psychometrically robust 19-item questionnaire that assesses burnout on three domains; personal (six items), work related (seven items), and client-related burnout (six items). Thus, it focusses more on personal exhaustion. The CBI is free to use.

DETERMINANTS AND MEDIATORS OF PHYSICIAN BURNOUT

The drivers of burnout include a host of personal and work-related factors. As physicians going through rigorous medical training, compulsivity, and attention to detail are a personality trait developed in us. Among physicians, culture and values include a sense of "patient comes first" and a culture of endurance in difficult situations. This may lead to professional isolation especially when there is no safe space to retreat or lack of social support at work. Increasing workload, varying job demands, as well as changing physician-patient dynamics and interactions have lately been contributing to emotional distress at work. Lack of control over the work schedule, inflexibility at work, and loss of autonomy based on the employer-employee relations are potential drivers of burnout.[8,9] Pressures of increased documentation time, especially using electronic medical records, and the resulting decreased face-to-face time with limited efficiency, and resources add to burnout.[10] It is to be noted that burnout is not the same as depression, though interestingly the diagnosis of physician burnout was recently added to the International Classification of Diseases (ICD)-10 codebook.[11] Depression has a well-established process of diagnosis and treatment. A high correlation exists between burnout and depression and it is speculated that drivers of severe burnout may lead to depression.[12]

Three major changes related to the healthcare scenario in India appear to contribute to the increasing trend of physician burnout. Firstly, the mushrooming of multispecialty corporate hospitals which have been likened to "shopping malls",[13] due to their offer of the entire bouquet of health services ranging from simple consultations to complex procedures such as organ transplants, all under one roof. These hospitals have a wide recruitment net and, as a result, it has become commonplace to find doctors working outside their home state.

What this means is that the earlier system, dominated by the local family physician who would enjoy a better rapport and understanding of the local culture and needs, has been gradually replaced by the corporate hospital culture which places a premium on patient volumes and is manned by physicians who do not share the same language and culture. This, in turn, has led to diminution in clinician autonomy as well as reduced connectedness with patients, both of which are key drivers of burnout.[14,15]

Second issue is the supply and demand mismatch of health care resources. This is especially true of public sector hospitals which, in India, attract high patient volumes due to the provision of subsidized health care. The available infrastructure, both in terms of manpower as well as physical infrastructure, is woefully inadequate to cater to the extant patient load. Over time, this leads to burnout because of poor working conditions.[8]

The third issue is the inequitable distribution of available health care resources. Multispeciality hospitals and even public sector teaching hospitals are mostly located in urban areas. As the rural-urban divide in the concentration of doctors increases, more and more doctors practicing in urban centers are forced to compete against each other for clientele. Consequently, they often end up doing freelancing in multiple hospitals in order to earn better. Even private practitioners and family physicians are not spared from this phenomenon. The result is long working hours, decreased family and social time, loneliness, and eventual burnout.[16]

STRATEGIES TO MANAGE BURNOUT

While numerous strategies have been proposed in research literature, a strategy that may work at a certain center may not work at another institution. Thus, it is best to work collaboratively with physician leaders and a wellness committee to identify local resources to address physician well-being. Below, we give a few suggestions to improve physician well-being, from an individual and systemic perspective:

1. *Develop work schedules to maintain work life balance*: It is important for a physician leader to acknowledge the value of the physician's time with patients; it is equally important too to understand their need to be with their families. Life events such as disability, death or illness in the family, maternity lead to the need for other physicians to provide coverage and may not be perceived as being cost effective. It is important to recognize that the life events are inevitable. Pre-emptive planning and ensuring that adequate full-time staffing is available can help tide over difficult times. Flexible or part-time work may offer adequate work-life balance and are being increasingly sought by physicians.[17]
2. *Right size documentation-related work*: Clinicians are overwhelmed about the need to establish and maintain connections with patients while time may be short and the productivity may be affected. Offloading nonclinical work such as order entry or use of scribes or medical assistants may relieve some of the pressure and improve the quality of the physician-patient interaction.

    Electronic medical records have changed the way we interact with our patients, documents, and billing. Organizations should be deliberate with electronic medical record training. Use of auto-text and autopopulation for certain documentation needs and having predefined order sets for common diagnosis would help to improve efficiency.
3. *Make physician wellness a priority*: It is often stated that if an employer takes care of their employees and remains invested in their well-being, employees will perform better with their clients. For organizations to maintain the workforce and prevent physician turnover, it is important

to make wellness a priority as this will lead to favorable patient, provider, and financial outcomes.

It is important for the physician to be able to take adequate care of himself or herself to facilitate optimal discharge of duties. This includes eating healthy meals, exercising regularly, having adequate sleep, mindfulness training, yoga, meditation, practicing relaxation techniques, and positive psychology, having diverse social interests, and building resilience. A physician needs to set limits to work and should not feel guilty to decline additional responsibilities especially when having other demands at work or their personal lives.

4. *Develop stellar leaders*: It is important for an organization to have leaders who value and model well-being and at the same time can engage and inspire physician employees. Having a strong leader who is invested in physician well-being is an important deterrent to burnout. There is a need to destigmatize depression especially for medical trainees, as many medical students and residents do not utilize professional mental health services when needed.[18,19] Programs emphasizing leadership and resource management skills ought to be a part of undergraduate and postgraduate training.

5. *Mentorship programs for early career teaching faculty*: Medical teachers are a unique group who have to juggle between the exacting demands of practicing medicine as well as teaching and researching. In most centers in India, there is no protected time for research activities and it has to be squeezed into the daily grind. This may engender feelings of professional stagnation. Evidence points to low levels of perceived achievement as a risk factor for burnout.[20,21] From this standpoint, it would help to have personalized mentorship programs for junior faculty. For resource constrained settings in low- and middle-income countries, a hybrid need driven mentoring model that incorporates matched and motivated mentor-protégé dyads, where available, as well as facilitated regular peer group mentorship meetings have been described.[22]

6. *Systems approach to prevention of burnout*: In a recent commentary based on their decade long experience with physician wellness programs, authors affiliated with the Mayo Clinic have highlighted nine organization-based strategies for prevention of physician burnout.[4] These include admitting and acknowledging the problem, harnessing the power of leadership, developing and implementing targeted interventions for specific drivers of burnout, enhancing peer support by cultivating work communities, incentivization of productivity among physicians, promoting flexibility at workplace so that physicians can adjust their timings to meet personal and professional obligations, implementing organizational programs that foster physician resilience and self-care and institutional investment in sustained programs.

A more workable and evidence-based solution could be to design interventions that enhance emotional intelligence (EI) and, potentially, prevent burnout. Inclusion of EI abilities in the curriculum, use of simulated patients to improve EI, and regular workshops to enhance EI, communication skills and emotion self-regulation[23] have all been suggested. EI is trainable and brief training programs have been found to induce sustainable changes in levels of EI.[24]

In summary, a combination of institutional and individual strategies are required, given the lack of evidence of superiority for any particular intervention in reducing burnout.[25]

CONCLUSION

Burnout is a growing problem in the practice of medicine and is best considered a long-term reaction to stress. Various predictors have been identified such as diminished clinician autonomy, poor medical infrastructure, impaired work life balance, reduced sense of personal accomplishment and lack of support, and empathy from senior colleagues. However, physician burnout is not inevitable. Understanding the predictors of burnout, implementing locally relevant strategies based on locally available resources and reassessing physician well-being can go a long way in addressing physician burnout and emotional well-being. We owe this effort to our physician brethren and our patients.

REFERENCES

1. Schaufeli WB. Burnout: A Short Socio-Cultural History. In: Neckel S, Schaffner A, Wagner G (Eds). Burnout, Fatigue, Exhaustion. Burnout, Fatigue, Exhaustion. Cham: Palgrave Macmillan; 2017. pp. 105-27.
2. Shanafelt TD, Hasan O, Dyrbye LN, Sinsky C, Satele D, Sloan J, et al. Changes in Burnout and Satisfaction With Work-Life Balance in Physicians and the General US Working Population Between 2011 and 2014. Mayo Clin Proc. 2015;90(12): 1600-13.
3. Menon V, Agrawal V, Joshi S, Ghosh AK. Physician burnout: Quo vadimus? Indian J Med Sci 2020;72:211-6
4. Shanafelt TD, Noseworthy JH. Executive Leadership and Physician Well-being: Nine Organizational Strategies to Promote Engagement and Reduce Burnout. Mayo Clin Proc. 2017;92:129-46.
5. Shanafelt TD, Dyrbye LN, West CP, Sinsky CA. Potential Impact of Burnout on the US Physician Workforce. Mayo Clin Proc. 2016;91:1667-8.
6. Linzer M, Poplau S, Babbott S, Collins T, Guzman-Corrales L, Menk J, et al. Worklife and Wellness in Academic General Internal Medicine: Results from a National Survey. J Gen Intern Med. 2016;31(9):1004-10.
7. Kristensen TS, Borritz M, Villadsen E, Christensen KB. The Copenhagen Burnout Inventory: A new tool for the assessment of burnout. Work Stress. 2005;19(3): 192-207.
8. Patel RS, Bachu R, Adikey A, Malik M, Shah M. Factors Related to Physician Burnout and Its Consequences: A Review. Behav Sci (Basel). 2018;8(11):98.
9. Del Carmen MG, Herman J, Rao S, Hidrue MK, Ting D, Lehrhoff SR, et al. Trends and Factors Associated With Physician Burnout at a Multispecialty Academic Faculty Practice Organization. JAMA Netw Open. 2019;2(3):e190554.

10. Sinsky C, Colligan L, Li L, Prgomet M, Reynolds S, Goeders L, et al. Allocation of Physician Time in Ambulatory Practice: A Time and Motion Study in 4 Specialties. Ann Intern Med. 2016;165(11):753-60.
11. World Health Organization. ICD-10 Classifications of Mental and Behavioural Disorder: Clinical Descriptions and Diagnostic Guidelines. Geneva: World Health Organization; 1992.
12. Bianchi R, Schonfeld IS, Laurent E. Physician burnout is better conceptualised as depression. Lancet. 2017;389(10077):1397-8.
13. Gadre A, Shukla A. Health Care becomes an industry: the Growing influence of Corporate and Multi-speciality Hospitals. In: Dissenting Diagnosis. Gurgaon: Random House Publishers India Pvt. Ltd; 2016. pp. 44-59.
14. Panagioti M, Geraghty K, Johnson J. How to prevent burnout in cardiologists? A review of the current evidence, gaps, and future directions. Trends Cardiovasc Med. 2018;28(1):1-7.
15. West CP, Dyrbye LN, Shanafelt TD. Physician burnout: contributors, consequences and solutions. J Intern Med. 2018;283(6):516-29.
16. Shapiro J, Zhang B, Warm EJ. Residency as a Social Network: Burnout, Loneliness, and Social Network Centrality. J Grad Med Educ. 2015;7:617-23.
17. Glauser W. Part-time doctors-reducing hours to reduce burnout. CMAJ 2018;190(35):E1055-6.
18. Guille C, Speller H, Laff R, Epperson CN, Sen S. Utilization and barriers to mental health services among depressed medical interns: a prospective multisite study. J Grad Med Educ. 2010;2:210-4.
19. Menon V, Sarkar S, Kumar S. Barriers to healthcare seeking among medical students: a cross sectional study from South India. Postgrad Med J. 2015;91(1079):477-82.
20. Pedersen AF, Andersen CM, Olesen F, Vedsted P. Risk of Burnout in Danish GPs and Exploration of Factors Associated with Development of Burnout: A Two-Wave Panel Study. Int J Family Med. 2013;2013:603713.
21. Zubairi AJ, Noordin S. Factors associated with burnout among residents in a developing country. Ann Med Surg. 2016;6:60-3.
22. Menon V, Muraleedharan A, Bhat BV. Mentoring for junior medical faculty: Existing models and suggestions for low-resource settings. Asian J Psychiatr. 2016;19:87-8.
23. Swami MK, Mathur DM, Pushp BK. Emotional intelligence, perceived stress and burnout among resident doctors: an assessment of the relationship. Natl Med J India. 2013;26(4):210-3.
24. Nelis D, Quoidbach J, Mikolajczak M, Hansenne M. Increasing emotional intelligence: (How) is it possible? Pers Individ Differ. 2009;47(1):36-41.
25. West CP, Dyrbye LN, Erwin PJ, Shanafelt TD. Interventions to prevent and reduce physician burnout: a systematic review and meta-analysis. Lancet. 2016;388(10057):2272-81.

2. Is Clinical Medicine a Forgotten Art?

MA Shekar

INTRODUCTION

Medicine is often described as the second oldest profession. The definition of clinical medicine: The study and practice of medicine based on direct observation of patients, in relation to the care of the patient.
- Is clinical medicine a forgotten art? Definitely NO!
- I would venture to say, the fading art of clinical medicine.
- Is clinical medicine a fading art? Probably YES!
- Now, clinical medicine or bedside medicine, what is the distinction?

In general, clinical medicine encompasses all! Bedside medicine is history and exam. So, fading practice of bedside medicine or the lost art of clinical skills would be more appropriate.

"Those who cannot remember the past are condemned to repeat it" or *"those who do not know the history are doomed to repeat it."*

There are so many physicians from history of medicine, some of them who lived their lives emphasizing the importance of clinical/bedside medicine are:
- Asclepius (Greek demigod) Imhotep (Kingdom of pharaohs), Susruta and Charaka (our own Hindu Saints), Avicenna (Persia) and of course, Hippocrates Asclepiades (Greek).

The following quotes from Sir William Osler exemplify the true essence of clinical/bedside medicine:

"Medicine is learned by the bedside and not in the classroom. Let not your conceptions of disease come from words heard in the lecture room or read from the book. See and then reason and compare and control. But see first."

"Medicine is science of uncertainty and an art of probability."

And speaking of art and science of medicine:
- The art of medicine:
  - The following quotes sum up the essence of art of medicine
    "One kind word can warm three winter months"
    —Japanese saying

    "Cure rarely, comfort mostly, but console always"
    —Hippocrates

> *"One kind word on the bedside can cure many ills"*
> —Anonymous

> *"Patient care is caring for the patient!"*
> —Sir Francis Peabody,
> Motto of Massachusetts General Hospital.

These quotes echo the quintessence of compassion, empathy, verbal, and nonverbal communication skills of a physician in the care of patients.

- The science of medicine:
  - Rapid advancements of medical technology have led to a belief that clinical skills are from bygone era and that advanced imaging techniques and laboratory tests have replaced age-old concept history-taking and physical examination.
  - Today, patients (google doctors) and healthcare professionals alike, think that the battery of investigations will invariably lead to correct diagnosis and management tips. And there is a tendency for some clinicians to rely more on laboratory reports and less on the history of the illness, the examination, behavior of the patient, and clinical judgment.
  - Certain top physicians do "chart rounds" in the ward/side rooms where the details of the patients, including al the laboratory-test results, are kept. Little time is spent with the patient in the bed side.
  - Unfortunately, technology is the "gold standard" for diagnosis instead of being an "adjunct/complementary tool" to clinical judgment.
  - The problem arises when healthcare professionals rush to order tests without first performing a thorough physical exam. While in many cases, laboratory findings are invaluable for reaching correct conclusions, one should never forget that "it takes a man, not a machine, to understand a man."

REINVENTING THE WHEEL

In an attempt to bring back the essence of clinical medicine, Medical Council of India (MCI), in their vision document in 2011–2012, created "competency-based undergraduate curriculum. Attitude, Ethics and Communication (AETCOM) module of medical education" which has been put into practice from 2018–2019 in all medical colleges.

The document stated that an Indian Medical Graduate (IMG) shall be a clinician, a leader, a communicator, a lifelong learner, and a professional.

In closing:

- In spite of the importance of history-taking and physical examination, medical education imparting clinical skills has decreased, the downslide beginning in medical colleges, and continuing through postgraduation and into practice.
- The AETCOM module of MCI vision document 2011–2012 has attempted to emphasize on over-all education of medical students.

- With the erosion of thorough history-taking and physical examinations, clinical reasoning has also decreased.
- Too often, illogical lab findings are accepted without question.
- Many documented evidences have shown that careful history and physical exam have been invaluable in making the correct diagnosis.
- High-quality medical care requires strong clinical skills and clinical reasoning, along with appropriate tests/technology.
- Today, the onus is on medical educators to dedicate themselves to teaching clinical skills but also emulating those skills in everyday work. They must integrate new technology into clinical education without diverting attention from patients.

3

Pedagogy in Medicine: How to be an Expert Medical Educator—Evidence-based Review

Amit K Ghosh

INTRODUCTION

The purpose of this review is to summarize the key evidence-based medical literature utilized in medical education to develop superb medical educators in 21st century. We will discuss the current review on pedagogy in medicine out to become an expert medical educator using three major headings:
1. Review key clinical teaching principles and strategies
2. Reflect on challenges and develop solutions
3. Reflect on new strategies that participants would like to adopt in own teaching

REVIEW KEY CLINICAL TEACHING PRINCIPLES AND STRATEGIES

With the changes in medical curriculum and the numerous venues for education, medical education can happen anywhere a patient care is being discussed. Hence, education can happen in the medical wards, medical outpatients, specialists' settings, structured patient education sessions, and grand rounds, he is paced conference and more importantly currently in a virtual says learning environment through zoom or other technological platforms.

The goal for medical education is to ensure that the learners are able to: (1) Interpret signs and symptoms, (2) Explain basics science behind signs and symptoms, (3) Formulate differential diagnosis based on clinical reasoning, (4) Describe pathological processes, (5) Interpret all clinical data to inform a diagnosis, (6) Discuss investigation plan for the patient, (7) Plan of management for the patient, and (8) Predict a prognosis.

It is essential to understand the principles of adult education so, bloom taxonomy regarding assessment in the knowledge, skills, and attitude required by all practitioners, and providing us safe space to enhance the educational climate of teaching using the Maslow's hierarchy (SPACE).

Principles of Adult Education—Learner Centric Approach

Adult education presumes that ever adult learner will assess their learning needs and identify topics for lifelong learning.[1] Background experience and prior learning of adults are critical in assessing how they interpret new information in their work situations and often needs to be taken into account. Malcolm Knowles[2,3] describes this form of learner centric adult learning as "andragogy", to differentiate it from teacher centric learning called "pedagogy".

Andragogy assumes that adults are independent and self-directed learners, who have already accumulated a great deal of experience. Adults are interested in an immediate problem centered approach and are driven to learn by internal demands to integrate learning with a problem at work. Hence, adult learning is often problem centered rather than subject centered.

Adult learning often are based on the following seven principles: (1) To promote effective environment for learning, adults should feel that the environment is safe where all opinions are respected, (2) Learners should be self-directed and involved in assessing their gaps in knowledge (3) Learners should be involved in planning their curriculum, (4) Learners accept responsibility for their own learning and design their own learning objectives, (5) Learners need to identify resources and devise strategies for using these sources to achieve their objectives, (6) They need to be supported in an informal and personal environment, and (7) Involved in self-reflection and evaluation of their own learning experience.[1]

Adults learn in different educational settings. However, research indicate that the efficacy of different modalities of education result in varying degree of retention of information. The retention of information is only 10% of what is read, 20% of what is heard, 30% of what is observed or demonstrated, 50% of what is discussed, 70% of what is practiced, and 90% of what is taught.[4] Hence, adults remember best when they actively involve themselves in learning, practicing, and teaching the material.

Bloom's Taxonomy of Testing Cognitive, Knowledge, and Affective Domains (Box 1)

Refer **Box 1**.

Box 1: Bloom's taxonomy.

Knowledge: Cognitive domain
- Medical decision-making
- Medical knowledge

Skills: Psychomotor domain
- Physical exam
- Procedures and surgeries
- Communication including case presentations, interactions with colleagues and phrasing of consult questions, patient interactions
- Note writing

Attitudes: Affective domain
- Professionalism, values, emotions, feelings

Education Climate of Teaching—SPACE—Maslow's Hierarchy

S—Safety: Safe place to learn, without bias. and discrimination
P—Physiological needs: Basic needs like air, water, food, shelter, and clothing are met
A—Actualization: Desire the most that one can be
C—Community: Friendship, belonging, intimacy, connection, and family
E—Esteem: Respect, self-esteem, status, recognition, strength, and freedom

REFLECT ON CHALLENGES AND DEVELOP SOLUTIONS

Challenges of Current Teaching[5]

- Time pressures
- Competing demands
- Often opportunistic
- Numbers/levels of trainees
- Fewer patients (short stays, too ill, or unwilling patients)
- Clinical settings not teaching friendly
- Rewards and recognition for teaching poor

Essential Strategies for Clinical Teacher's

This includes planning, teaching, evaluating, and reflecting.[6]

Planning includes: (1) Direct and oriented hours, (2) A positive learning environment, (3) Pre-select patient's, (4) Brief the learners.

Teaching includes teaching from clinical cases, using questions to diagnose learners, asking advanced learners to participate teaching, using the illness scripts, and teaching scripts going to the bedside of exam room, role model, and observe.

Evaluating and reflecting include evaluate learners, provide feedback, and promote self-assessment and self-directed learning.

The Six Areas of Activity of a Teacher[7]

1. Teacher as an information provider—lecturer and clinical teacher
2. Teachers as a role model—on the job role model and teaching role model
3. Teachers as an assessor—student assessor and curriculum evaluator
4. Teachers as a planner—curriculum planner and course organizer
5. Teacher as a resource developer—study guide producer and resource material creator
6. Teacher as a facilitator—mentor and learning facilitator

Solutions—One Minute Preceptor Model—Six Micro Skills

1. Get a commitment—What do you think is going on?
2. Probe for supporting evidence—What led you to that conclusion?

3. Teach general rules—When this happens, do this....
4. Reinforce what was right—Specifically, you did an excellent job of....
5. Correct mistakes—Next time this happens, try this....
6. Identify next learning steps—What do we need to learn more about?

Solutions—SNAPPS[8]

S—Summarize briefly the history and findings
N—Narrow the differential to two or more possibilities
A—Analyze the differential
P—Probe the preceptor by asking questions
P—Plan management
S—Select a case-related issue for self-directed learning

REFLECT ON NEW STRATEGIES THAT PARTICIPANTS WOULD LIKE TO ADOPT IN OWN TEACHING

Experience-based Learning—The SPaRC (Support, Participation, Real Patient Learning, and Capability) Model[9]

Experience-based learning specifies the unique capabilities that medical student acquire from practical experience with patients. It shows how clinician behavior help students gain experience, and shows how by reflection students converts real patient leaning into capability. Desirable features of learning environment are identified. Experiences based learning are a concept of supporting students while learning from medial patients within clinical practice. Students are prepared to become doctors who are ready to deliver safe, effective, and compassionate care.

Effective Feedback of Students

Feedback should be viewed from a learner perspective. It is effective only when it is assimilated and leads to behavior change.
Three questions need to be asked about feedback.[10]
1. Where am I? Assessment of performance, strength, and areas of improvement
2. Where do I need to be? Outcome to be achieved-knowledge skills and attitudes
3. How do I get there? Reflection, self-assessment, and action plan

From the Unique Models Minute been use to Provide Feedback to Learners is the R2C2 Model[11]

The R2C2 model[11]
R—Build relationship and rapport
R—React then reflect
C—Confirm understanding of content
C—Cocreate action plans and changes

Educators should also routinely attend Professional Development Courses dealing specifically with medical education

CONCLUSION

- Medical educator should be aware of the different domains of education using Bloom taxonomy.
- Medical educator should provide an excellent climate for teaching.
- Adult learning techniques should be used for education.
- Educators need to adopt learning strategies based on their assessment of their learners.
- Providing evaluation and feedback is an essential function of educators.
- Medical educators should attend Professional Development Courses dealing specifically with medical education.

REFERENCES

1. Kaufman DM. Applying education theory in practice. BMJ. 2003;326(7382):213-6.
2. Knowles MS. The modern practice of adult education: andragogy versus pedagogy. New York, NY: Association Press; 1970.
3. Knowles MS. Introduction: the art and science of helping adults learn. Andragogy in action: applying modern principles of adult learning. San Francisco, Calif: Jossey–Bass; 1984.
4. Collins J. Education techniques for lifelong learning: principles of adult learning. Radiographics. 2004;24:1483-9.
5. Spencer J. Learning and teaching in the clinical environment. BMJ. 2003;326(7389):591-4.
6. Irby DM, Bowen JL. Time-efficient strategies for learning and performance. Clin Teach. 2004;1(1):23-8.
7. Harden RM, Crosby J. AMEE Guide No 20: The good teacher is more than a lecturer - the twelve roles of the teacher. Med Teach. 2009;22(4):334-47.
8. Wolpaw TM, Wolpaw DR, Papp KK. SNAPPS: a learner-centered model for outpatient education. Acad Med. 2003;78(9):893-8.
9. Dornan T, Conn R, Monaghan H, Kearney G, Gillespie H, Bennett D. Experience Based Learning (ExBL): Clinical teaching for the twenty-first century. Med Teach. 2019;41(10):1098-105.
10. Ramani S. Reflections on feedback: Closing the loop. Med Teach. 2015;38(2):206-7.
11. Sargeant J, Mann K, Manos S, Epstein I, Warren A, Shearer C, et al. R2C2 in Action: Testing an Evidence-Based Model to Facilitate Feedback and Coaching in Residency. J Grad Med Educ. 2017;9(2):165-70.

Acute Rheumatic Fever

Anil Modak, Sunanda Chaoji, Tanuja Manohar

INTRODUCTION

Acute rheumatic fever (ARF) is a type of autoimmune disease following group A streptococcal (GAS) upper respiratory tract infection (URI). Jones established clinical diagnostic criteria (1944) for ARF, which were subsequently modified by American Heart Association (AHA), but still failed to diagnose asymptomatic patients of ARF.[1] Such patients may not receive secondary prophylaxis and ultimately progressed to severe form of rheumatic heart disease (RHD), hence, new echocardiographic guidelines were developed which are more sensitive to pickup disease, so patients can be treated early.

EPIDEMIOLOGY

Although there is global decline in RHD burden[2] but prevalence is still significant in South-East Asia, Africa, and Oceania[2] where RHD is endemic. ARF is a disease of childhood between 5 and 14 years, recurrence is common in adolescents and young adults that is why RHD peaks between 25 and 40 years.

PATHOPHYSIOLOGY[3]

Acute rheumatic fever is caused by URI due to GAS. Susceptibility is inherited. Some human leukocyte antigen (HLA) alleles, HLA-DR7 and HLA-DR4, are more susceptible. The pathogenesis is based on the concept of molecular mimicry. In this model, antibodies against streptococcal antigen crossreact with endothelial cells of heart valves inducing immune response leading to damage.

NATURAL HISTORY OF ACUTE RHEUMATIC FEVER AND RHEUMATIC HEART DISEASE

There is a latent period of 1–5 weeks between onset of URI and ARF. Most of the symptoms due to ARF recover fully over a period of time, except RHD.

There is a transition from rheumatic carditis to RHD in the subsequent years after ≥1 episodes of ARF, although ARF is recognized only in 30–50% of cases, suggesting that the diagnosis of ARF is frequently missed (**Fig. 1**).

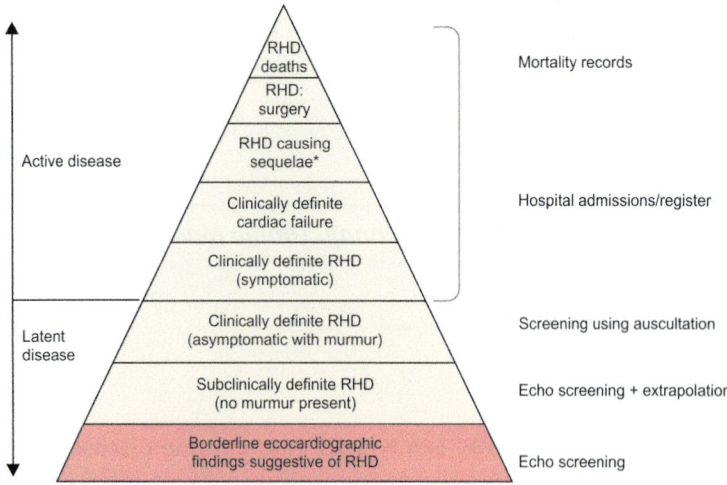

*Atrial fibrillation (AF), stroke, infective endocarditis.

FIG. 1: Showing rheumatic heart disease (RHD) burden in society.[4]

Severity of the disease increases as the time passes due to repeated attacks of clinical or subclinical ARF. This subclinical disease which is seven times more common and forms a major bulk which is detectable by echocardiography[2] only.

CLASSIFICATION OF ACUTE RHEUMATIC FEVER[4]

Definite ARF: Acute presentation which fulfills Jones diagnostic criteria for ARF.

Probable ARF: Acute presentation which does not fulfill Jones diagnostic criteria for ARF, missing one major or one minor criterion or lacking evidence of preceding streptococcal infection, but ARF is still considered the most likely diagnosis.

Possible ARF: Acute presentation which does not fulfill Jones diagnostic criteria for ARF, missing one major or one minor criterion or lacking evidence of preceding streptococcal infection, and ARF is considered uncertain but cannot be ruled out.

CLINICAL FEATURES OF ACUTE RHEUMATIC FEVER

Most common features are polyarthritis (60–75%) and carditis (50–60%), chorea (<3–30%), erythema marginatum, and subcutaneous nodules are rare (<5%).

Heart involvement: Mitral valve is almost always affected, it may be associated with aortic valve involvement. Symptoms of RHD develop very late. More than 50% may not give history of ARF. Auscultation may not be very effective in diagnosis of RHD. Acute rheumatic valvulitis manifests as valvular regurgitation, over a time, chronic inflammation leads to valve stenosis with or without associated regurgitation. Many times RHD may be diagnosed for the first time during pregnancy or after a complication such as acute heart failure, atrial arrhythmia, an embolic event, or infective endocarditis. Most patients have heart failure symptoms at the time of clinical diagnosis with pathological heart murmurs on auscultation.[2]

Joint involvement: Large joints migratory polyarthritis/polyarthralgia is common presentation. Sometimes aseptic monoarthritis may be present. ARF polyarthritis resolves completely without any residual damage.

Skin manifestations: The erythema marginatum rash is pink macular rash, centrally clear, and disappears within short time. It is seen often on trunk and sometimes on limbs. It appears 2–3 weeks after the onset of disease and may last for few days to 3 weeks. Subcutaneous nodules are rarely seen.

Chorea: Sydenham's chorea has very prolonged latent period and is commonly seen in females. It is manifested as quasipurposive movements commonly affecting head, neck, face, and upper extremities.

Fever: Fever ($\geq 38°C$) is seen associated with raised acute phase reactants.

Evidence of gas infection: Most patients do not have positive throat swab culture but demonstration of ASO and antideoxyribonuclease B (ADB) titers are important.

ECHOCARDIOGRAPHY SCREENING

Rationale for screening: Aims at identification of asymptomatic individuals with latent RHD. Echocardiographic screening is more sensitive than clinical. It is found that subclinical cases are seven times more prevalent than overt cases.[2] School going children are most likely to be benefited from secondary prophylaxis, if detected early by echocardiographic screening.

DEFINITIONS OF RHEUMATIC HEART DISEASE[4]

Latent RHD: Asymptomatic RHD diagnosed through echocardiographic screening which may be clinical (pathological murmur) or subclinical (no clinical signs).

Subclinical RHD: RHD without audible murmur or other clinical symptoms or signs. Subclinical RHD is only diagnosed by echocardiography (**Box 1**) and is typically less advanced than clinical RHD.

Clinical RHD: RHD with clinical symptoms or signs including pathological heart murmur. Echocardiography is required to confirm the diagnosis.

Confirmation of ARF is based upon evidence of typical clinical features of ARF by applying modified Jones criteria (**Tables 1** and **2**).[1] Often there may be subclinical ARF which can be diagnosed by World Heart Federation (WHF) criteria (**Box 1**) based on echocardiography.[4] Evidence of GAS infection may be established by estimating antistreptolysin O (ASO), ADB titers, and rapid antigen detection test (RADT).[3]

> **Box 1: World Heart Federation (WHF) criteria for echocardiographic diagnosis of rheumatic heart disease (RHD) in individuals <20 years.[5]**
>
> - *Definite RHD (either A, B, C, or D)*:
>   - Pathologic MR and at least two morphologic features of RHD of mitral valve (MV)
>   - MS mean gradient of ≥4 mm Hg
>   - Pathologic AR and at least two morphologic features of RHD of AV
>   - Borderline disease of both MV and AV
> - *Borderline RHD (either A, B, or C)*:
>   - At least two morphologic features of RHD of MV without pathological MR or MS
>   - Pathologic MR
>   - Pathologic AR
> - *Pathologic regurgitation*:
>   - Pathologic MR: All of the following is seen in two views: Jet length ≥2 cm, peak velocity ≥3 m/s and pansystolic jet
>   - Pathologic AR: All of the following is seen in two views: Jet length ≥1 cm, peak velocity ≥3 m/s and pandiastolic jet
> - Morphological findings on echo in rheumatic valvulitis
>   - Acute mitral valve changes:
>   - Annular dilation
>   - Chordal elongation
>   - Chordal rupture resulting in flail leaflet with severe mitral regurgitation
>   - Anterior (or less commonly posterior) leaflet tip prolapse and beading/nodularity of leaflet tips
>   - Chronic mitral valve changes: Not seen in acute carditis
>   - Leaflet thickening ≥3 mm
>   - Chordal thickening and fusion
>   - Restricted leaflet motion
>   - Calcification
> - Aortic valve changes in either acute or chronic carditis
>   - Irregular or focal leaflet thickening
>   - Coaptation defect
>   - Restricted leaflet motion
>   - Leaflet prolapse

(AR: aortic regurgitation; AV: aortic valve; MR: mitral regurgitation; MS: mitral stenosis; MV: mitral valve)

TREATMENT[4]

Primary prevention: This consists of treatment of GAS infection for which phenoxymethylpenicillin 500 mg BID or amoxycillin 50 mg/kg or maximum 500 mg BID for 10 days, or single dose of 1.2 million units of benzathine penicillin G (BPG) given intramuscular (IM).

TABLE 1: Diagnostic criteria for acute rheumatic fever (ARF).[1,4]

For all patient populations with evidence of preceding group A streptococcal infection (GAS)

Diagnosis: Initial ARF	Two major manifestations or one major plus two minor manifestations
Diagnosis: Recurrent ARF	Two major or one major and two minor or three minor criteria
Probable or possible ARF (first episode or recurrence)[4]	A clinical presentation in which ARF is considered a likely diagnosis but falls short in meeting the criteria by either: • One major or one minor manifestation, or • No evidence of preceding GAS infection. Such cases should be further categorized according to the level of confidence with which the diagnosis is made • Probable ARF • Possible ARF

(ARF: acute rheumatic fever)

TABLE 2: T. Duckett Jones modified criteria 2020.[1,4]

Major criteria	
Low-risk population	High-risk population
Carditis: Clinical or subclinical	Carditis: clinical or sub clinical
Arthritis	Arthritis
Polyarthritis only	Monoarthritis or polyarthritis/polyarthralgia
Chorea	Chorea
Erythema marginatum	Erythema marginatum
Subcutaneous nodules	Subcutaneous nodules
Minor criteria	
Low-risk population	High-risk population
Polyarthralgia	Monoarthralgia
Fever ≥38°C	Fever ≥ 37.5°C (Oral)
ESR > 60 mm and CRP > 3 mg/dL	ESR > 30 mm and/or CRP > 3 mg/dL
Prolonged PR interval	Prolonged PR interval

Note: High-risk groups are those living in communities with high rates of ARF (incidence >30/100,000 per year in 5–14-year-old) or RHD (all-age prevalence > 2/1,000).[4]

(ARF: acute rheumatic fever; CRP: C-reactive protein; ESR: erythrocyte sedimentation rate; RHD: rheumatic heart disease)

Treatment of Acute Rheumatic Fever

- Salicylates and nonsteroidal anti-inflammatory drugs (NSAIDs): Aspirin is the drug of choice for arthritis, dose is 50–60 mg/kg/day, in 4–6 divided doses to be given for 2–4 weeks. Or Naproxen 10–20 mg/kg/day in two doses.
- *Glucocorticoids*: Role of steroids in carditis is controversial. If used, the dose is 1–2 mg/kg/day.

TABLE 3: Recommendations for secondary prophylaxis.[2,4]

Category of patients	Duration of prophylaxis
RF without carditis	• 5 years after last attack; or • Up to 21 years of age, whichever is longer
RF with carditis, but no residual valvular disease	• 10 years after last attack; or • Up to 21 years of age, whichever in longer
RF with RHD evident clinically or on echocardiography	• 10 years after last attack; or • Up to 40 years of age, whichever is longer; or • Sometimes lifelong

(RF: rheumatic fever; RHD: rheumatic heart disease)

Chorea: Carbamazepine or sodium valproate are preferred drugs for control of abnormal movements to be continued for 2–3 weeks after control of symptoms.

Prednisolone is also effective in the dose of 0.5 mg/kg/day for chorea.

Intravenous immunoglobulin (IVIg) leads to more rapid resolution of chorea but not effective for carditis.

Secondary prevention: Injection benzathine penicillin G (BPG) is injected 1.2 million units every month or more often. If injection is contraindicated, oral penicillin V 250 mg BID or erythromycin 250 mg BID, can be given. Duration of secondary prophylaxis depends upon many factors (**Table 3**).

CONCLUSION

- Rheumatic heart disease burden is still high, mostly in poor population.
- Echocardiography screening based on WHF criteria holds promise to identify patients earlier, when prophylaxis is more likely to be effective particularly in school going children.

REFERENCES

1. Gewitz MH, Baltimore RS, Tani LY, Sable CA, Shulman ST, Carapetis J, et al. Revision of the Jones criteria for the diagnosis of acute rheumatic fever in the era of Doppler echocardiography: a scientific statement from the American Heart Association. Circulation. 2015;131(20):1806-18.
2. Kumar RK, Antunes MJ, Beaton A, Mirabel M, Nkomo VT, Okello E, et al. Contemporary Diagnosis and Management of Rheumatic Heart Disease: Implications for Closing the Gap: A Scientific Statement From the American Heart Association. Circulation. 2020;142(20):e337-57.
3. Carapetis JR, Beaton A, Cunningham MW, Guilherme L, Karthikeyan G, Mayosi BM, et al. Acute rheumatic fever and rheumatic heart disease. Nat Rev Dis Primers. 2016;2:15084.
4. Ralph AP, Noonan S, Wade V, Currie BJ. The 2020 Australian guideline for prevention, diagnosis and management of acute rheumatic fever and rheumatic heart disease. Med J Aust. 2021;214(5):220-7.
5. Remenyi B, Wilson N, Steer A, Ferreira B, Kado J, Kumar K, et al. World Heart Federation criteria for echocardiographic diagnosis of rheumatic heart disease—an evidence-based guideline. Nat Rev Cardiol. 2012;9(5):297-309.

5
Angiotensin Receptor Blocker and Angiotensin-converting Enzyme Inhibitors: Newer Insights

Nihar Mehta, Yogesh Solanki

INTRODUCTION
- Angiotensin-converting enzyme (ACE) inhibitors and angiotensin receptor blockers (ARBs) are widely prescribed for the treatment of primary hypertension (HTN).
- Angiotensin-converting enzyme inhibitors and ARBs inhibit the renin-angiotensin system (RAS) but have different sites of action.
- Angiotensin-converting enzyme inhibitors inhibit the conversion of angiotensin I (AT1) to angiotensin II (AT2).
- Angiotensin receptor blockers antagonize receptor binding of AT2 to AT1 receptors.

Therefore, it is often assumed that the two drug classes have similar efficacy in cardiovascular (CV) disease prevention.

EVIDENCE
- Current evidence analyzing ACE inhibitors, and the other ARBs, has shown similar efficacy in lowering the blood pressure (BP).
- The efficacy of a drug in lowering BP cannot be taken as a definitive indicator of its efficacy in reducing mortality and morbidity.
- Evidence exists for ACE inhibitors and ARBs in preventing CV events.

OLMESARTAN VERSUS RAMIPRIL IN HYPERTENSION
A study by Stefano Ombani et al. in December 2012, antihypertensive efficacy and safety of olmesartan medoxomil and ramipril in elderly mild to moderate essential hypertensive patients with or without metabolic syndrome showed that olmesartan provides more effective BP control than ramipril in elderly hypertensive patients with and without metabolic syndrome.[1]

DIABETICS EXPOSED TO TELMISARTAN AND ENALAPRIL (DETAIL) STUDY
It was a double-blind, randomized, noninferiority, controlled trial of 250 patients aged 35–80 years with type 2 diabetes mellitus (T2DM) and HTN taking an ACE inhibitor.

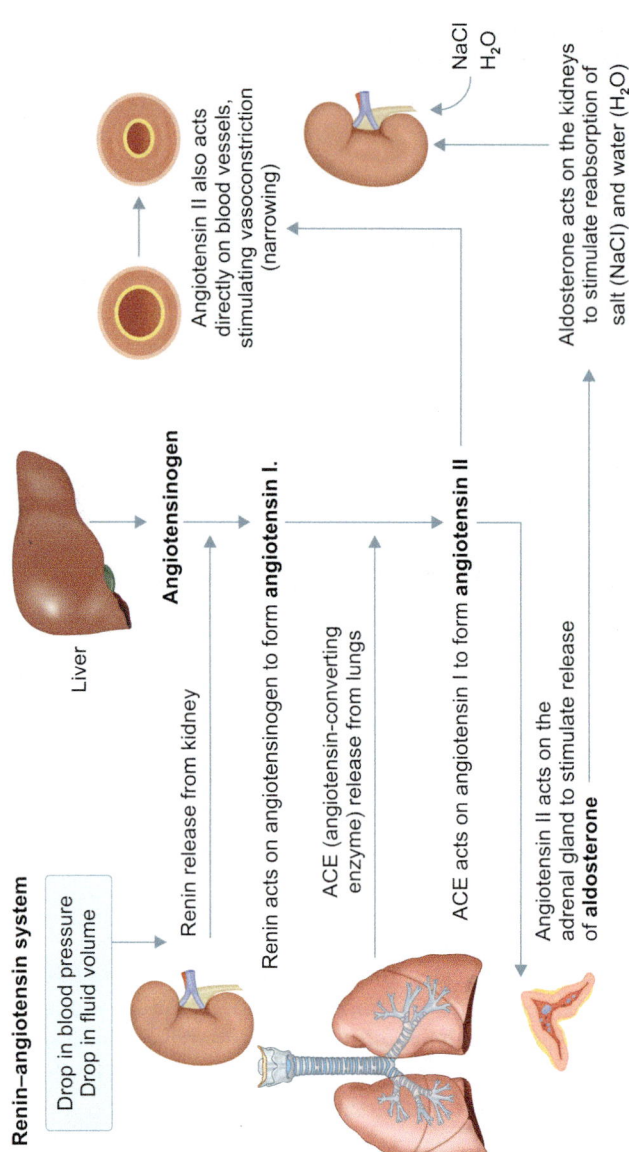

FIG. 1: The renin–angiotensin–aldosterone system.[17]

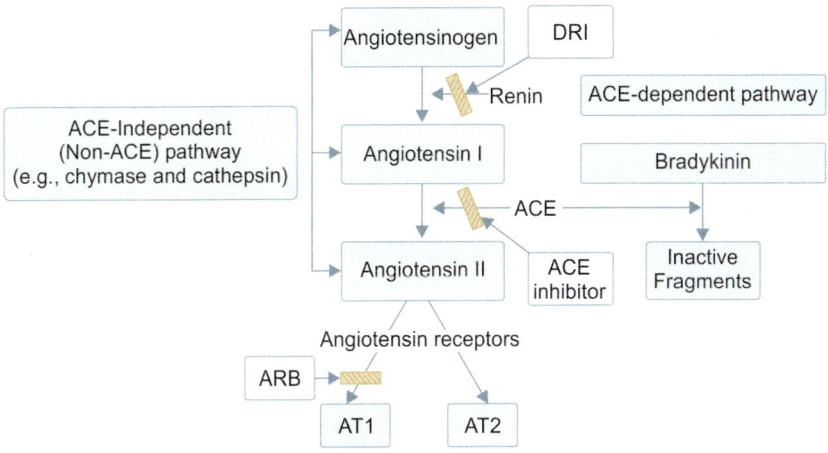

(AT: angiotensin; DRI: direct renin inhibitor)

FLOWCHART 1: Mechanism of action of angiotensin-converting enzyme (ACE) inhibitor and angiotensin receptor blocker (ARB).[18]

TABLE 1: Comparison of angiotensin receptor blockers (ARBs) versus angiotensin-converting enzyme (ACE) inhibitor.

Property	ARB	ACE inhibitor
Major site of block	AT1 receptor	Converting enzyme
Major claims and basic science	• More complete AT1 block • AT2 activity increased; latter may be beneficial (not certain)	Block of two receptors: AT1, AT2. Inhibition of breakdown of protective bradykinin
Side effects	• Generally similar to placebo • Cough unusual • Angioedema very rare but reported	Dry cough; angioedema higher in black (1.6%) than nonblack patients (0.6%)
Compelling indications, modified from JNC 7	Heart failure, diabetes, chronic renal disease, and recurrent stroke	As for ARB plus post-MI, high coronary risk, recurrent stroke (with diuretic)
Major clinical claims in hypertension	Equal BP reduction to ACE inhibitors, little or no cough, excellent tolerability, well tested in LVH and in diabetic nephropathy	Well tolerated, years of experience especially in CHF, good quality of life; used in coronary prevention trials (HOPE, EUROPA, and PEACE)
Outcome trials (death, stroke, coronary events, etc.)	• LIFE (losartan better than atenolol, stroke less, deaths less in diabetics) • VALUE (valsartan vs. amlodipine; about equal); JIKEI-heart (valsartan)	• Enalapril > diuretic • Diuretic > lisinopril in ALLHAT

(AT: angiotensin; BP: blood pressure; CHF: congestive heart failure; JNC: Joint National Committee; LVH: left ventricular hypertrophy; MI: myocardial infarction)

TABLE 2: Studies of angiotensin receptor blockers (ARBs) versus angiotensin-converting enzyme (ACE) inhibitor/placebo.

Trial	Condition	n	Follow-up	ARB	Outcome	Results
OPTIMAAL[19]	Acute MI and HF	5,477	6 month	Losartan vs. captropril	All-cause mortality, nonfatal MI, SCD	No difference, ↑ mortality with losartan
VALIANT[20]	Acute MI and HF	14,703	2.1 years	Valsartan vs. captopril or both	All-cause mortality, CV death, MI and CHF hospitalization	No difference
ValHeFT[21]	CHF	5,010	4 years	Valsartan vs. placebo	All-cause mortality	No change in mortality, ↓ hospitalization
ELITE II[22]	CHF	3,152	1.6 years	Losartan vs. captopril	Composite	No difference
CHARM-Added[23]	CHF	2,548	3.4 years	Candesartan vs. placebo	Composite	15% RRR
CHARM-Alternate[24]	CHF	2,028	2.8 years	Candesartan vs. placebo	Composite	23% RRR
CHARM-Preserved[25]	CHF	3,023	3 years	Candesartan vs. placebo	CV death	11% RRR
CHARM overall[26]	CHF	7,601	2 years	Candesartan vs. placebo	All-cause mortality	17% RRR
ONTARGET[4]	CAD, diabetes, hypertension	25,620	4.8 years	Telmisartan vs. ramipril or both	Composite, CV death, stroke, MI, hospitalization	Noninferiority to ramipril, ↑ adverse effects with combination

(CAD: coronary artery disease; CHF: congestive heart failure; CV: cardiovascular; HF: heart failure; MI: myocardial infarction; RRR: relative risk reduction; SCD: sudden cardiac death)

Both groups experienced a decrease in glomerular filtration rate (GFR) but it was found that telmisartan was not inferior to enalapril in preventing the progression of renal disease.[2]

TELMISARTAN VERSUS RAMIPRIL IN HYPERTENSION

- *PRISMA I and II* trials 1,613 patients enrolled in this study of 14 weeks duration with primary end points change from baseline in mean ambulatory systolic BP (SBP) and diastolic BP (DBP) during the final 6 hours of the 24-hour dosing cycle.
- Telmisartan 80 mg/day versus ramipril 5–10 mg/day
- Telmisartan is more effective than ramipril throughout the 24-hour period and during the early morning.[3]

ANGIOTENSIN RECEPTOR BLOCKERS VERSUS ANGIOTENSIN-CONVERTING ENZYME-I IN CARDIOVASCULAR RISK

Ontarget Trial

- In ONTARGET, 25,620 patients were randomized to receive telmisartan 80 mg/day, ramipril 10 mg/day, or the combination of both drugs, and were followed for 56 months.
- Telmisartan was equivalent to ramipril for the primary outcome [telmisartan 16.7%, ramipril 16.5%, RR 1.01; 95% confidence interval (CI) 0.94–1.09].
- Renin–angiotensin–aldosterone system (RAAS) blockade with either telmisartan or ramipril is optimal for CV risk reduction and that telmisartan is comparable to ramipril in patients with vascular disease or high-risk diabetes, with fewer cough and angioedema events.[4]

Transcend Trial

- About 5,926 high-risk patients intolerant to ACE inhibitors but otherwise similar to ONTARGET population were randomized to receive telmisartan 80 mg/day or placebo.
- Telmisartan reduced the secondary composite outcome of CV death, myocardial infarction (MI), and stroke [telmisartan 13%, placebo 14.8%; odds ratio (OR) 0.86; 95% CI 0.74–1.00; $p = 0.045$] which was the HOPE composite outcome.
- Therefore, TRANSCEND validates the role of ARBs in reducing CV risk in high-risk patients and does not contradict ONTARGET.[5]

Orient Trial

Trial conducted in Japan and Hongkong involving 556 patients with diabetic nephropathy, the addition of olmesartan to pre-existing antihypertensive treatment was associated with a higher rate of death from CV causes (10 cases vs. three cases).[6]

Roadmap Trial

- ROADMAP (Randomized Olmesartan and Diabetes Microalbuminuria Prevention) study was a randomized, double-blind, placebo-controlled, multicenter trial conducted in Europe.
- The trial included 4,447 patients with T2DM and at least one additional CV risk factor but without overt evidence of nephropathy.
- Patients were randomized to receive either 40 mg of olmesartan or placebo daily.
- But in the study showed that olmesartan group has high CV death compare to placebo group (15 vs. 3).
- Food and Drug Administration (FDA's) review is ongoing and the agency has not concluded that olmesartan increases the risk of death. FDA currently believes that the benefits of olmesartan in patients with high BP continue to outweigh its potential risk.[7]

PREVENTION REGIMEN FOR EFFECTIVELY AVOIDING SECOND STROKES

- It is another large randomized controlled trial (RCT) that enrolled 20,322 patients older than 50 years of age who had an ischemic stroke in the previous 120 days and were clinically and neurologically stable.
- Patients were randomized to receive telmisartan 80 mg/day versus placebo, and were followed for 2.5 years.
- Therapy with telmisartan initiated soon after an ischemic stroke and continued for 2.5 years did not significantly lower the rate of recurrent stroke, major CV events, or diabetes.
- Post hoc analyses showed that from 6 months on, recurrent stroke rate was lower in the telmisartan group (5.3% vs. 6.0%; HR 0.88; 95% CI 0.78–0.99).
- This finding suggests a time-dependent benefit of telmisartan and that the trial duration may have been too short to detect a difference.[8]

AMONG ANGIOTENSIN RECEPTOR BLOCKERS—WHICH ONE?

- Among available ARBs, there is growing evidence of the higher efficacy of the long-lasting compounds, such as olmesartan and telmisartan, in achieving an early and sustained BP control.
- Comparison of the effects of telmisartan and olmesartan on home BP, glucose, and lipid profiles in patients with HTN, chronic heart failure, and metabolic syndrome, a trial by Tatsuya Sasaki et al. in 2008 concluded that telmisartan was more beneficial than olmesartan for controlling BP in the early morning, as well as for improving glucose and lipid profiles in patients with HTN, chronic heart failure, and metabolic syndrome.[9]
- Olmesartan is more effective than other angiotensin receptor antagonists in reducing proteinuria in patients with chronic kidney disease (CKD) other than diabetic nephropathy study by Takashi et al. in 2013

retrospectively examine the protective effect of ARBs (olmesartan, losartan, candesartan, and valsartan) on CKD patients without a history of diabetic nephropathy. From this, it was concluded that olmesartan is more effective in reducing urinary protein than other ARBs, suggesting that the renal protective effects of olmesartan may be better than those of other ARBs.[10]

- Antihypertensive effects of olmesartan compared with other ARBs: A meta-analysis study by Long Wang et al. (**Fig. 2**) reports of RCTs of olmesartan versus other ARBs were identified through a systematic search of PubMed (up to July 2010), EMBASE (1980 to July 2010), SinoMed (up to July 2010), and the Cochrane Central Register of Controlled Trials (CENTRAL) (Cochrane Library Issue 7, 2010). 22 studies with data from 4,892 patients were considered for analyses. Olmesartan provided greater DBP and SBP reductions compared with losartan (DBP: 95% CI 0.59, 2.62; SBP: 95% CI 0.46, 5.92). Olmesartan provided greater SBP reductions compared with valsartan (95% CI 0.29, 3.16). Similar BP response rates and incidence of adverse events were found with losartan, valsartan, candesartan, and irbesartan.[11]
- Several studies have demonstrated that a greater percentage of patients treated with olmesartan achieved BP targets, compared to those who received initial doses of losartan, candesartan, valsartan, and irbesartan, with a significant greater reduction of both clinical and ambulatory SBP and DBP levels, already after 1, 2, 4, and 8 weeks of therapy, both in naïve and previously treated patients and independently from the grade of HTN.[11]

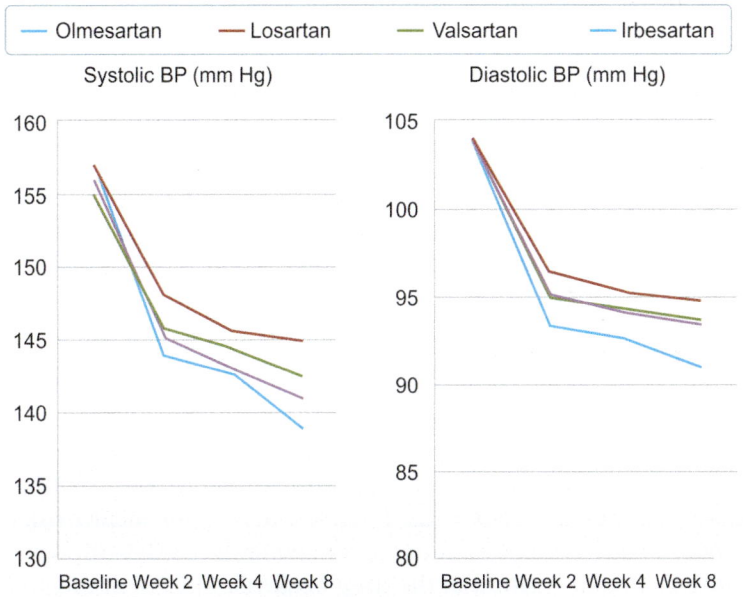

FIG. 2: Comparison between various ARBs in blood pressure lowering efficacy.[27]

WHICH ANGIOTENSIN RECEPTOR BLOCKER? COMBINATION THERAPY

- The efficacy and safety profile of olmesartan has been demonstrated also in combination therapies with both calcium channel blocker (CCB) and diuretics, producing faster and larger reductions in both SBP and DBP compared to associations based on irbesartan, telmisartan, and valsartan
- Similar results have been obtained in the BP CRUSH and the TRINITY (the Triple Therapy with Olmesartan Medoxomil, Amlodipine, and Hydrochlorothiazide in Hypertensive Patients Study) trials which have demonstrated that both seated SBP and DBP reductions were faster and greater with triple combination therapy of olmesartan, amlodipine, and hydrochlorothiazide (HCTZ), compared with those of dual combination therapies.[12,13]
- Other long-lasting compounds in the class, such as azilsartan, appear to have a similar effective profile in effectively reducing BP in hypertensives in a fast and sustained fashion.

Azilsartan

- Azilsartan is newer ARB with 60% bioavailability and not affected by food and its peak plasma concentration reaches within 1.5-3 hour after ingestion with $t_{1/2}$ of 11 hours and excreted via hepatic metabolism.
- Azilsartan 80 mg reduced the mean SBP by an additional 2.1 mm Hg as compared to olmesartan 40 mg or 320 mg of valsartan daily.[14]

Fimasartan

- It is a newer long-acting armament to fight HTN via selective AT2 type I receptor antagonist.
- Usually given in dosage of 60-120 mg OD with $t_{1/2}$ of 5-16 hours and excreted via fecal and biliary root and only 2% via renal route.
- No dose adjustment required in mild to moderate renal failure but in the creatinine clearance <30 mL/min starting dose should be 30 mg OD.
- It is not recommended in moderate to severe hepatic failure.[15]
- SAFE-KANARB study has established efficacy, safety, and tolerability of fimasartan in patients potentially at higher risk for adverse events.[16]

SIDE EFFECTS

- *Hypotension*: Hypotension appears to be more common with ARBs than ACE inhibitors. The magnitude of this effect was illustrated in the ONTARGET trial cited above in which hypotensive symptoms severe enough to require permanent discontinuation occurred significantly more often with telmisartan (2.7 vs. 1.7% with ramipril, relative risk 1.54).
- *Reduced GFR*: An elevation in serum creatinine sufficiently severe to warrant discontinuation of the drug occurred in 0.7% of the patients who received ramipril in the ONTARGET trial. A doubling of the serum creatinine in this trial occurred in 1.9%.

Renal function should be checked at 3–5 days when an ACE inhibitor is begun in a patient who has renal artery stenosis or who is at high risk for this problem (as in an older patient with severe HTN and atherosclerotic vascular disease).
- *Hyperkalemia*: In prospective study of 251 hemodialysis patients in which there was an association between a predialysis serum potassium concentration of ≥5.5 mEq/L and the use of an ACE inhibitor or ARB.

  Use of these agents was associated with an increased risk of hyperkalemia (OR 2.2, 95% CI 1.4–3.4) which was observed in patients with and without residual renal function.

  Dietary measures were the only intervention required to manage the hyperkalemia.
- *Cough*: The best data come from a meta-analysis of 29 trials in which cough was noted in 9.9% of patients treated with ACE inhibitors. In the ONTARGET trial, cough sufficiently severe to discontinue the drug was observed in 4.2% of the patients treated with ramipril. Cough is much less common with ARBs.
- *Anemia*: ACE inhibitors (and ARBs) can suppress the production of erythropoietin.

  This is more likely to occur in the presence of CKD due to accumulation of N-acetyl-seryl-aspartyl-lysyl-proline which inhibits stem cell multiplication.
- *Angioedema/Anaphylactoid reaction*: Angioedema is a rare but potentially fatal complication of ACE inhibitors that, in the largest clinical trial (ONTARGET), occurred in 0.3% of the >8,500 patients treated with ramipril.

  Angioedema—available evidence suggests the rate of angioedema with ARB therapy is low.
- *Enteropathy*: Enteropathy with olmesartan—In 2013, the FDA reported that olmesartan can produce a "sprue-like enteropathy" characterized by severe chronic diarrhea and weight loss, occurring months to years after initiation of the drug.

The condition resolved after discontinuation of olmesartan but rechallenge with the drug sometimes reproduced the symptoms.

ANGIOTENSIN RECEPTOR BLOCKERS UNDER DEVELOPMENT

Several nonpeptide ARBs are in various phases of development:
- Embusartan
- Fimasartan
- Pratosartan (seven times affinity for AT1 receptor than losartan)

SUMMARY

- Angiotensin receptor blockers are first line drugs used in the treatment of HTN.
- Although they both are RAAS blockers, there are some differences.

- Current evidence shows that ARBs have similar efficacy in reducing BP.
- Compelling indications to use ARBS are in left ventricular hypertrophy (LVH), post MI, heart failure, diabetes mellitus (DM), nephropathy, and high CV risk.
- Fine tuning our selection of ARBs in more optimal treatment of HTN could result in better control.
- Longer acting agents should be preferred.
- Single pill combination therapy should be considered.
- Amongst side effects, ARBs are better tolerated in terms of cough.

REFERENCES

1. Omboni S, Malacco E, Mallion JM, Volpe M. Antihypertensive efficacy and safety of olmesartan medoxomil and ramipril in elderly mild to moderate essential hypertensive patients with or without metabolic syndrome: a pooled post hoc analysis of two comparative trials. Drugs Aging. 2012;29(12):981-92.
2. Barnett AH. Preventing renal complications in diabetic patients: the Diabetics Exposed to Telmisartan And enalaprIL (DETAIL) study. Acta Diabetol. 2005;42(1):S42-9.
3. Williams B, Lacourciere Y, Schumacher H, Gosse P, Neutel JM. Antihypertensive efficacy of telmisartan vs ramipril over the 24-h dosing period, including the critical early morning hours: a pooled analysis of the PRISMA I and II randomized trials. J Hum Hypertens. 2009;23(9):610-9.
4. Mann JF, Anderson C, Gao P, Gerstein HC, Boehm M, Ryden L, et al. Dual inhibition of the renin–angiotensin system in high-risk diabetes and risk for stroke and other outcomes: results of the ONTARGET trial. J Hypertens. 2013;31(2):414-21.
5. Kappert K, Böhm M, Schmieder R, Schumacher H, Teo K, Yusuf S, et al. Impact of sex on cardiovascular outcome in patients at high cardiovascular risk: analysis of the telmisartan randomized assessment study in ACE-intolerant subjects with cardiovascular disease (TRANSCEND) and the ongoing telmisartan alone and in combination with ramipril global end point trial (ONTARGET). Circulation. 2012;126(8):934-41.
6. Imai E, Ito S, Haneda M, Chan JC, Makino H. Olmesartan reducing incidence of endstage renal disease in diabetic nephropathy trial (ORIENT): rationale and study design. Hypertens Res. 2006;29(9):703-9.
7. Ruilope L, Izzo J, Haller H, Waeber B, Oparil S, Weber M, et al. Prevention of microalbuminuria in type 2 diabetes: what do we know? J Clin Hypertens. 2010;12(6):422-30.
8. Diener HC, Sacco RL, Yusuf S, Cotton D, Ôunpuu S, Lawton WA, et al. Effects of aspirin plus extended-release dipyridamole versus clopidogrel and telmisartan on disability and cognitive function after recurrent stroke in patients with ischaemic stroke in the Prevention Regimen for Effectively Avoiding Second Strokes (PRoFESS) trial: a double-blind, active and placebo-controlled study. Lancet Neurol. 2008;7(10):875-84.
9. Sasaki T, Noda Y, Yasuoka Y, Irino H, Abe H, Adachi H, et al. Comparison of the effects of telmisartan and olmesartan on home blood pressure, glucose, and lipid profiles in patients with hypertension, chronic heart failure, and metabolic syndrome. Hypertens Res. 2008;31(5):921-9.
10. Ono T, Sanai T, Miyahara Y, Noda R. Olmesartan is more effective than other angiotensin receptor antagonists in reducing proteinuria in patients with chronic kidney disease other than diabetic nephropathy. Curr Ther Res Clin Exp. 2013;74:62-7.
11. Wang L, Zhao JW, Liu B, Shi D, Zou Z, Shi XY. Antihypertensive effects of olmesartan compared with other angiotensin receptor blockers: a meta-analysis. Am J Cardiovasc Drugs. 2012;12(5):335-44.

12. Nesbitt SD, Shojaee A, Maa JF, Weir MR. Efficacy of an amlodipine/olmesartan treatment algorithm in patients with or without type 2 diabetes and hypertension (a secondary analysis of the BP-CRUSH study). J Hum Hypertens. 2013;27(7):445-52.
13. Oparil S, Melino M, Lee J, Fernandez V, Heyrman R. Triple therapy with olmesartan medoxomil, amlodipine besylate, and hydrochlorothiazide in adult patients with hypertension: the TRINITY multicenter, randomized, double-blind, 12-week, parallel-group study. Clin Ther. 2010;32(7):1252-69.
14. Jones JD, Jackson SH, Agboton C, Martin TS. Azilsartan medoxomil (Edarbi): the eighth angiotensin II receptor blocker. P T. 2011;36(10):634-40.
15. Pradhan A, Gupta V, Sethi R. Fimasartan: A new armament to fight hypertension. J Family Med Prim Care. 2019;8(7):2184-8.
16. Park JB, Sung KC, Kang SM, Cho EJ. Safety and efficacy of fimasartan in patients with arterial hypertension (safe-kanarb study): an open-label observational study. Am J Cardiovasc Drugs. 2013;13(1):47-56.
17. Britannica, The Editors of Encyclopaedia. Renin-angiotensin system. Encyclopedia Britannica, 14 Aug. 2017, https://www.britannica.com/science/renin-angiotensin-system. Accessed 2 October 2021.
18. Haroon-Ur R. Renoprotection, renin inhibition, and blood pressure control: the impact of aliskiren on integrated blood pressure control. Integrated blood pressure control. 2010;3:133-44. 10.2147/IBPC.S12407.
19. Dickstein K. OPTIMAAL Steering Committee of the OPTIMAAL Study Group. Effects of losartan and captopril on mortality and morbidity in high-risk patients after acute myocardial infarction: the OPTIMAAL randomised trial. Optimal Trial in Myocardial Infarction with Angiotensin II Antagonist Losartan. Lancet. 2002;360:752-60.
20. Velazquez EJ, Pfeffer MA, McMurray JV, Maggioni AP, Rouleau JL, Van de Werf F, et al. VALsartan In Acute myocardial iNfarcTion (VALIANT) trial: baseline characteristics in context. European Journal of Heart Failure. 2003;5(4):537-44.
21. Jong P, Demers C, McKelvie RS, Liu PP. Angiotensin receptor blockers in heart failure: meta-analysis of randomized controlled trials. Journal of the American College of Cardiology. 2002;39(3):463-70.
22. Berry C, Norrie J, McMurray JJ. Are angiotensin II receptor blockers more efficacious than placebo in heart failure? Implications of ELITE-2. Evaluation of Losartan In The Elderly. The American journal of cardiology. 2001 Mar 1;87(5):606-7.
23. Weir RA, McMurray JJ, Puu M, Solomon SD, Olofsson B, Granger CB, Yusuf S, Michelson EL, Swedberg K, Pfeffer MA, CHARM Investigators. Efficacy and tolerability of adding an angiotensin receptor blocker in patients with heart failure already receiving an angiotensin-converting inhibitor plus aldosterone antagonist, with or without a beta blocker. Findings from the Candesartan in Heart failure: Assessment of Reduction in Mortality and morbidity (CHARM)-Added trial. European journal of heart failure. 2008;10(2):157-63.
24. Randy Wexler MD, David Feldman MD, Chavey WE, Nicklas JM. Combination of ARB and ACE Inhibitors in Heart Failure Patients/IN REPLY. American Family Physician. 2009;79(6):454.
25. Tan LB, Williams SG, Goldspink DF. From CONSENSUS to CHARM—how do ACEI and ARB produce clinical benefits in CHF?. International journal of cardiology. 2004;94(2-3):137-41.
26. Chang SM, Granger CB, Johansson PA, Kosolcharoen P, McMurray JJ, Michelson EL, Murray DR, Olofsson B, Pfeffer MA, Solomon SD, Swedberg K. Efficacy and safety of angiotensin receptor blockade are not modified by aspirin in patients with chronic heart failure: a cohort study from the Candesartan in Heart failure–Assessment of Reduction in Mortality and morbidity (CHARM) programme. European journal of heart failure. 2010;12(7):738-45.
27. Volpe M, Gallo G, Tocci G. Is early and fast blood pressure control important in hypertension management?. International journal of cardiology. 2018;254:328-32.

6 Subclinical Hyperthyroidism

Jimit Vadgama

INTRODUCTION

Subclinical hyperthyroidism (SHyper) is one of the rarely discussed topics, as it is very rare to find as an isolated etiology. Though it has similar features to overt hyperthyroidism; but it has slightly subtle clinical features. Similar to subclinical hypothyroidism (SHypo) definition, SHyper is defined as normal levels of thyroid hormones and a suppressed thyroid-stimulating hormone (TSH) level. Though less weighted till last few decades, newer and consistent evidences and meta-analysis now indicates that "subclinical" hyperthyroidism reduces the quality of life, affecting both the psycho and somatic components of well-being. More concerned are the association between SHyper and its cardiovascular effects and excess fracture risk.

DEFINITION OF SUBCLINICAL HYPERTHYROIDISM

European Thyroid Association[1] (ETA) has defined SHyper, not by any clinical criteria but exclusively biochemically by; persistently subnormal TSH concentration along with normal levels of free thyroxine (FT4), triiodothyronine (TT3), and/or free triiodothyronine (FT3).

That's why one should be very cautious while labeling any patient SHyper based on any clinical features. Only exclusively by biochemical results of thyroid function tests.

CLASSIFICATION, GRADING, AND ETIOLOGY

Subclinical hyperthyroidism can be classified into two different categories—endogenous and exogenous SHyper (**Flowchart 1**).

Endogenous SHyper is most commonly due to Graves' disease (GD), toxic adenoma (TA), and toxic multinodular goiter (MNG). While GD is the most common cause in younger patients (<65 years) in iodine-replete areas, TA and toxic MNG are relatively more frequent in iodine-deficient areas and in older persons (≥65 years).

Exogenous SHyper is due to thyroid hormone overtreatment, either intentionally (in patients with thyroid cancer), unintentionally (in patients on hypothyroidism treatment) or sometimes by factitial use of the hormone.

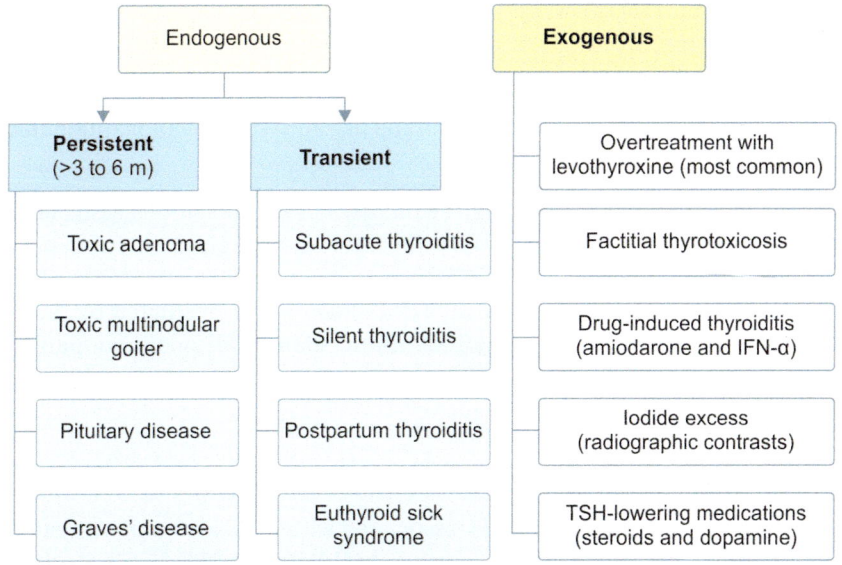

(IFN: interferon; TSH: thyroid-stimulating hormone)

FLOWCHART 1: Common causes of subclinical hyperthyroidism.

Sometimes transient SHyper can also occur. The etiology for such transient cases can be either treatment of overt hyperthyroidism with ATDs/radioiodine or sometimes thyroiditis can present with such picture, e.g., subacute thyroiditis, postpartum thyroiditis, painless, and silent thyroiditis. It becomes necessary to identify causes of low TSH that are not actual SHyper. Such as pituitary or hypothalamic insufficiency, some psychiatric illness, and sometimes drugs like iodide excess by radiographic contrasts; dopamine or high doses of glucocorticoids, somatostatin analogs, dobutamine, amphetamine, bromocriptine, etc.

European Thyroid Association has done severity grading of SHyper in two grades:
- *Grade 1*—which has low but detectable serum TSH levels; TSH value 0.1–0.39 mIU/L
- *Grade 2*—which has suppressed serum TSH levels; TSH value <0.1 mIU/L

APPROACH TO DIAGNOSIS OF SUBCLINICAL HYPERTHYROIDISM (EUROPEAN THYROID ASSOCIATION GUIDELINES)[1]

Whenever we are suspecting patient with SHyper, a proper approach must be followed to reach the diagnosis. ETA 2015 guidelines[1] have given different levels of investigations for the same. We should rule out causes of transient TSH variations or subnormal serum TSH not associated with SHyper. All Initial subnormal serum TSH with thyroid hormone levels within or at the upper limit of the normal range should be retested within 2–3 months because SHyper is defined as a persistently subnormal TSH.

Level 1 investigations to establish the persistent SHyper diagnosis by thyroid profile, first low TSH value screening and then FT4, TT3, or FT3.

Level 2 investigations should establish the etiology of SHyper; e.g., thyroid scan or ultrasonography and blood workup like anti-TSH receptor antibodies (TSHR-Abs).

Level 3 investigations should identify the risks or complications associated with SHyper and also to determine treatment requirements; e.g., electrocardiogram (ECG) and Holter monitoring and 2D Echo for cardiac involvement. Bone mineral density (BMD) should be evaluated by dual-energy X-ray absorptiometry (DEXA) bone scan in all postmenopausal patients, in elderly patients, and in those patients with some established fracture risk factors.

RISKS-ASSOCIATED SUBCLINICAL HYPERTHYROIDISM

As newer evidences emerge, risks-associated with persistent and untreated endogenous SHyper are also getting highlighted. The most studied complications are cardiac and osteoporotic complications and newer evidences on overall mortality, quality of life derangements, and even cognitive effects and mood changes.

Cardiovascular Effects

Thyroid hormone plays an essential part in both development of heart and also functioning of heart-like positive chronotropic effects.[2] They are also responsible for coronary arteriolar angiogenesis and even reduction of vascular resistance.[2] Direct effect of thyroid hormone on heart leads to positive chronotropic effect leading to tachycardia. Thyroid hormone also increases total blood volume, stroke volume, cardiac output, and ejection fraction. Peripheral action of thyroid hormone leads to increase oxygen demands and can result in peripheral vasodilation and consequent reduction in peripheral resistance by around half.[3-5] Increased stroke volume and tachycardia leads to increase cardiac output and cardiac workload. These effects can lead to altered left ventricular mass, tachycardia, hear rate variability, and also arrythmias.[2] These changes are predominantly due to electrophysiological effects of thyroid hormones.[6]

A big meta-analysis of five prospective cohort studies which had showed an increased risk of atrial fibrillation in patients with TSH levels <0.1 mIU/L with hazard ratio (HR) of 2.54 (95% CI 1.08–5.99) and 0.1–0.44 mIU/L with HR = 1.63 (95% CI 1.10–2.41).[7] This study included a total of 8,711 participants and it indicated that atrial fibrillation risk correlates inversely with the serum TSH levels. One cohort study[8] of 2,007 elderly patients crossing 60 years with TSH levels <0.1 mIU/L had a Higher relative risk of 3.1 for atrial fibrillation over 10 years, compared with other persons with normal TSH.

Even for heart failure analysis of six prospective cohort studies found higher risk of heart failure in those with TSH levels <0.1 mIU/L than euthyroid participants. This analysis included around 25,390 participants with a mean follow-up of 10 years.[9]

Subclinical hyperthyroidism was also associated with overall increased all-cause mortality and also major adverse cardiovascular events (MACE) with heart failure as the leading cause of increased cardiovascular mortality. This was shown in a large Danish study which was retrospective population based.[10] On the contrary, there were no major trials found which have accessed effect of treatment of SHyper over cardiovascular effects.

Bone Metabolism

We all know about overt hyperthyroidism causes increased bone turnover, reduction in bone density, and overall-increased fracture risk. In elderly and postmenopausal women, SHyper can cause similar effects, but little or no evidence exist for these studies in men or premenopausal women.[11] And no studies have evaluated effect of treating SHyper on prevention of fractures.

Quality of Life and Cognition

As the definition of SHyper is only biochemical, many patients can have clinical features of adrenergic overactivity. In one study, lower TSH levels was found to be more associated with nervousness, palpitations, heat intolerance, tremor, and sweating then euthyroid persons. Thus, it indicated lower functional health and well-being.[12] Another systematic review of 23 studies showed an association between SHyper and cognitive impairment.[13]

WHEN AND HOW TO TREAT?

American Thyroid Association (ATA) recommends[14] that treatment should be based on the underlying etiology of SHyper, e.g., toxic MNG or a solitary autonomous nodule cases, radioactive iodine ablation should be a definitive treatment and it is also a preferred choice because of unlikely spontaneous remission. In patients with GD, antithyroid drugs and radioactive iodine both

TABLE 1: Recommendations from American Thyroid Association[14] for subclinical hyperthyroidism treatment.		
	TSH < 0.1 mIU/L	TSH 0.1 to lower limit
Age ≥ 65 years	Treat	Consider treating
Age < 65 years in asymptomatic patient	Consider treating	Observe
Age < 65 years with comorbidities		
CV disease	Treat	Consider treating
Symptomatic for hyperthyroidism	Treat	Consider treating
Osteoporosis	Treat	Consider treating
Postmenopausal (not on estrogen or bisphosphonate treatment)	Treat	Consider treating

(CV: cardiovascular; TSH: thyroid-stimulating hormone)

are appropriate treatment options as per clinical judgment and patient's preferences.

The major question arises is when to consider treatment for SHyper. ATA recommends treatment in 65 years or older patients with persistent low TSH levels below 0.1 mIU/L. Also treat in younger than 65 years patients either symptomatic or with comorbidities like CV disease or osteoporosis; or if they are postmenopausal.

American Thyroid Association also recommends considering treatment for 65 years and older patients who have TSH levels of 0.1–0.4 mIU/L. The ATA says in such mildly reduced TSH, you can consider treating in younger patients with comorbidities but without comorbidities you can just observe them.

REFERENCES

1. Biondi B, Bartalena L, Cooper D, Hegedüs L, Laurberg P, Kahaly GJ. The 2015 European Thyroid Association Guidelines on Diagnosis and Treatment of Endogenous Subclinical Hyperthyroidism. Eur Thyroid J. 2015;4(3):149-63.
2. Grais IM, Sowers JR. Thyroid and the heart. Am J Med. 2014;127(8):691-8.
3. Ertek S, Cicero AF. Hyperthyroidism and cardiovascular complications: a narrative review on the basis of pathophysiology. Arch Med Sci. 2013;9(5):944-52.
4. Klein I, Danzi S. Thyroid disease and the heart. Circulation. 2007;116(15):1725-35.
5. Fadel B, Ellahham S, Lindsay J, Ringel M, Wartofsky L, Burman K. Hyperthyroid heart disease. Clin Cardiol. 2000;23(6):402-8.
6. Biondi B, Palmieri EA, Lombardi G, Fazio S. Effects of subclinical thyroid dysfunction on the heart. Ann Intern Med. 2002;137(11):904-14.
7. Collet TH, Gussekloo J, Bauer DC, den Elzen WP, Cappola AR, Balmer P, et al. Subclinical hyperthyroidism and the risk of coronary heart disease and mortality. Arch Intern Med. 2012;172(10):799-809.
8. Sawin CT, Geller A, Wolf PA, Belanger AJ, Baker E, Bacharach P, et al. Low serum thyrotropin concentrations as a risk factor for atrial fibrillation in older persons. N Engl J Med. 1994;331(19):1249-52.
9. Gencer B, Collet TH, Virgini V, Bauer DC, Gussekloo J, Cappola AR, et al. Subclinical thyroid dysfunction and the risk of heart failure events: an individual participant data analysis from 6 prospective cohorts. Circulation. 2012;126(9):1040-9.
10. Selmer C, Olesen JB, Hansen ML, von Kappelgaard LM, Madsen JC, Hansen PR, et al. Subclinical and overt thyroid dysfunction and risk of all-cause mortality and cardiovascular events: a large population study. J Clin Endocrinol Metab. 2014;99(7):2372-82.
11. Uzzan B, Campos J, Cucherat M, Nony P, Boissel JP, Perret GY. Effects on bone mass of long term treatment with thyroid hormones: a meta-analysis. J Clin Endocrinol Metab. 1996;81(12):4278-89.
12. Biondi B, Palmieri EA, Fazio S, Cosco C, Nocera M, Saccà L, et al. Endogenous subclinical hyperthyroidism affects quality of life and cardiac morphology and function in young and middle-aged patients. J Clin Endocrinol Metab. 2000;85(12):4701-5.
13. Gan EH, Pearce SH. Clinical review: The thyroid in mind: cognitive function and low thyrotropin in older people. J Clin Endocrinol Metab. 2012;97(10):3438-49.
14. Ross DS, Burch HB, Cooper DS, Greenlee MC, Laurberg P, Maia AL, et al. 2016 American Thyroid Association guidelines for diagnosis and management of hyperthyroidism and other causes of thyrotoxicosis. Thyroid. 2016;26(10):1343-1421.

7. Approach to Sleep Apnea

Hathur Basavanagowdappa, KS Lokesh

INTRODUCTION

The sleep apnea syndrome is very common disorder, characterized by intermittent cessation of airflow at the nose or mouth lasting for >10 seconds, with >5 episodes per hour. The cessation of airflow may occur due to collapse or obstruction of upper airway, which is called as obstructive apnea (OA), or it may occur due to decreased central trigger for breathing, i.e., lack of ventilator drive and effort, which is termed as central apnea (CA). Mixed apnea (MA) is the apnea which is due to both the causes. The OA is predominant in most of the individuals with sleep apnea and, hence, the condition is commonly called as obstructive sleep apnea (OSA).

Prevalence of OSA in India varies between 4 and 14% in various studies and more in presence of comorbidities. The OSA will not only affects a person's quality of life, but it may result in very serious events such as road traffic accidents, workplace accidents with heavy machinery leading to huge losses of life and infrastructure. These accidents results from impaired judgment, impaired response time, and excessive daytime sleepiness due to OSA. In United States of America (USA), mandatory evaluation for OSA is required for the people working in these areas. OSA is recognized as one of the cause for divorce in western countries which is not only due to loud snoring but also due to impaired memory, behavior, and personality changes.

RISK FACTORS FOR OBSTRUCTIVE SLEEP APNEA

In adults: Obesity, hypothyroidism, acromegaly, structural defects in upper airway which leads to its narrowing, macroglossia, retrognathia, and use of substances that reduce muscle tone such as alcohol, sedatives, or hypnotics increase the risk for OSA.

In children: The presence of enlarged adenoid (age 2-4 years), tonsils (age 5-7 years), polyps, history of allergic rhinitis, Down's syndrome, cleft palate, connective tissue disorders (Marfan's syndrome), and obesity are the risks for OSA.

PATHOPHYSIOLOGY

The upper airway obstruction which manifests during sleep, not only leads to alveolar hypoventilation, it also leads to negative intrathoracic pressure and increases cardiac after load. The alveolar hypoventilation leads to impaired gas exchange where it manifests as hypoxemia, hypercapnia, and respiratory acidosis which results in pulmonary vasoconstriction, pulmonary hypertension, and may lead to corpulmonale. There can be risk for arrhythmia, myocardial infarction (MI), and sudden cardiac deaths. There will be systemic vasoconstriction and risk for systemic hypertension. The increased respiratory drive and increased activity of respiratory muscles in response to alveolar hypoventilation results in frequent arousals leading to poor quality sleep. This leads to excessive day time sleepiness, impaired cognition and intellectual function, behavioral, and personality changes. The arousal will increase the tone of the pharyngeal muscles which restores the upper airway patency and airflow resumes. The vicious cycle repeats.

CLINICAL FEATURES

The history of recurrent or chronic loud snoring, gasping, or choking episodes during sleep is suggestive of OSA. The poor quality of sleep leads to excessive day time sleepiness, headache, easy fatigability, and personality changes. The hypoxemia and hypercapnia can add to declining cognition and memory, easy fatigability, and breathlessness on exertion. Some patients may give history of dozing episodes or history of automobile or work-related accidents. The presence of cor pulmonale, cardiac failure, resistant hypertension and brittle diabetes, and unexplained pulmonary hypertension should alert clinician to look for possible OSA (**Table 1**).

In critical care settings, OSA can create challenges to clinician, there can be prolonged apnea with sedatives or delayed recovery, or there can be difficulty in weaning from ventilation.

On clinical examination, presence of overweight and obesity, large neck size of >17 inches in men and 16 inches in women, presence of nasal obstruction, high and narrow nose, elongated soft palate, massive uvula, enlarged adenoids, enlarged tonsils, and large tongue should prompt

TABLE 1: The common clinical profile.

Patient's expressions	Opinion by spouse	Clinician's viewpoints
• Poor quality of sleep • Daytime sleepiness • Tiredness • Impotence • Headaches • Enuresis • GORD	• Excessive snoring • Apneas • Daytime sleepiness • Behavioral changes • Altered memory • Impotence	• Somnolent while waiting for consultation • Resistant hypertension • Glycemic variability • Unexplained right heart failure • Pulmonary hypertension • Obesity, hypothyroidism, acromegaly, macroglossia, and upper-airway abnormalities

(GORD: gastro-oesophageal reflux disease)

the clinician to suspect OSA. The visualization of soft palate and grading according to Mallampati grading also helps to identify the higher risk of OSA.

Some of the scoring systems which are available for assessing the risk of OSA are STOP BANG [snoring, tiredness, observed event, pressure (hypertension), body mass index (BMI) >35, age >50, neck size >16 inch, gender (male)], Sleep Apnea Clinical Score (SACS), and Berlin Questionnaire (BQ). The Epworth Sleepiness Scale (ESS) questionnaire helps in assessing the presence of excessive daytime sleepiness.

DIAGNOSIS

The diagnosis of OSA is made according to the American Academy of Sleep Medicine criteria:
- Excessive daytime sleepiness that is not better explained by other factors.
- Two or more of the following that are not better explained by other factors—choking during sleep, recurrent awakenings, nonrefreshing sleep, daytime fatigue, and impaired concentration.
- Apnea Hypopnea Index (AHI) five or more events per hour during sleep.

The gold standard test for diagnosis of OSA is polysomnography which includes electroencephalogram (EEG) for sleep staging, chest, and abdominal movements for respiratory efforts, airflow sensors, ocular sensors, limb sensors, position sensors, pulse oximetry, and electrocardiogram (ECG). The events are identified as apnea, hypopnea (central, obstructive, or mixed). In apnea, there is total cessation of airflow lasting for 10 seconds. In hypopnea, there is a decrease of airflow for at least 10 seconds, a 30% reduction in ventilation, and a decrease in oxygen saturation by 4% from baseline. The AHI is the number of apnea + hypopnea events occurring per hour during the sleep and the Respiratory Disturbance Index (RDI) is apnea + hypopnea + respiratory event-related arousals per hour of sleep. These indices are used for grading sleep apnea. If the AHI or RDI is <5 per hour it is normal, mild OSA if it is between 5 and 15 per hour, moderate OSA if it is between 15 and 30 per hour, and severe OSA if AHI or RDI ≥ 30.

Upper airway evaluation by ear-nose-throat (ENT) specialist and dentist is required to identify the site of obstruction and evaluation for need for the oral appliances. The individuals should be evaluated for hypothyroidism, cardiac status-right sided pressures and brain natriuretic peptide (BNP), cognitive function, and exercise testing. These parameters will help in monitoring the prognosis and response to therapy.

TREATMENT

Multidisciplinary treatment is needed for managing OSA. Early treatment improves the quality of sleep and life and reduces the risk of complications.

Lifestyle modification and individualized treatment plan are required. Optimal treatment of comorbidities and regular follow-up improves the treatment outcomes of OSA.

The general measures in management of OSA involves attaining an ideal body weight, to sleep on the side instead of supine, elevating the head end of the bed, avoid sedative medication, avoid overindulging in alcohol, and avoid large meals before bedtime. The presence of atopy is to be evaluated and its treatment will reduce the upper airway resistance. Smoking cessation helps in preventing the complications of OSA. Identification of risk factors (like obesity) and addressing them are very important.

Positional therapy: Sleeping sideward will reduce the upper airway obstruction and improves sleep quality. Patients can be provided positional support with the help of pillows or specialized cots. Especially designed t-shirts and devices can be used to prevent involuntary supine posture during sleep.

Cervical pillows: Provides support for neck, limits the over extension, and prevent the collapse of upper airway.

Oral appliances: The tongue retaining devices prevent the tongue falling back and reducing the obstruction can be used in patients who are not fit for surgery or where there is a relapse after surgery. Common disadvantage is poor compliance. Patients with retrognathism get benefited by mandibular advancement devices.

Nasal dilators: When the OSA is due to narrowing of nasal openings, these devices can reduce the obstruction.

Positive airway pressure (PAP) therapy: The PAP splints the airway from collapsing and reduces the obstruction. It is the gold standard in treatment of OSA. Continuous PAP (CPAP) devices are most commonly used and are effective in >90% of patients. The CPAP titration sleep study identifies the pressures required for preventing the airway collapse and improving the success rates. The counseling, proper type of mask/interface, its size, and settings improve the compliance to this therapy. Patients with predominant central sleep apneas, increased work of breathing, get benefited by bilevel PAP.

Surgical management for OSA: When the specific site of upper airway is identified, the surgical correction can be a better therapeutic option for OSA. The surgeries can be nasal surgeries such as polypectomy, reduction of turbinate size, and correction of deviated nasal septum. The adenoidectomy and uvulopalatopharyngoplasty (UPPP) can be done to relieve the obstruction in the site of retropalatal pharynx. Tongue size reduction, linguloplasty and resection, mandibular advancement, and mandibular osteotomy can be done when the obstruction is in the level of retrolingual pharynx. The position of tongue can be corrected with genioglossus advancement and hyoid myotomy (GAHM) and suspension. Maxillary and mandibular advancement osteotomy (MMO) can be done in highly selective patients to decrease the obstruction in pharynx.

CONCLUSION

High index of suspicion, early diagnosis, addressing the common risk factors, grading of OSA and appropriate corrective procedures, and proper counseling to use CPAP will improve the diagnosis and treatment outcomes of OSA. Multidisciplinary approach is required for management of OSA.

SUGGESTED READINGS

1. Sharma SK, Katoch VM, Mohan A, Kadhiravan T, Elavarasi A, Ragesh R, et al. Consensus and evidence-based Indian initiative on obstructive sleep apnea guidelines 2014 (first edition). Lung India. 2015;32(4):422-34.
2. Obstructive Sleep Apnoea. In: Barbe F, Pepin JL (eds). Eur Respir Soc. 2015:336.
3. Kryger MH, Roth T, Dement WC. Principles and practice of sleep medicine. Sixth edition. Philadelphia: Elsevier; 2017. p. 1730.
4. Kapur VK, Auckley DH, Chowdhuri S, Kuhlmann DC, Mehra R, Ramar K, et al. Clinical Practice Guideline for Diagnostic Testing for Adult Obstructive Sleep Apnea: An American Academy of Sleep Medicine Clinical Practice Guideline. J Clin Sleep Med. 2017;13(3):479-504.
5. Benjafield AV, Ayas NT, Eastwood PR, Heinzer R, Ip MSM, Morrell MJ, et al. Estimation of the global prevalence and burden of obstructive sleep apnoea: a literature-based analysis. Lancet Respir Med. 2019;7(8):687-98.

8. Jaundice in Pregnancy

Tanuja Manohar

INTRODUCTION

Pregnancy is a fascinating physiological condition usually having pleasant outcome, however, when it gets complicated by liver dysfunction, it can lead to adverse obstetric outcome. The challenge lies in the need to consider the safety of both the expectant mother and the unborn fetus in the clinical management decisions. Pregnancy encompasses a wide variety of physiological changes even in liver function tests (LFTs) but elevations of transaminases, bilirubin, and prothrombin time almost always indicate a pathologic state. Jaundice in pregnancy is a relatively rare condition accounting for 0.4–0.9/1,000 deliveries. Abnormal LFT occurs in 3–5% of pregnancies. Initial assessments of liver jaundice in pregnancy should primarily done by laboratory studies and ultrasonography. If further assessment is needed, magnetic resonance imaging without gadolinium contrast is the preferred modality. Use of computed tomography (CT) scan and fluoroscopy in pregnancy should be carefully weighed against the risks of ionizing radiation to the fetus.

ETIOLOGY

Broadly jaundice in pregnancy can be classified as liver diseases unique to pregnancy, liver diseases coincidental to pregnancy, and pregnancy in patients with pre-existing liver disease (**Table 1**). Accurate identification of the condition and its impact on both maternal and fetal health is of utmost importance.

LIVER DISEASES UNIQUE TO PREGNANCY

Hyperemesis Gravidarum (HG)

It is relatively benign condition occurring in the first trimester of pregnancy. Persistent vomiting accompanied by weight loss exceeding 5% of prepregnancy body weight is the classical presentation. It is associated with dehydration, electrolyte imbalance, and nutritional deficiencies. Liver involvement is seen in 50–60% of hospitalized patients. LFT reveal transaminitis with alanine aminotransferase (ALT) > aspartate aminotransferase (AST). Bilirubin is often normal and usually does not

TABLE 1: Classification of jaundice in pregnancy.

Liver diseases unique to pregnancy	Liver diseases coincidental to pregnancy	Pregnancy in patients with pre-existing liver disease
Hyperemesis gravidarum	Viral hepatitis A,B,C, and E	Autoimmune hepatitis
Intrahepatic cholestasis of pregnancy	Cytomegalovirus or herpes simplex hepatitis	Cirrhosis of liver
Pre-eclampsia and eclampsia	Budd–Chiari syndrome	Chronic hepatitis B and C
HELLP syndrome	Gallstone disease	Primary biliary cirrhosis
Acute fatty liver of pregnancy	Alcohol and pregnancy	Primary sclerosing cholangitis
		Wilson's disease

(HELLP: hemolysis, elevated liver enzymes and low platelets)

exceed beyond 4 mg%. Risk factors include obese/underweight female, nonsmokers, multiple gestations, gastroesophageal reflux disease, history of in previous pregnancy or family history and *H. pylori* infection. Treatment is mainly supportive in the form of intravenous fluids, antiemetics, and vitamin (thiamine, pyridoxine, and folic acid) supplementation. Patient is advised to take small frequent high carbohydrate and low-fat diet.

Intrahepatic Cholestasis of Pregnancy

Intrahepatic cholestasis of pregnancy (ICP) is a reversible condition of cholestasis occurring in second or third trimester of pregnancy. Genetic predisposition/family tendency along with hormonal changes is thought to contribute to ICP. Advanced age, multiparity, and previous history of cholestasis after oral contraceptive use are the risk factors for ICP. Clinically, it is characterized by intense pruritus involving whole body especially palms and soles. It has tendency to recur in subsequent pregnancy. Rise in serum bile acid >10 mmol/L and increase in AST/ALT is diagnostic investigations. Management includes ursodeoxycholic acid 10–20 mg/kg/day and bile acid sequestrants like cholestyramine. ICP is relatively benign for mother but is associated with significant fetal complications like preterm birth, meconium-stained amniotic fluid, fetal distress, and stillbirth. Delivery planning by 37th week of gestation is definitely shown to improve obstetric outcome.

Hemolysis, Elevated Liver Enzymes and Low Platelets Syndrome

Hemolysis, elevated liver enzymes and low platelets syndrome is a rare serious third trimester pregnancy-related disorder considered as one of the presentations of pre-eclampsia syndrome and occurring in 0.2–0.9% of all pregnancies but almost in 10–20% patients of pre-eclampsia/eclampsia.

It is associated with significant (7.4–34%) maternal and fetal mortality. Placental changes secondary to genetic and immunological factors are supposed to cause this syndrome. Pre-eclampsia, antiphospholipid antibody positivity, diabetes, hypertension, advanced maternal age, hypertensive disorder in previous pregnancy, and family history are the important risk factors. Clinically, patient can present with right hypochondriac pain, nausea, vomiting, edema, and jaundice. Liver hematoma, spontaneous hepatic rupture, and acute liver failure are life threatening complications. Extrahepatic manifestations include renal failure, neurological-like cerebral edema, cerebral infarction, or intracerebral bleed, permanent vision loss, acute pulmonary edema, bleeding or disseminated intravascular coagulopathy (DIC), placental abruption, and fetal loss. Tennessee or Mississippi classification is used for diagnosis. Management includes low dose aspirin, $MgSO_4$, other antihypertensive drugs for hypertension, corticosteroids, platelet transfusion if required, and surgical intervention for hepatic complications. Delivery is the only curative treatment and should be advised in accordance with expected duration of pregnancy and severity or rate of deterioration of patient.

Acute Fatty Liver of Pregnancy

Acute fatty liver of pregnancy (AFLP) is a rare predominantly third trimester disorder of pregnancy with prevalence of 1 in 7,000–16,000 pregnancies. It is considered as mitochondrial hepatopathy and occurs as a result of inherited deficiency of enzyme long-chain 3-hydroxyacyl-coenzyme-A dehydrogenase (LCHAD). Risk factors for AFLP are multiple gestations, underweight female, primipara, male child, pre-eclampsia, and twin pregnancy. It is associated with high maternal (10–15%) and fetal (20%) mortality. Clinically, it presents with nausea, vomiting, right upper quadrant (RUQ) pain, jaundice, and bleeding. It is associated with wide array of complications like acute liver failure, acute renal failure, DIC, ascites, pancreatitis, and transient diabetes insipidus. Diagnosis is done by demonstrating LFT abnormalities, hypoglycemia, rise in S ammonia and amino acids, hyperuricemia, deranged coagulation profile, leukocytosis and thrombocytopenia, and abnormal USG. Microvesicular fatty infiltration in perivenular hepatocyte is the histological hallmark. Swansea criteria which are based on clinical, laboratory, radiographic, and histological features are used for diagnosis of AFLP. Prompt suspicion, early recognition, and emergent careful delivery of the baby remain cornerstone of management of AFLP (**Table 2**). Associated complications should be treated appropriately. Newborns should be monitored closely for liver failure, hypoglycemia, cardiomyopathy, myopathy, and neuropathy.

LIVER DISEASE COINCIDENTAL TO PREGNANCY

As such any liver disease can occur in pregnancy but conditions which can have deleterious effects on pregnancy are viral hepatitis B and E, hepatitis caused by herpes simplex virus and gall stone disease.

TABLE 2: Management of liver diseases unique to pregnancy.		
Disorder	**Trimester**	**Management**
HG	First up to 20 weeks	Supportive management
IHCP	Second/third	• UDCA 10–15 mg/kg • Early delivery at 37 weeks
Eclampsia and pre-eclampsia	After 20 weeks	After 36 weeks, women with severe pre-eclampsia should be delivered promptly
HELLP	After 22 weeks	• Delivery after 34 weeks • Platelet transfusion to 40,000–50,000 cells/μL should be considered before delivery, especially if cesarean section is likely
AFLP	Third	Women with AFLP should be delivered promptly. Infant should be monitored for manifestations of deficiency of LCHAD including hypoketotic hypoglycemia and fatty liver

(AFLP: acute fatty liver of pregnancy; HELLP: hemolysis, elevated liver enzymes and low platelets; HG: hyperemesis gravidarum; IHCP: intrahepatic cholestasis of pregnancy; LCHAD: long-chain 3-hydroxyacyl-coenzyme-A dehydrogenase; UDCA: ursodeoxycholic acid)

Source: ACG Clinical Guideline 2016: Liver Disease and Pregnancy. Official journal of the American College of Gastroenterology ACG. 2016;111(2):176-94.

Acute Viral Hepatitis

Acute viral hepatitis (AVH) is the most common cause of jaundice in pregnancy. An acute attack of hepatitis B usually has same course in the pregnant as in the nonpregnant woman. In poor resource countries, the mortality is high and fetal wastage and stillbirths are increased. There are high chances of vertical/perinatal transmission of infection worldwide. Immunoprophylaxis in the form of hepatitis B immune globulin (HBIG) and starting of hepatitis B vaccine schedule within 12 hours of birth is the preferred modality for preventing vertical transmission. Lamivudine, tenofovir, and telbivudine are the drugs which can be used to halt vertical transmission.

Acute hepatitis E is relatively benign infection, however, if occurs in third trimester of pregnancy is associated with severe hepatitis, acute fulminant hepatic failure in mother, and preterm labor. It is associated with 20–30% maternal and about 50% fetal mortality. There is high risk of vertical transmission ranging from 46 to 50%. Further large studies are required to know exact prevalence of vertical transmission. Treatment is mainly supportive.

Pancreaticobiliary Disease

Symptomatic gallstone disease is common in pregnancy and pose significant risk to both mother and fetus. Choledocholithiasis is a serious condition and have grave consequences during pregnancy. Evaluation is same as in nonpregnant women. Endoscopic retrograde cholangiopancreatography (ERCP) can be performed when indicated for pregnant women presenting with biliary diseases like biliary pancreatitis, symptomatic choledocholithiasis, and/or cholangitis. However, it should be performed with judicious use of fluoroscopy. *Symptomatic cholecystitis* should be managed with early surgical intervention with laparoscopic cholecystectomy which can be done safely in second trimester.

PREGNANCY IN PRE-EXISTING LIVER DISEASE

As such to conception in patients with pre-existing liver disease, especially cirrhosis is uncommon, however, the liver disease is not an indication for termination of pregnancy. Pregnancy as such is not contraindicated in patients with primary biliary cirrhosis, autoimmune hepatitis, or Wilson's disease but these conditions are associated with significant fetal loss. Patients having bleeding esophageal varices are treated on the same lines as nonpregnant woman.

SUMMARY

Liver disease in pregnancy may present as a disorder that is unique to pregnancy or as an acute or chronic liver disease occurring coincidentally in pregnancy. While managing jaundice in pregnancy, it is very important to balance maternal and fetal well-being which can be clinically challenging. Many of the clinical features and investigations overlap between these conditions, hence, high index of suspicion, prompt diagnosis based on clinical, laboratory, and radiological features is of vital importance. Diagnosing these conditions at the earliest is important because decision regarding continuation of pregnancy can be taken at appropriate time thereby reducing adverse obstetric events. The gestational age of the pregnancy is a vital determinant deciding management of jaundice.

SUGGESTED READINGS

1. Saha S, Reau N. Approach to Gastrointestinal and liver disease in pregnancy. In: Podolsky DK, Camilleri M, Fitz JG (eds). Yamada's Textbook of Gastroenterology, 6th edition. New Jersey: John Wiley & Sons, Ltd.; 2016.
2. Brady CW. Liver Disease in Pregnancy: What's New. Hepatol Commun. 2020;4(2): 145-56.
3. Sherlock S, and Dooley J. The Liver in Pregnancy. In: Sherlock S, Dooley J (eds). Diseases of the liver and biliary system, 11th edition. Blackwell Science Ltd.; 2002. pp. 471-9.
4. Tran TT, Ahn J, and Reau NS. ACG clinical guideline: Liver disease and pregnancy. Am J Gastroenterol. 2016;111(2):176-94.
5. Bensan A, Oren R. The liver in pregnancy. In Boyer T, Lindor K (eds). Zakim and Boyer's hepatology: A textbook of liver disease, 7th edition Elsevier; 2016. pp. 817–36.
6. Sharma S, Kumar A, Kar P, Agarwal S, Ramji S, Husain SA, et al. Risk factors for vertical transmission of hepatitis E virus infection. J Viral Hepat. 2017;24(11):1067-75. doi: 10.1111/jvh.12730. Epub 2017 Jul 12. PMID: 28570034.

9

Cardiometabolic-based Chronic Disease; Is it Adiposity-based Chronic Disease and Dysglycemic-based Chronic Disease?

Kamal Sharma

BACKGROUND

Cardiovascular disease (CVD) is the leading cause of death worldwide.[1,2] Primordial and primary prevention strategies decrease CVD despite increased total CVD deaths due to aging population and increased burden of obesity and type 2 diabetes mellitus (T2DM) warranting more effective prevention strategies as atherosclerosis begins as early as first decade of life creating opportunities for primary, secondary, and tertiary prevention to mitigate the CV events.[2-4]

The chronic disease process often involves T2DM and obesity, distinct from end-stage CVD, even though both are risk factors of chronic CVD. In the "state-of-the-art" review article in Journal of the American College of Cardiology (JACC), Jeffrey Mechanick et al. first proposed a model addressing pathophysiology, inter-relationships amongst obesity, T2DM, and CVD for comprehensive approaches for primary, secondary, and tertiary prevention focused on CVD [specifically coronary heart disease (CHD), heart failure (HF), and atrial fibrillation (AF)] as end-stage developments in these chronic processes.[5]

DEFINITIONS[5]

- *Adiposity-based chronic disease (ABCD)* has two parts: Adiposity-based abnormalities in the mass, function, and distribution of adipose tissue; and chronic disease which reflects the risk, presence, and severity of its complications.
- *Dysglycemia-based chronic disease (DBCD)* is a general term that includes all forms of diabetes (but only T2DM and prediabetes, including states of increased molecular risk for T2DM, such as insulin resistance). The cardinal manifestations of insulin resistance being normoglycemia/hyperglycemia with hyperinsulinemia.
- *Cardiometabolic-based chronic disease (CMBCD)* dwells into inter-relationships between obesity, T2DM, and CVD outlining approaches for primary, secondary, and tertiary prevention focused on CVD (specifically CHD, HF, and AF) as end-stage developments in this chronic disease process with the central abnormality being insulin resistance. Multiple studies have shown that the residual risk despite statin therapy is largely be attributed to insulin resistance.[6-12]

ETIOPATHOLOGICAL DRIVERS OF CARDIOMETABOLIC-BASED CHRONIC DISEASE

- *Genetics*: Familial inheritance is as much dependent on modifiable risks as on heredity.[13] The use of system genetics to identify molecular drivers through these complex interaction of genes, environment, and behavior ultimately determining risk and disease phenotypes is partially known (**Table 1**). As minority of gene variants may explain CHD, disease drivers corresponding to hub genes at the top of a regulatory network represent a stronger mechanism of genetic drivers.[14] Data suggests gene regulatory networks in the atherosclerotic arterial wall and abdominal adipose tissue are main disease drivers for CHD even though these lack risk score models for clinical prediction for diagnosis and prognosis.[14]

Epigenetic modifications in utero with maternal gestational diabetes may confer insulin resistance phenotype in offspring which if persists into adulthood leads to T2DM, obesity, and CVD.[15-18] In a meta-analysis, childhood obesity has shown to be a risk factor for CVD due to its associations with adult risk factors viz. systolic and diastolic blood pressure (SBP/DBP), total cholesterol, high-density lipoprotein (HDL), low-density lipoprotein (LDL), non-HDL, and triglycerides.[19] In fact, newborns of obese women have shown to have thicker intraventricular septa and decreased left ventricular (LV) function.[20]

TABLE 1: Some important molecular factors associated with CMBCD.[5]		
Factor	**Phenotypic trait**	**Cardiometabolic effect**
BCL2	Regulates apoptosis	Insulin resistance
eNOS	Hypermethylation and nitric oxide	Adult MetS
FAM19A2	Brain chemokine	Insulin resistance
HLA-B, HLA-DRB1, HLA-C	Major histocompatibility complex	Adiposity
IGF1	Insulin-like growth factor 1	Insulin resistance
IRS1	Insulin receptor substrate 1	Insulin resistance
KCNQ1	K voltage-gated channel subfamily Q member 1	β-Cell function
NAT2	N-acetyltransferase 2	Lipids and insulin resistance
Netrin	Angiogenesis pathway	Vascular
p66Shc	Hypomethylation and free radicals	Adult MetS
PON1 Q192R/L55M	Paraoxonase 1 gene variants	Insulin resistance
PPARG	Peroxisome proliferator-activated receptor γ	Insulin resistance
RYR2	Ryanodine receptor 2	β-cell function
SLIT-ROBO	Angiogenesis pathway	Vascular
TCF7L2	Transcription factor 7 like 2	β-cell function

- *Environment*: Man-made and cultural environment provide facilitate the expression of genetic cardiometabolic risk factors.[21] Lower socioeconomic strata and decreased access to quality health care, low education and literacy levels, regions of high alcohol intake, both urban and rural living, air and noise pollution, and poor quality of drinking water are known as environmental risk factors.[22] Environment toxins or endocrine disruptors can affect the risk for T2DM by modulating gene expression, as well as interacting with molecular trafficking and other pathophysiological pathways to influence CV outcomes.
- *Metabolic drivers*:
  - *Adiposity-based chronic disease:* Terminology has been adopted by both the American Association of Clinical Endocrinologists and the European Association for the Study of Obesity.[23] Not all patients with obesity are insulin resistant and lean individuals may also exhibit an insulin-resistant state with increased risk of T2DM and CVD. The relationship between generalized increase in adiposity and insulin sensitivity indicates that only about 11% of individual variability in insulin sensitivity can be attributed to BMI.[24] The leg and thigh, but not arm fat, have significant protective cardiometabolic benefits.[25,26] Adipokines influence various interactions within these CV pathways.[27] Patients with high body mass index (BMI) may be insulin sensitive and not at increased risk of T2DM or CVD referred to as the "*metabolically healthy obese*" accounting for 15-20% in National Health and Nutrition Examination Survey (NHANES) cohort in United States (US).[28-30] This modestly increased BMI with lower risks of CVD is referred to as *"the obesity paradox"*.[31,32]

EFFECTS OF ADIPOSITY ON CARDIOVASCULAR DISEASE

In the Korean Genome and Epidemiology Study, visceral adipose tissue was associated with increased LV mass index and decreased LV diastolic function.[33] In the Iranian CASPIAN-V study,[34] anthropometric parameters in normal-weight children and adolescents were predictive for CV risk factors. Epicardial and visceral adipose tissue are positively associated with atherosclerotic burden whereas subcutaneous adipose tissue had a negative association.[35] Epicardial adipose tissue secretes more phospholipase A2 II with ischemia, resulting in more phospholipid hydrolysis and generation of local free fatty acids (FFA) which impairs nerve impulse propagation and increases risk of arrhythmias.[36]

DYSGLYCEMIA-BASED CHRONIC DISEASE

This is more accurate term than diabetes for the spectrum of events stemming from insulin resistance, prediabetes, T2DM, and CVD. The effects of insulin resistance include:
- Defects in glucose metabolism and mitochondrial dysfunction;
- Increased inflammation and free oxidative radicals;

- Alterations in lipoproteins;
- Impaired lipid storage in adipocytes
- Dysregulation of vasoregulation due to a reduced endothelial nitric oxide synthase (eNOS) and nitric oxide (NO)
- Acetylcholine-induced coronary artery spasm without frank T2DM.[37-44]

The Insulin Resistance Atherosclerosis Study (IRAS) and the Bezafibrate Infarction Prevention (BIP) Trial demonstrated that insulin resistance was associated with the development of CVD events.[45-51] The changes in lipids and lipoproteins that occur due to insulin resistance are atherogenic, accelerate atherosclerosis independent of overall LDL-C, and begins early in CMBCD often being implicated to elevated small dense LDL levels.

EFFECT OF INSULIN RESISTANCE ON INFLAMMATION

The inflamed adipose tissue releasing proinflammatory cytokines is hallmark of insulin resistance causing cell adhesion molecule expression, monocyte margination, macrophages conversion, and accumulation of small dense LDL (sdLDL) particles that are prone to modification by oxidation, acetylation, and glycation inducing an immune response compounding atherogenicity by foam cell formation and fatty streak and plaque development.[52]

EFFECT OF INSULIN RESISTANCE ON CARDIAC METABOLISM

The lipotoxicity due to increased accumulation of ectopic lipid in the cardiomyocyte with elevated serum FFA and impaired insulin signaling through the insulin receptor, insulin receptor substrate 1 (IRS-1), and activation of nuclear factor kappa B (NF-κB) pathways amplifies myocyte inflammation.[53] These reduce the ability of insulin to stimulate glucose uptake and oxidation in the heart. The myocardium uses fatty acids as its preferred fuel choice, except in the presence of pacing or ischemia when the heart relies on glucose for fuel. Due to defects in insulin action and mitochondrial function, this flexibility to convert to glucose metabolism is impaired. The result is HF with preserved ejection fraction accompanied by increased left atrial size, LV mass, and development of diastolic dysfunction and later on systolic dysfunction as well.[54]

PREDIABETES/TYPE 2 DIABETES MELLITUS AND CARDIOVASCULAR DISEASE

The United Kingdom Prospective Diabetes Study (UKPDS) established an epidemiological link between hyperglycemia and CHD by showing a linear relationship between hemoglobin A1c (HbA1c) and CVD events including myocardial infarction.[55] The association of increased CVD risk in patients with T2DM is well established.[56-59] The risk of hospitalization for HF is also higher with T2DM, though decreased with advanced age (>75 years) and target A1c (<7%), or without albuminuria.[60]

The overall impact of glucose lowering on macro-vascular complications in T2DM is still an open issue despite the publication of UKPDS subgroup analyses (UKPDS-35).

The subsequent studies of intensification including, Action in Diabetes and Vascular disease: PreterAx and Diamicron-MR Controlled Evaluation (ADVANCE), Action to Control Cardiovascular Risk in Diabetes (ACCORD), and the Veterans Affairs Diabetes Trial (VADT), also showed a decrease in the risk of microvascular end points but not in the primary cardiovascular end point.[61-63]

CLINICAL IMPLICATIONS AND RECENT TRIALS

- *REDUCE-IT Trial*: Patients with established CVD or with diabetes and other risk factors, on statin therapy with fasting triglyceride level of 135–499 mg% and LDL of 41–100 mg% were randomly assigned to receive 2 g of icosapent ethyl twice daily (total daily dose 4 g) or placebo. The rates of additional ischemic end points, as assessed according to a prespecified hierarchical schema, were significantly lower in the icosapent ethyl group than in the placebo group, including the rate of cardiovascular death (4.3% vs. 5.2%; hazard ratio 0.80; 95% CI 0.66–0.98; $p = 0.03$).[64]
- *HOPE-3 trial*: In one comparison from a two-by-two factorial trial, 12,705 patients who did not have CVD and were at intermediate risk received rosuvastatin at a dose of 10 mg/day or placebo. The overall mean LDL was 26.5% lower in the rosuvastatin group than in the placebo arm. The incremental benefit was observed with statins and antihypertensive arm as compared to single arm with 40% reduction as compared to 30% reduction in statin arm.[65]
- *Sodium-glucose cotransporter-2 (SGLT-2) inhibitors and glucagon-like peptide1 (GLP-1) analogs*: CV outcome reducing therapies in management of diabetes with therapies-like SGLT-2 inhibitors (EMPA-REG, DECLARE-TIMI 58, and CANVAS) and GLP-1 analogs (LEADERS and SUSTAIN-6) have shown promise to further reinforce the management strategies directed toward CMBCD rather than just managing ABCD or DBCD including HF reduction trials even in prediabetics and nondiabetics (DAPA-HF and EMEROR-REDUCED).

MITOCHONDRIAL MODULATION—NOVEL APPROACH FOR CMBCD

- Recent evidence suggests that the phenomenon of derangement of metabolic flexibility or metabolic inflexibility plays a central role in accelerating the development and progression of T2DM.
- Metabolic flexibility, which refers to the ability to efficiently adapt the utilization of substrates such as glucose and fatty acids based on nutrient availability and requirements, may be compromised due to the continuous mismatch between metabolic load and metabolic 'capacity'.
- The resultant nutrient overload may cause mitochondrial dysfunction characterized by ineffective substrate switching and incomplete substrate

utilization. Thus, modulation of mitochondria seems to be a promising pharmaceutical target for the treatment of T2DM and its associated vascular complications.
- Restoration of metabolic fuel switching towards additional glucose substrate disposal or utilization (i.e., glucoefficiency) improves pancreatic β-cell dysfunction, insulin resistance, obesity while preventing progression towards vascular complications.[66,67]

REFERENCES

1. Townsend N, Nichols M, Scarborough P, Rayner M. Cardiovascular disease in Europe–epidemiological update 2015. Eur Heart J. 2015;36(40):2696-705.
2. Mensah GA, Roth GA, Sampson UK, Moran AE, Feigin VL, Forouzanfar MH, et al. Mortality from cardiovascular diseases in sub-Saharan Africa, 1990-2013: a systematic analysis of data from the Global Burden of Disease Study 2013. Cardiovasc J Afr. 2015;26(2):S6-10.
3. Roth GA, Forouzanfar MH, Moran AE, Barber R, Nguyen G, Feigin VL, et al. Demographic and epidemiologic drivers of global cardiovascular mortality. N Engl J Med. 2015;372(14):1333-41.
4. Roth GA, Johnson C, Abajobir A, Abd-Allah F, Abera SF, Abyu G, et al. Global, regional, and national burden of cardiovascular diseases for 10 causes, 1990 to 2015. J Am Coll Cardiol. 2017;70(1):1-25.
5. Mechanick JI, Farkouh ME, Newman JD, Garvey WT. Cardiometabolic-Based Chronic Disease, Adiposity and Dysglycemia Drivers: JACC State-of-the-Art Review. J Am Coll Cardiol. 2020;75(5):525-38.
6. Howard G, O'Leary DH, Zaccaro D, Haffner S, Rewers M, Hamman R, et al. Insulin sensitivity and atherosclerosis. The Insulin Resistance Atherosclerosis Study (IRAS) Investigators. Circulation. 1996;93(10):1809-17.
7. Saad MF, Rewers M, Selby J, Howard G, Jinagouda S, Fahmi S, et al. Insulin resistance and hypertension: the Insulin Resistance Atherosclerosis study. Hypertension. 2004;43(6):1324-31.
8. Gast KB, Tjeerdema N, Stijnen T, Smit JW, Dekkers OM. Insulin resistance and risk of incident cardiovascular events in adults without diabetes: meta-analysis. PLoS One. 2012;7(12):e52036.
9. Rewers M, Zaccaro D, D'Agostino R, Haffner S, Saad MF, Selby JV, et al. Insulin Resistance Atherosclerosis Study Investigators. Insulin sensitivity, insulinemia, and coronary artery disease: the Insulin Resistance Atherosclerosis Study. Diabetes Care. 2004;27(3):781-7.
10. Tenenbaum A, Motro M, Fisman EZ, Tanne D, Boyko V, Behar S. Bezafibrate for the secondary prevention of myocardial infarction in patients with metabolic syndrome. Arch Intern Med. 2005;165(10):1154-60.
11. Tenenbaum A, Fisman EZ, Boyko V, Benderly M, Tanne D, Haim M, et al. Attenuation of progression of insulin resistance in patients with coronary artery disease by bezafibrate. Arch Intern Med. 2006;166(7):737-41.
12. Tenenbaum A, Motro M, Fisman EZ, Adler Y, Shemesh J, Tanne D, et al. Effect of bezafibrate on incidence of type 2 diabetes mellitus in obese patients. Eur Heart J. 2005;26(19):2032-8.
13. Bjorkegren JLM, Kovacic JC, Dudley JT, Schadt EE. Genome-wide significant loci: how important are they? Systems genetics to understand heritability of coronary artery disease and other common complex disorders. J Am Coll Cardiol. 2015;65(8):830-45.

14. Zeng L, Talukdar HA, Koplev S, Giannarelli C, Ivert T, Gan LM, et al. Contribution of gene regulatory networks to heritability of coronary artery disease. J Am Coll Cardiol. 2019;73(23):2946-57.
15. Yang IV, Zhang W, Davidson EJ, Fingerlin TE, Kechris K, Dabelea D. Epigenetic marks of in utero exposure to gestational diabetes and childhood adiposity outcomes: the EPOCH study. Diabet Med. 2018;35(5):612-20.
16. Ruchat SM, Houde AA, Voisin G, St-Pierre J, Perron P, Baillargeon JP, et al. Gestational diabetes mellitus epigenetically affects genes predominantly involved in metabolic diseases. Epigenetics. 2013;8(9):935-43.
17. Kang J, Lee CN, Li HY, Hsu KH, Lin SY. Genome-wide DNA methylation variation in maternal and cord blood of gestational diabetes population. Diabetes Res Clin Pract. 2017;132:127-36.
18. Sobngwi E, Boudou P, Mauvais-Jarvis F, Leblanc H, Velho G, Vexiau P, et al. Effect of a diabetic environment in utero on predisposition to type 2 diabetes. Lancet. 2003;361(9372):1861-5.
19. Umer A, Kelley GA, Cottrell LE, Giacobbi P Jr, Innes KE, Lilly CL, et al. Childhood obesity and adult cardiovascular disease risk factors: a systematic review with meta-analysis. BMC Public Health. 2017;17(1):683.
20. Nyrnes SA, Garnæs KK, Salvesen Ø, Timilsina AS, Moholdt T, Ingul CB. Cardiac function in newborns of obese women and the effect of exercise during pregnancy. A randomized controlled trial. PLoS One. 2018;13(6):e0197334.
21. Mechanick JI, Adams S, Davidson JA, Fergus IV, Galindo RJ, McKinney KH, et al. Transcultural diabetes care in the United States: a position statement by the American Association of Clinical Endocrinologists. Endocr Pract. 2019;25(7):729-65.
22. Mena C, Sepulveda C, Fuentes E, Ormazábal Y, Palomo I. Spatial analysis for the epidemiological study of cardiovascular diseases: a systematic literature search. Geospat Health. 2018;13(1):587.
23. Fruhbeck G, Busetto L, Dicker D, Yumuk V, Goossens GH, Hebebrand J, et al. The ABCD of obesity: an EASO position statement of a diagnostic term with clinical and scientific implications. Obes Facts. 2019;12(2):131-6.
24. Garvey WT, Lara-Castro C. Diet, insulin resistance, and obesity: zoning in on data for Atkins dieters living in South Beach. J Clin Endocrinol Metab. 2004;89:4197-205.
25. Sanchez-Lopez M, Ortega FB, Moya-Martinez P, López-Martínez S, Ortiz-Galeano I, Gómez-Marcos MA, et al. Leg fat might be more protective than arm fat in relation to lipid profile. Eur J Nutr. 2013;52(2):489-95.
26. Snijder MB, Visser M, Dekker JM, Goodpaster BH, Harris TB, Kritchevsky SB, et al. Low subcutaneous thigh fat is a risk factor for unfavourable glucose and lipid levels, independently of high abdominal fat. The Health ABC Study. Diabetologia. 2005;48(2):301-8.
27. Mechanick JI, Zhao S, Garvey WT. The adipokine-cardiovascular-lifestyle network. J Am Coll Cardiol. 2016;68:1785-803.
28. Guo F, Moellering DR, Garvey WT. The progression of cardiometabolic disease: validation of a new cardiometabolic disease staging system applicable to obesity. Obesity. 2014;22:110-8.
29. Guo F, Garvey WT. Cardiometabolic disease risk in metabolically healthy and unhealthy obesity: Stability of metabolic health status in adults. Obesity. 2016;24:516-25.
30. Guo F, Garvey WT. Trends in cardiovascular health metrics in obese adults: National Health and Nutrition Examination Survey (NHANES), 1988-2014. J Am Heart Assoc. 2016;5:e003619.
31. Elagizi A, Kachur S, Lavie CJ, Carbone S, Pandey A, Ortega FB, et al. An overview and update on obesity and the obesity paradox in cardiovascular diseases. Prog Cardiovasc Dis. 2018;61(2):142-50.

32. Matinrazm S, Ladejobi A, Pasupula DK, Javed A, Durrani A, Ahmad S, et al. Effect of body mass index on survival after sudden cardiac arrest. Clin Cardiol. 2018;41(1):46-50.
33. Park J, Kim NH, Kim SH, Kim JS, Kim YH, Lim HE, et al. Visceral adiposity and skeletal muscle mass are independently and synergistically associated with left ventricular structure and function: the Korean Genome and Epidemiology Study. Int J Cardiol. 2014;176(3):951-5.
34. Ahadi Z, Bahreynian M, Qorbani M, Heshmat R, Motlagh ME, Shafiee G, et al. Association of anthropometric measures and cardio-metabolic risk factors in normal-weight children and adolescents: the CASPIAN-V study. J Pediatr Endocrinol Metab. 2018;31(8):847-54.
35. Rodriguez-Granillo GA, Reynoso E, Capunay C, Carpio J, Carrascosa P. Pericardial and visceral, but not total body fat, are related to global coronary and extra-coronary atherosclerotic plaque burden. Int J Cardiol. 2018;260:204-10.
36. Manzella D, Barbieri M, Rizzo MR, Ragno E, Passariello N, Gambardella A, et al. Role of free fatty acids on cardiac autonomic nervous system in noninsulin-dependent diabetic patients: effects of metabolic control. J Clin Endocrinol Metab. 2001;86(6):2769-74.
37. Petersen MC, Shulman GI. Roles of diacylglycerols and ceramides in hepatic insulin resistance. Trends Pharmacol Sci. 2017;38:649-65.
38. Festa A, D'Agostino R, Howard G, Mykkanen L, Tracy RP, Haffner SM. Chronic subclinical inflammation as part of the insulin resistance syndrome: the Insulin Resistance Atherosclerosis Study (IRAS). Circulation. 2000;102(1):42-7.
39. Luo N, Chung BH, Wang X, Klein RL, Tang CK, Garvey WT, et al. Enhanced adiponectin actions by over-expression of adiponectin receptor 1 in macrophages. Atherosclerosis. 2013;228(1):124-35.
40. Boden G, She P, Mozzoli M, Cheung P, Gumireddy K, Reddy P, et al. Free fatty acids produce insulin resistance and activate the proinflammatory nuclear factor-kappaB pathway in rat liver. Diabetes. 2005;54(12):3458-65.
41. Nigro J, Osman N, Dart AM, Little PJ. Insulin resistance and atherosclerosis. Endocr Rev. 2006;27(3):242-59.
42. Steinberg D. Low density lipoprotein oxidation and its pathobiological significance. J Biol Chem. 1997;272:20963-6.
43. Garvey WT, Kwon S, Zheng D, Shaughnessy S, Wallace P, Hutto A, et al. Effects of insulin resistance and type 2 diabetes on lipoprotein subclass particle size and concentration determined by nuclear magnetic resonance. Diabetes. 2003;52(2):453-62.
44. Kang KW, Choi BG, Rha SW. Impact of insulin resistance on acetylcholine-induced coronary artery spasm in non-diabetic patients. Yonsei Med J. 2018;59:1057-63.
45. Howard G, O'Leary DH, Zaccaro D, Haffner S, Rewers M, Hamman R, et al. Insulin sensitivity and atherosclerosis: the Insulin Resistance Atherosclerosis Study (IRAS) Investigators. Circulation. 1996;93(10):1809-17.
46. Saad MF, Rewers M, Selby J, Howard G, Jinagouda S, Fahmi S, et al. Insulin resistance and hypertension: the Insulin Resistance Atherosclerosis study. Hypertension. 2004;43(6):1324-31.
47. Gast KB, Tjeerdema N, Stijnen T, Smit JW, Dekkers OM. Insulin resistance and risk of incident cardiovascular events in adults without diabetes: meta-analysis. PLoS One. 2012;7(12):e52036.
48. Rewers M, Zaccaro D, D'Agostino R, Haffner S, Saad MF, Selby JV, et al. Insulin sensitivity, insulinemia, and coronary artery disease: the Insulin Resistance Atherosclerosis Study. Diabetes Care. 2004;27(3):781-7.
49. Tenenbaum A, Motro M, Fisman EZ, Tanne D, Boyko V, Behar S. Bezafibrate for the secondary prevention of myocardial infarction in patients with metabolic syndrome. Arch Intern Med. 2005;165(10):1154-60.

50. Tenenbaum A, Fisman EZ, Boyko V, Benderly M, Tanne D, Haim M, et al. Attenuation of progression of insulin resistance in patients with coronary artery disease by bezafibrate. Arch Intern Med. 2006;166(7):737-41.
51. Tenenbaum A, Motro E, Fisman EZ, Adler Y, Shemesh J, Tanne D, et al. Effect of bezafibrate on incidence of type 2 diabetes mellitus in obese patients. Eur Heart J. 2005;26(19):2032-8.
52. Tertov VV, Orekhov AN, Kacharava AG, Sobenin IA, Perova NV, Smirnov VN. Low density lipoprotein-containing circulating immune complexes and coronary atherosclerosis. Exp Mol Pathol. 1990;52(3):300-8.
53. Zhou YT, Grayburn P, Karim A, Shimabukuro M, Higa M, Baetens D, et al. Lipotoxic heart disease in obese rats: implications for human obesity. Proc Natl Acad Sci U S A. 2000;97(4):1784-9.
54. Williams LJ, Nye BG, Wende AR. Diabetes-related cardiac dysfunction. Endocrinol Metab (Seoul). 2017;32:171-9.
55. Turner RC, Millns H, Neil HA, Stratton IM, Manley SE, Matthews DR, et al. Risk factors for coronary artery disease in non-insulin dependent diabetes mellitus: United Kingdom Prospective Diabetes Study (UKPDS: 23). Br Med J. 1998;316(7134):823-8.
56. Assmann G, Schulte H. The Prospective Cardiovascular Munster (PROCAM) study: prevalence of hyperlipidemia in persons with hypertension and/or diabetes mellitus and the relationship to coronary heart disease. Am Heart J. 1988;116:1713-24.
57. Fujishima M, Kiyohara Y, Kato I, Ohmura T, Iwamoto H, Nakayama K, et al. Diabetes and cardiovascular disease in a prospective population survey in Japan: the Hisayama study. Diabetes. 1996;45(Suppl 3):S14-6.
58. Yokoyama H, Matsushima M, Kawai K, Hirao K, Oishi M, Sugimoto H, et al. Low incidence of cardiovascular events in Japanese patients with Type 2 diabetes in primary care settings: a prospective cohort study (JDDM 20). Diabet Med. 2011;28(10):1221-8.
59. Haffner SM, Lehto S, Ronnemaa T, Pyörälä K, Laakso M. Mortality from coronary heart disease in subjects with Type 2 diabetes and in nondiabetic subjects with and without prior myocardial infarction. N Engl J Med. 1998;339(4):229-34.
60. Rosengren A, Edqvist J, Rawshani A, Sattar N, Franzén S, Adiels M, et al. Excess risk of hospitalization for heart failure among people with type 2 diabetes. Diabetologia. 2018;61(11):2300-9.
61. Patel A, MacMahon S, Chalmers J, et al. Intensive blood glucose control and vascular outcomes in patients with type 2 diabetes. N Engl J Med 2008;358: 2560-72.
62. Gerstein HC, Miller ME, Byington RP, et al. Effects of intensive glucose lowering in type 2 diabetes. N Engl J Med 2008; 358:2545-59.
63. Duckworth W, Abraira C, Moritz T, et al. Glucose control and vascular complications in veterans with type 2 diabetes. N Engl J Med 2009;360:129-39.
64. Bhatt DL, Steg PG, Miller M, Brinton EA, Jacobson TA, Ketchum SB, et.al. Cardiovascular Risk Reduction with Icosapent Ethyl for Hypertriglyceridemia. N Engl J Med. 2019;380(1):11-22.
65. Yusuf S, Bosch J, Dagenais G, Zhu J, Xavier D, Liu L, et.al. Cholesterol Lowering in Intermediate-Risk Persons without Cardiovascular Disease. N Engl J Med. 2016;374(21):2021-31.
66. Kwak SH, Park KS, Lee K-U, Lee HK. Mitochondrial metabolism and diabetes. J Diabetes Investig 2010;1(5):161-9.
67. Maack C, Lehrke M, Backs J, et al. Heart failure and diabetes: metabolic alterations and therapeutic interventions: a state-of-the-art review from the Translational Research Committee of the Heart Failure Association–European Society of Cardiology. Eur Heart J 2018;39:4243-54.

10 Endocrine Hypertension

L Sreenivasamurthy

INTRODUCTION

Secondary hypertension, a term used for the hypertension for which there is an identifiable cause, accounts for 10% of all patients with hypertension.[1,2] Endocrine conditions as a cause of secondary hypertension comprise 5–10% of all patients with hypertension.[2]

This form of hypertension, although uncommon, is potentially treatable conditions. Hence, an early identification and prompt treatment initiated to the underlying cause can lead to cure or significant improvement of the hypertension, hence, decreasing the incidence of cardiovascular morbidities and mortality associated with hypertension.

Endocrine Causes of Hypertension

- Adrenal causes:
    - Pheochromocytoma and sympathetic paraganglioma
    - Primary aldosteronism
    - Congenital adrenal hyperplasia
        - Hyperdeoxycorticosteronism
            - 11β-hydroxylase deficiency
            - 17α-hydroxylase deficiency
        - Deoxycorticosterone-producing tumor
        - Primary cortisol resistance
    - Cushing syndrome
- Apparent mineralocorticoid excess (AME)/11β-hydroxysteroid dehydrogenase deficiency
    - Genetic
    - Acquired
- Pituitary causes
    - Acromegaly
    - Cushing's syndrome
- Thyroid causes
    - Hypothyroidism
    - Hyperthyroidism
- Parathyroid causes
    - Hyperparathyroidism

When to Suspect?

- Severe or resistant hypertension. Resistant hypertension is defined as the persistence of hypertension despite concurrent use of adequate doses of three antihypertensive agents from different classes, including a diuretic.
- An acute rise or increased lability in blood pressure developing in a patient with previously stable values.
- Nonobese patient with age <30 years with a negative family history of hypertension and no other risk factors (e.g., obesity) for hypertension.
- Malignant or accelerated hypertension (e.g., patients with severe hypertension and signs of end-organ damage such as acute kidney injury or papilledema, neurologic disturbance, heart failure, or retinal hemorrhages.
- When hypertension is associated with electrolyte disorders including hypokalemia and metabolic alkalosis.
- Proven age of onset before puberty.

PHEOCHROMOCYTOMA

Pheochromocytoma and paragangliomas are catecholamine secreting neural crest cell tumors arising from the sympathetic (e.g., adrenal medulla or sympathetic trunk) or parasympathetic (e.g., carotid body, glomus tympanicum, and glomus jugulare). Although some practitioners use this term interchangeably, World Health Organization (WHO) restricts the term pheochromocytoma to adrenal tumors and applies the term paraganglioma to tumors arising from other site.

Incidence: About 60% of these tumors are sporadic seen equally distributed among men and women[3,4] both the sexes in the fourth to fifth decade, remaining 40% cases are familial, usually presents much earlier than the former. Familial pheochromocytoma are often associated with the following syndromes:
- Multiple endocrine neoplasia type 2 (MEN2)
- Von Hippel–Lindau (VHL) disease
- Neurofibromatosis-1 (NF1)
- SDHB, SDHC, and SDHD (sub units of succinate dehydrogenase enzyme)

Clinical Features

Due to its highly variable clinical presentation it's also termed as "the *great masquerader*". It can be asymptomatic tumor that grows over many years to dilated cardiomyopathy or heart failure. The most common clinical presentation is as "panic attacks", although it neither a specific or sensitive sign. The classical triad of pheochromocytoma consists of *episodic headache, profuse sweating, and tachycardia* are not always present in most patients;[5,6] other symptoms includes nausea, abdominal pain, weakness, weight loss, polyuria, and polydipsia. The most common sign, found in about 80–90% of patients with pheochromocytoma, is hypertension.[7] Types of hypertension in pheochromocytoma:[3,8] (1) Sustained hypertension—found in about 50%

of the patients with pheochromocytoma; (2) Paroxysmal hypertension—found in 45% of the patients; (3) Normotension in 5–15% of the patients.

Diagnosis

Biochemical: Demonstration of elevated plasma and urinary levels of catecholamines and metanephrines forms the cornerstone of diagnosis. Most pheochromocytomas have fluctuating levels of catecholamines, but the metabolism of catecholamines into metanephrines is constant.[3,9,10] 24 hour urinary fractionated metanephrine is the screening test that is commonly employed, due to its very good specificity and sensitivity. However, if in a patient with high clinical suspicion of pheochromocytoma, negative 24 hour urinary fractionated metanephrine does not completely rule out the disease. In such a case, measurement of plasma fractionated metanephrine has to be done.

Imaging: Adrenal pheochromocytomas with a size >0.5 cm as well as metastatic pheochromocytomas can be detected by computed tomography (CT) scan with high sensitivity of 85–94%.[11] Approximately, two-thirds of pheochromocytomas are solid and the rest is complex or cystic.[12] Hemorrhage and calcifications in a pheochromocytoma can be found in approximately 10% of all pheochromocytomas and it may increase the density of the pheochromocytoma.[12]

Although CT is the primary adrenal imaging modality, magnetic resonance imaging (MRI) has advantages in certain clinical situations.[13] MRI gadolinium enhancement on MRI is variable depending on the presence of cystic-necrotic areas, which do not enhance.[14]

In patients with large (>10 cm) pheochromocytomas, extra adrenal tumor, metastatic disease functional imaging is indicated with either ^{68}Ga-DOTATATE PET/CT or scintigraphy with iodine-123-metaio-dobenzylguanidine (^{123}I-MIBG) scintigraphy.

Treatment

The ultimate therapeutic goal is the complete removal of tumor.

Preoperative Management

Appropriate and optimal pharmacological therapy to block the effects of released catecholamines is of critical importance in the preoperative phase of the surgical management of pheochromocytoma.[15]

Phenoxybenzamine is the preferred drug to control the blood pressure and arrhythmia in the preoperative period. It is a long acting, irreversible, and nonspecific alpha-adrenergic blocking agent that is usually started at a dose of 10 mg bid. It is increased by 10–20 mg every 2–3 days as needed to control clinical symptoms of pheochromocytoma.

After achieving an optimal alpha blockade, beta-blockers are used to control the tachycardia that is associated with both high circulating catecholamines and alpha blockade. If it is used prior to alpha adrenergic blockade, unopposed alpha-adrenergic blockade would result in severe hypertension and cardiopulmonary decompensation. Propranolol (20-40 mg TID) is the most commonly used agent.

Calcium channel blockers are the second line antihypertensive medications use to supplement alpha-blockers.[16] They block noradrenaline-mediated calcium influx into vascular smooth muscle, thus controlling hypertension and tachyarrhythmias. Amlodipine (10-20 mg), nicardipine (60-90 mg), and nifedipine (30-90 mg) are commonly used.

Surgery

The laparoscopic approach to the adrenal gland is currently the procedure of choice for patients with solitary intra-adrenal pheochromocytomas smaller than 8 cm in diameter.[17-19] If the pheochromocytoma is in the adrenal gland, the entire gland should be removed. Laparoscopic adrenalectomy for pheochromocytoma should be converted to open adrenalectomy in cases of difficult dissection, invasion, adhesions, or surgeon inexperience.[19]

PRIMARY HYPERALDOSTERONISM

Pulmonary arterial hypertension is one of the most common causes of secondary hypertension and is an increasing recognized disease.[20] As the word suggests, it is associated with excess production of aldosterone. PAH exists in several forms. This includes idiopathic hyperaldosteronism (bilateral adrenal hyperplasia) that is more commonly seen than aldosterone producing adenoma (unilateral adrenal adenoma). The latter is also known as Conn's syndrome. Seen in the second decade of life with equal incidence in both males and females.

Clinical Features

The clinical features of PAH is due to the excess mineralocorticoid receptor (MR) activation produced by the aldosterone, resulting in potassium depletion and sodium water retention. This results in hypokalemia and hypertension—the clinical hallmark of PAH. Increased activity of epithelial Na channel (ENac) channel also results in hydrogen depletion leading to metabolic alkalosis. The patients can present with symptoms associated with hypokalemia such as muscle cramps, muscle weakness to overt proximal myopathy.

Biochemical Tests

Screening for PAH should be considered for hypertensive patients with the following presentation: hypokalemia, difficult to control hypertension on three or more antihypertensive drugs or hypertension of ≥160 mm Hg systolic and ≥100 mm Hg diastolic, or those with hypertension and an incidental adrenal mass, young onset of hypertension, or those being evaluated for other causes of secondary hypertension.[20]

$$\text{Plasma aldosterone concentration (PAC)} > 10 \text{ ng/dL}$$
$$\text{OR}$$
$$\text{Plasma renin activity (PRA)} < 1 \text{ ng/mL}$$

Impact of medications on screening: If patient is on spironolactone it has to be stopped 6 weeks prior to the test and use other medications to control hypertension.[21] Ideally, hypertensive drugs which interfere with renin and aldosterone measurements should be discontinued for atleast 2 weeks prior.

Confirmatory Test

Saline infusion test: 2 L of normal saline is infused over 4 hours. The resultant increase intravascular volume would suppress renin–angiotensin–aldosterone system (RAAS) axis and decreases aldosterone as a normal response. After infusion of saline we have to repeat serum aldosterone level which if still high is confirmatory.

Treatment

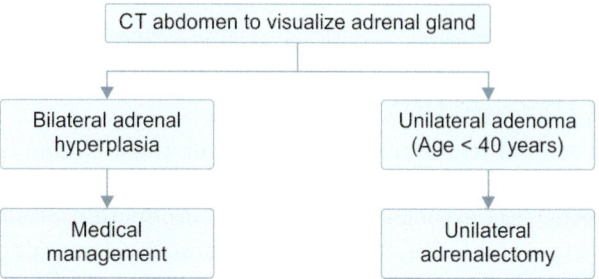

The mainstay of treatment of PAH is spironolactone, a competitive aldosterone receptor antagonist.[22] It can be started at 12.5–50 mg BD and can be increased up to maximum of 400 mg/day to control BP and normalize potassium. Side effects include gynecomastia, menstrual irregularity and decreased libido breast engorgement, decreased libido, muscle cramps, erectile dysfunction, menstrual irregularities, and loss of axillary hair.[23] Eplerenone, which is a more selective (MR) antagonist is preferred. It can be started at a dose of 25 mg BD and can be increased up to 200 mg/day.

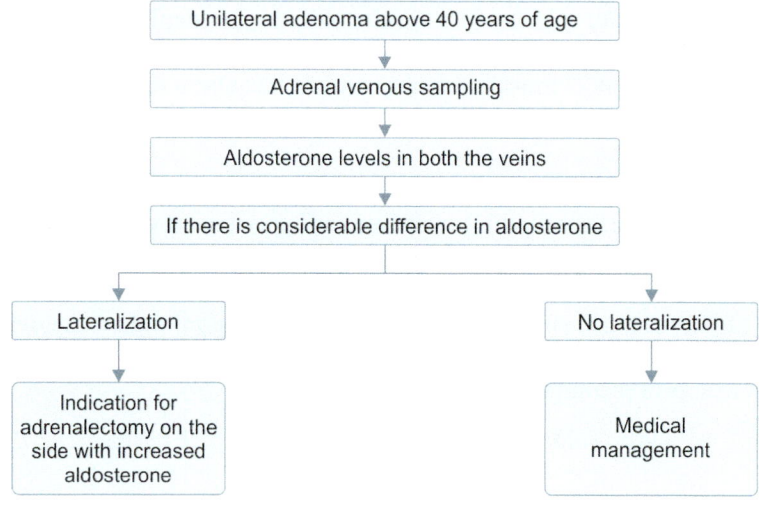

HYPERDEOXYCORTICOSTERONISM

- *Congenital adrenal hyperplasia*: These are the group of autosomal recessive disorders caused by enzymatic defects in adrenal steroidogenesis, resulting in deficient secretion of cortisol. Among the enzymatic defects, deficiencies of 11β-hydroxylase or 17α-hydroxylase results in hypertension and hypokalemia due to hypersecretion of the mineralocorticoid 11-deoxycorticosterone.
    - *11β-hydroxylase deficiency*: More than 40 mutations have been described in CYP11B1, the gene encoding 11β-hydroxylase.[24] The impaired conversion of 11-deoxycorticosterone to corticosterone leads to high levels of 11-deoxycorticosterone and 11-deoxycortisol; resulting in increased levels of adrenal androgens. Females in infancy or childhood with hypertension, hypokalemia, acne, hirsutism, and virilization. Males present with hypertension, hypokalemia, and pseudoprecocious puberty. Approximately, two-thirds of patients have mild to moderate hypertension.
    - *17α-hydroxylase deficiency*: 17α-hydroxylase is crucial for the synthesis of cortisol and gonadal hormones. Deficiency causes decreased production of cortisol and sex steroids. Genetic 46,XY males present with either pseudohermaphroditism or as phenotypic females and 46,XX females present with primary amenorrhea. Hence, individuals with this disorder may not come to medical attention until puberty. Children, adolescents, and young adults present with hypertension and spontaneous hypokalemia and low levels of aldosterone and renin.
- *Deoxycorticosterone-producing tumor*: This is one of the rare conditions, typically presenting as a rapid onset of marked hypertension with hypokalemia and low blood levels of aldosterone and renin. May be associated with other signs and symptoms depending on the other hormones produced by the tumor, e.g., virilization by androgens in females.
- *Primary cortisol resistance*: Caused by the genetic defects in glucocorticoid receptor and the steroid receptor complex.

APPARENT MINERALOCORTICOID EXCESS SYNDROME

Apparent mineralocorticoid excess is the result of impaired activity of the microsomal enzyme HSD11B2, which normally inactivates cortisol in the kidney by converting it to the inactive 11-keto compound, cortisone.[25] As a result of this impaired activity, high levels of cortisol accumulate in the kidney and it exerts a potent mineralocorticoid action. Congenital AME typically presents in childhood with hypertension, hypokalemia, low birth weight, failure to thrive, hypertension, polyuria and polydipsia, and poor growth.[24] Acquired AME due to licorice root ingestion presents with hypertension and hypokalemia.

CUSHING SYNDROME

Hypertension occurs in 75-80% of patients with Cushing syndrome.[26] The mechanisms of hypertension include increased production of 11-deoxycorticosterone, increased pressor sensitivity to endogenous vasoconstrictors (e.g., epinephrine and angiotensin II), activation of the renin angiotensin aldosterone system by increased hepatic production of angiotensinogen, increased cardiac output, and cortisol activation of the mineralocorticoid receptor.

THYROID DYSFUNCTION

Hyperthyroidism

Excessive amounts of circulating thyroid hormones interact with thyroid hormone receptors on peripheral tissues, increasing the sensitivity of circulating catecholamines, and also the metabolic activity. Thyrotoxic patients usually have tachycardia, high cardiac output, increased stroke volume, decreased peripheral vascular resistance, and increased systolic blood pressure.[27] The initial management in patients with hypertension and hyperthyroidism includes use of a β-adrenergic blocker to treat hypertension, tachycardia, and tremor. The definitive treatment of hyperthyroidism is cause-specific.[28]

Hypothyroidism

The frequency of hypertension (usually diastolic) is increased threefold in hypothyroid patients and may account for as many as 1% of cases of diastolic hypertension in the general population.[29,30] The mechanisms for the elevation in blood pressure include increased systemic vascular resistance and extracellular volume expansion. Treatment of thyroid hormone deficiency decreases blood pressure in most patients with hypertension and in one-third of patients it normalizes blood pressure.

Hypercalcemia and Primary Hyperparathyroidism

Hypercalcemia is associated with an increased frequency of hypertension.[31] The frequency of hypertension in patients with primary hyperparathyroidism varies from 10 to 60%.[32] The mechanisms of hypertension are unclear because there is no direct correlation with the elevated parathyroid hormone or calcium levels.

Acromegaly

Hypertension occurs in 20-40% of the patients with acromegaly and is associated with sodium retention and extracellular volume expansion.[33,34] The hypertension of acromegaly is treated most effectively by curing the excess of growth hormone.[34]

REFERENCES

1. Vega J, Bisognano JD. The prevalence, incidence, prognosis, and associated conditions of resistant hypertension. Semin Nephrol. 2014;34(3):247-56.
2. Velasco A, Vongpatanasin W. The evaluation and treatment of endocrine forms of hypertension. Curr Cardiol Rep. 2014;16(9):528.
3. Manger WM. The protean manifestations of pheochromocytoma. Horm Metab Res. 2009;41(9):658-63.
4. Guerrero MA, Schreinemakers JM, Vriens MR, Suh I, Hwang J, Shen WT, et al. Clinical spectrum of pheochromocytoma. J Am Coll Surg. 2009;209:727-32.
5. Lenders JW, Eisenhofer G, Mannelli M, Pacak K. Phaeochromocytoma. Lancet. 2005;366:665-75.
6. Baguet JP, Hammer L, Mazzuco TL, Chabre O, Mallion JM, Sturm N, et al. Circumstances of discovery of phaeochromocytoma: a retrospective study of 41 consecutive patients. Eur J Endocrinol. 2004;150:681-6.
7. Calhoun DA, Jones D, Textor S, Goff DC, Murphy TP, Toto RD, et al. Resistant hypertension: diagnosis, evaluation, and treatment. A scientific statement from the American Heart Association Professional Education Committee of the Council for High Blood Pressure Research. Hypertension. 2008;51:1403-19.
8. Zelinka T, Eisenhofer G, Pacak K. Pheochromocytoma as a catecholamine producing tumor: implications for clinical practice. Stress. 2007;10:195-203.
9. Chen H, Sippel RS, O'Dorisio MS, Vinik AI, Lloyd RV, Pacak K. The North American Neuroendocrine Tumor Society consensus guideline for the diagnosis and management of neuroendocrine tumors: pheochromocytoma, paraganglioma, and medullary thyroid cancer. Pancreas. 2010;39:775-83.
10. Lenders JW, Pacak K, Walther MM, Linehan WM, Mannelli M, Friberg P, et al. Biochemical diagnosis of pheochromocytoma: which test is best? JAMA. 2002;287:1427-34.
11. Ilias I, Pacak K. Current approaches and recommended algorithm for the diagnostic localization of pheochromocytoma. J Clin Endocrinol Metab. 2004;89:479-91.
12. Park BK, Kim CK, Kwon GY, Kim JH. Re-evaluation of pheochromocytomas on delayed contrast-enhanced CT: washout enhancement and other imaging features. Eur Radiol. 2007;17:2804-9.
13. Brink I, Hoegerle S, Klisch J, Bley TA. Imaging of pheochromocytoma and paraganglioma. Fam Cancer. 2005;4:61-8.
14. Krestin GP, Steinbrich W, Friedmann G. Adrenal masses: evaluation with fast gradient-echo MR imaging and Gd-DTPA-enhanced dynamic studies. Radiology. 1989;171:675-80.
15. Pacak K, Eisenhofer G, Ahlman H, Bornstein SR, Gimenez-Roqueplo AP, Grossman AB, et al. Pheochromocytoma: recommendations for clinical practice from the First International Symposium. October 2005. Nat Clin Pract Endocrinol Metab. 2007;3(2):92-102.
16. Lebuffe G, Dosseh ED, Tek G, Tytgat H, Moreno S, Tavernier B, et al. The effect of calcium channel blockers on outcome following the surgical treatment of phaeochromocytomas and paragangliomas. Anaesthesia. 2005;60:439-44.
17. Assalia A, Gagner M. Laparoscopic adrenalectomy. Br J Surg. 2004;91:1259-74.
18. Agarwal G, Sadacharan D, Aggarwal V, Chand G, Mishra A, Agarwal A, et al. Surgical management of organ-contained unilateral pheochromocytoma: comparative outcomes of laparoscopic and conventional open surgical procedures in a large single-institution series. Langenbecks Arch Surg. 2012;397(7):1109-16.
19. Shen WT, Sturgeon C, Clark OH, Duh QY, Kebebew E. Should pheochromocytoma size influence surgical approach? A comparison of 90 malignant and 60 benign pheochromocytomas. Surgery. 2004;136(6):1129-37.

20. Young WF. Primary aldosteronism: renaissance of a syndrome. Clin Endocrinol (Oxf). 2007;66:607-18.
21. Funder JW, Carey RM, Fardella C, Gomez-Sanchez CE, Mantero F, Stowasser M, et al. Case detection, diagnosis, and treatment of patients with primary aldosteronism: an endocrine society clinical practice guideline. J Clin Endocrinol Metab. 2008;93:3266-81.
22. Karagiannis A, Tziomalos K, Kakafika AI, Athyros VG, Harsoulis F, Mikhailidis DP. Medical treatment as an alternative to adrenalectomy in patients with aldosterone-producing adenomas. Endocr Relat Cancer. 2008;15:693-700.
23. Ghose RP, Hall PM, Bravo EL. Medical management of aldosterone-producing adenomas. Ann Intern Med. 1999;131:105-8.
24. New MI, Geller DS, Fallo F, Wilson RC. Monogenic low renin hypertension. Trends Endocrinol Metab. 2005;16:92-7.
25. Chapman K, Holmes M, Seckl J. 11beta-hydroxysteroid dehydrogenases: intracellular gate-keepers of tissue glucocorticoid action. Physiol Rev. 2013;93:1139-206.
26. Baid S, Nieman LK. Glucocorticoid excess and hypertension. Curr Hypertens Rep. 2004;6:493-9.
27. Danzi S, Klein I. Thyroid hormone and blood pressure regulation. Curr Hypertens Rep. 2003;5:513-20.
28. Bahn RS, Burch HB, Cooper DS, Garber JR, Greenlee MC, Klein I, et al. Hyperthyroidism and other causes of thyrotoxicosis: management guidelines of the American Thyroid Association and American Association of Clinical Endocrinologists. Endocr Pract. 2011;17(3):456-520.
29. Streeten DH, Anderson GH Jr, Howland T, Chiang R, Smulyan H. Effects of thyroid function on blood pressure. Recognition of hypothyroid hypertension. Hypertension. 1988;11(1):78-83.
30. Jian WX, Jin J, Qin L, Fang WJ, Chen XR, Chen HB, et al. Relationship between thyroid-stimulating hormone and blood pressure in the middle-aged and elderly population. Singapore Med J. 2013;54(7):401-5.
31. Han D, Trooskin S, Wang X. Prevalence of cardiovascular risk factors in male and female patients with primary hyperparathyroidism. J Endocrinol Invest. 2012;35:548-52.
32. Richards AM, Espiner EA, Nicholls MG, Ikram H, Hamilton EJ, Maslowski AH. Hormone, calcium and blood pressure relationships in primary hyperparathyroidism. J Hypertens. 1988;6(9):747-52.
33. Terzolo M, Matrella C, Boccuzzi A, Luceri S, Borriero M, Reimondo G, et al. Twenty-four hour profile of blood pressure in patients with acromegaly. Correlation with demographic, clinical and hormonal features. J Endocrinol Invest. 1999;22(1):48-54.
34. Berg C, Petersenn S, Lahner H, Herrmann BL, Buchfelder M, Droste M, et al. Cardiovascular risk factors in patients with uncontrolled and long-term acromegaly: comparison with matched data from the general population and the effect of disease control. J Clin Endocrinol Metab. 2010;95(8):3648-56.

11 GINA 2020: What's New and Why?

Pratibha Singhal, Iram Syed

INTRODUCTION

The Global Initiative for Asthma (GINA) report is an integrated evidence-based strategy focusing on clinical practice. It is not a guideline in the true sense of the word. Recommendations are framed to prevent asthma deaths and exacerbations and improve symptom control. The GINA report has been updated in 2020 after the twice-yearly cumulative review of the literature by the GINA Scientific Committee. We will discuss the key changes and what's new in GINA 2020.

For new therapies, the GINA Science Committee makes recommendations after approval for asthma by at least one major regulatory agency [e.g., European Medicines Agency, and Food and Drug Administration (FDA)]. However, decisions by GINA to make or not make a recommendation about any therapy are based on the best available peer-reviewed evidence and not on labeling directives from regulators. Since, GINA is a global strategy and regulatory indications vary between countries, GINA 2020 states that specific therapies are no longer stated to be "off-label". Clinicians should use their own professional judgment in assessing and treating individual patients based on eligibility of patient, licensed drug dosages, financial implications, and national guidelines when prescribing a particular therapy.

INTERIM GUIDANCE ABOUT ASTHMA AND COVID-19

Brief advice has been added about management of asthma during the coronavirus disease 2019 (COVID-19) pandemic, with a focus on safety of patients and healthcare workers.[1]

Spirometry

Spirometry can disseminate viral particles and expose staff and patients to risk of infection hence, spirometry is to be avoided in patients with confirmed/suspected COVID-19. With ongoing community transmission of the virus, postpone spirometry and peak flow measurement within healthcare facilities unless urgently needed.

Treatment

Patients with asthma are advised to continue taking their prescribed asthma medications, particularly inhaled corticosteroids (ICS), and oral corticosteroids (OCS), as prescribed for use on regular basis. Discontinuing ICS suddenly often leads to potentially dangerous worsening of asthma. For patients with severe asthma biologic therapy and or OCS should be continued as prescribed and not discontinued. Patients should be counseled to consult their doctor prior to making changes in their treatment.

All patients should have a written asthma action plan with instructions about increasing controller and reliever medication when asthma worsens.[1] In severe asthma exacerbations short course of OCS can be taken. Patients should be advised when to seek medical help (**Flowchart 1**).

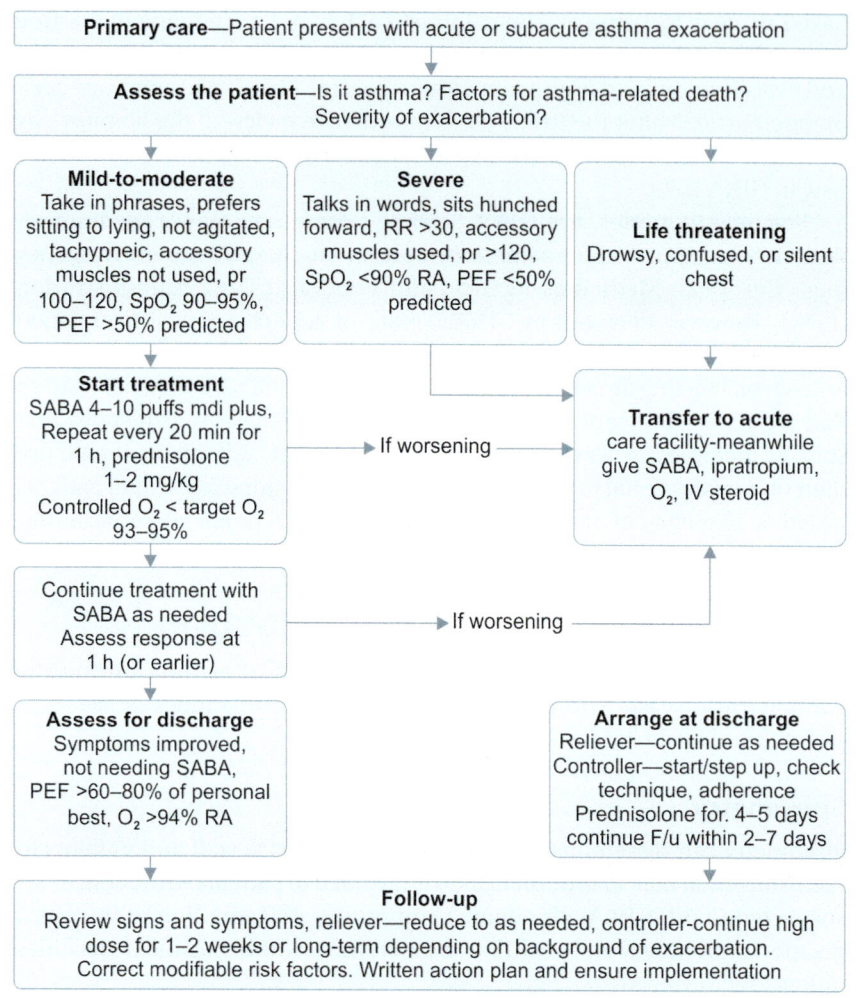

FLOWCHART 1: Management of asthma exacerbation.

Nebulizers can transmit viral particles up to 1 m, hence, it is advisable to avoid nebulizers where possible to reduce the risk of disseminating virus to other patients and healthcare professionals.

Pressurized metered dose inhaler (pMDI) via a spacer is the preferred treatment during severe exacerbations with a mouthpiece or tightly fitting face mask if required and sharing inhalers or spacers with family members to be avoided.

Infection Control Measures

If spirometry is needed urgently, all contact and droplet precautions are to be followed. Follow strict infection control procedures for other aerosol-generating procedures such as nebulization, oxygen therapy (including with nasal prongs), sputum induction, manual ventilation, noninvasive ventilation, and intubation. Use of personal protective equipment should be followed as per the local and national recommendations.

TREATMENT OF ASTHMA IN ADULTS AND ADOLESCENTS

The major change in 2019 GINA recommendation was use of as-needed ICS-formoterol in mild asthma compared to previous recommendation of SOS short-acting beta-agonist (SABA).[1] This is additionally supported by the results of two randomized controlled trials (RCTs) in adults of as-needed low dose budesonide-formoterol in mild asthma. These 12-month novel START (n = 668) and PRACTICAL (n = 885) study[2,3] showed significant reduction in severe exacerbations in study group versus SABA alone, and versus maintenance ICS, with small or no difference in symptom control. Lower average ICS dose was needed. Reduction in risk of severe exacerbations with as-needed ICS-formoterol was independent of baseline characteristics, including blood eosinophils and exhaled nitric oxide. FeNO was significantly reduced by SOS ICS-formoterol (with average 3–5 doses per week) Based on past and current evidence, GINA recommends treatment with daily low dose ICS or as-needed low dose ICS-formoterol (**Fig. 1**) for all patients with mild asthma, to reduce the risk of serious exacerbations.[1]

Maximum Daily Dose of Inhaled Corticosteroids Formoterol

For patients on maintenance and reliever treatment with ICS-formoterol, the maximum recommended total dose in a day is 48 µg formoterol for beclometasone-formoterol and 72 µg formoterol for budesonide-formoterol. Although applicable to SOS use of budesonide-formoterol in mild asthma. RTCs in mild asthma have demonstrated that average use was around lesser, 3–4 doses per week.[3,4]

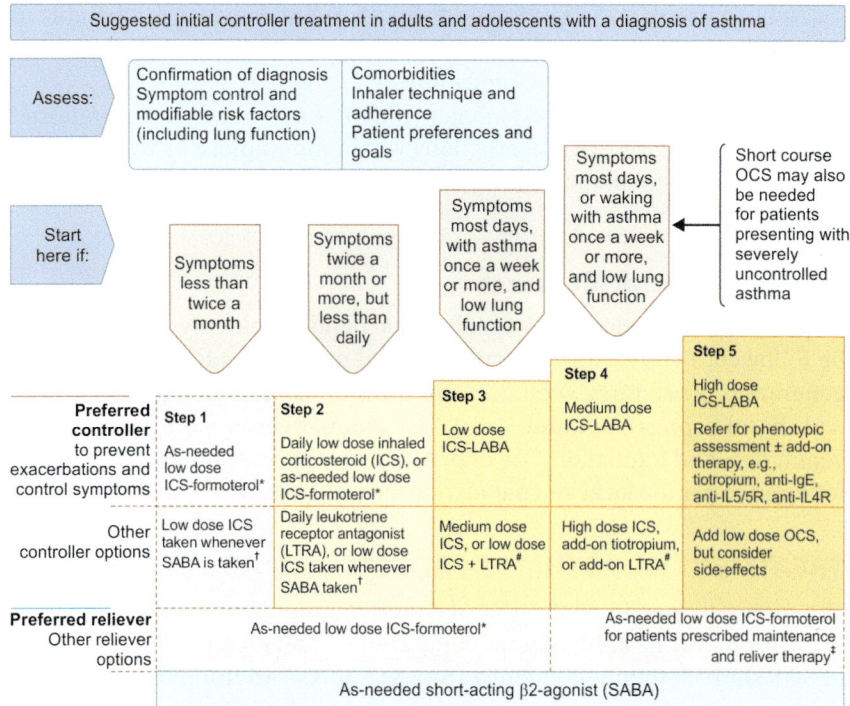

*Data only with budesonide-formoterol (bud-form).
†Separate or combination ICS and SABA inhalers.
‡Low-dose ICS-form is the reliever only for patients prescribed bud-form or BDP-form maintenance and reliever therapy.
#Consider adding HDM SLIT for sensitized patients with allergic rhinitis and FEV1 >70% predicted.

(OCS: oral corticosteroids)

FIG. 1: Initial treatment in adults and adolescents.

Low, Medium, and High Dose Inhaled Corticosteroids

This is not an equivalence table, instead represents suggested doses of various ICS formulations included in treatment recommendations (**Table 1**). Doses and regulatory labeling will vary in different countries, e.g., mometasone is not available in India.

ASTHMA IN CHILDREN

Factors Contributing to Development of Asthma

New evidence suggests that 13% of global asthma incidence in children may be attributable to traffic-related air pollution and obesity may be a risk factor for developing asthma.[5]

TABLE 1: Inhaled corticosteroids (ICS) doses.

	Adults and adolescents (12 years and older)		
	Total daily ICS dose (µg)		
Inhaled corticosteroid	Low	Medium	High
Beclomethasone dipropionate (pMDI, standard particle, and HFA)	200–500	>500–1,000	>1,000
Beclomethasone dipropionate (pMDI, extrafine particle, and HFA)	100–200	>200–400	>400
Budesonide (DPI)	200–400	>400–800	>800
Ciclesonide (pMDI, extrafine particle, and HFA)	80–160	>160–320	>320
Fluticasone furoate (DPI)		100	200
Fluticasone propionate (DPI)	100–250	>250–500	>500
Fluticasone propionate (pMDI, standard particle, and HFA)	100–250	>250–500	>500
Mometasone furoate (DPI)		200	400
Mometasone furoate (pMDI, standard particle, and HFA)		200–400	>400

(DPI: dry powder inhaler; HFA: hydrofluoroalkane; pMDI: pressurized metered dose inhaler)

Treatment

Recommendation to take ICS (separate inhalers) whenever SABA is taken in mild asthma is supported by a RCT in African-American children (ASIST) study.[1]

New evidence added in 2020 includes a systematic review showing that school-based programs including asthma self-management reduced emergency visits, hospitalizations, and days of reduced activity; and that in preschoolers with asthma, daily ICS is more effective than leukotriene receptor antagonists (LTRA) for symptom control and exacerbation reduction.[6]

Assessment of severe exacerbations in children no longer includes chest retractions, respiratory rate has been added in GINA 2020. New tables for treatment have been added (**Figs. 2** and **3**).

Low, Medium, and High Dose Inhaled Corticosteroids

Like for adults this is not an equivalence table, doses, and regulatory labeling will vary in different countries (**Table 2**).

Mepolizumab in Children

This biologic agent has been approved for children ≥6 years with severe eosinophilic asthma. Long-term safety, pharmacodynamic, and efficacy data supports a positive benefit-risk profile for mepolizumab in children with severe asthma with an eosinophilic phenotype, similar to data in studies in adults and adolescents.[7]

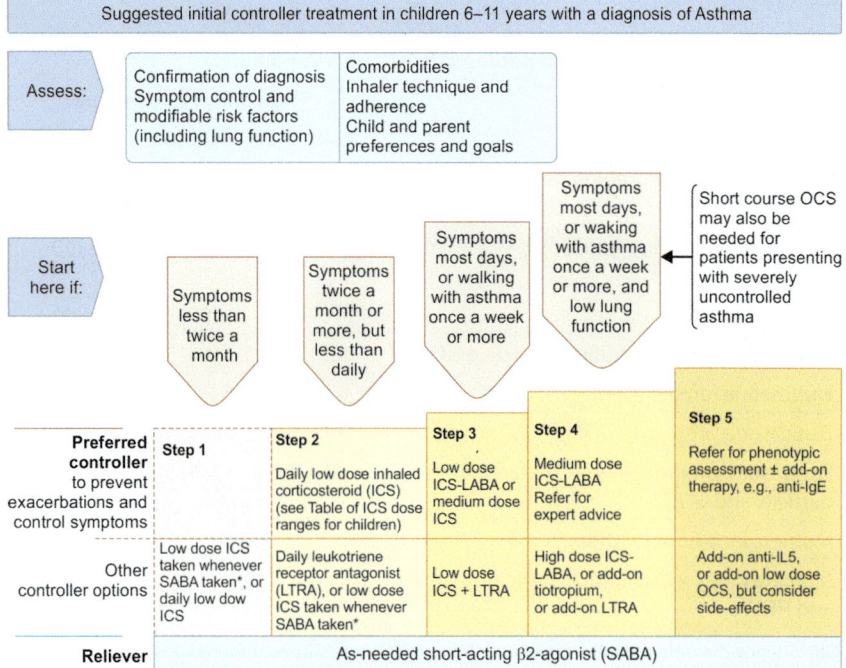

*Separate ICS and SABA inhalers.

(OCS: oral corticosteroids)

FIG. 2: Initial treatment in children 6–11 years.

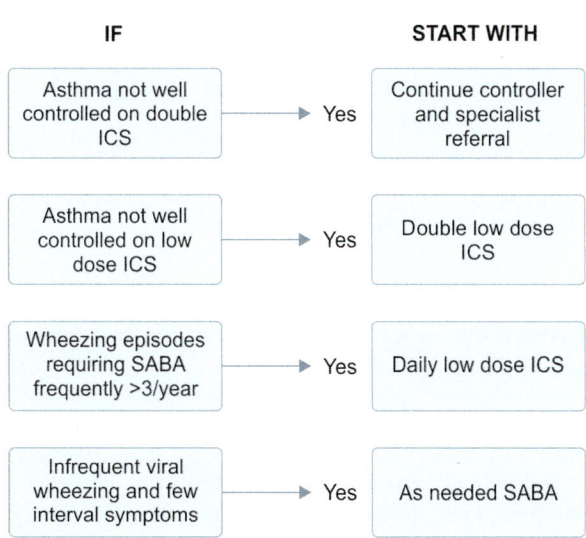

(ICS: inhaled corticosteroids; SABA: short-acting beta-agonist)

FIG. 3: Initial treatment in children ≤5 years.

TABLE 2: Inhaled corticosteroids doses.

Inhaled corticosteroid	Low total daily dose (µg) (age-group with adequate safety and effectiveness data)
BDP (pMDI, standard particle, and HFA)	100 (ages 5 years and older)
BDP (pMDI, exrtrafine particle, and HFA)	50 (ages 5 years and older)
Budesonide nebulized	500 (ages 1 years and older)
Fluticasone propionate (pMDI, standard particle, and HFA)	50 (ages 4 years and older)
Fluticasone furoate (DPI)	Not sufficiently studied in children 5 years and younger
Momotasone furoate (pMDI, standard particle, and HFA)	100 (ages 5 years and older)
Ciclesonide (pMDI, extrafine particle, and HFA)	Not sufficiently studied in children 5 years and younger)

(BDP: beclomethasone dipropionate; DPI: dry powder inhaler; HFA: hydrofluoroalkane; pMDI: pressurized metered dose inhaler)

RISK OF ADVERSE EFFECTS OF MONTELUKAST

Alerts have been added with montelukast, including the requirement by the FDA for a boxed warning in March 2020 about risk of serious neuropsychiatric events, including suicidality in adults and adolescents and nightmares and behavioral problems in children. Health professionals should consider its benefits and risks, and patients should be counselled.[1]

ASTHMA AND CHRONIC OBSTRUCTIVE PULMONARY DISEASE

Differentiating asthma from chronic obstructive pulmonary disease (COPD) is challenging. Chapter 5 in GINA is about patients with features of both asthma and COPD, also described as '"asthma-COPD overlap" or '"asthma + COPD" (**Fig. 4**). It advices clinicians in view of available with available evidence that patients with diagnoses of both asthma and COPD are more likely to die or to be hospitalized, if treated with LABA versus ICS-LABA.[8]

ASSESSMENT OF SYMPTOM CONTROL

It is clarified that the reliever use criterion forming part of the assessment of asthma symptom control relates to as-needed SABA. GINA 2020 states that their current view is that frequency of as-needed ICS-formoterol should not be included in the assessment of symptom control, particularly for patient's not taking maintenance ICS as it is providing the patients controller therapy. Further, data are awaited to be reviewed again next year.

Clinical phenotype—Adults with chronic respiratory symptoms (dyspnea, cough, chest tightness and wheeze)		
Highly likely to be asthma If several of the following features **Treat as asthma**	**Features of both asthma + COPD** **Treat as asthma**	**Likely to be COPD** If several of the following features **Treat as COPD**

History
• Symptoms vary over time in intensity
  – Triggers may include laughter, exercise, allergens, and seasonal
  – Onset before age 40 years
  – Symptoms improve spontaneously or with bronchodilators (minutes) or ICS (days to weeks)
• Current asthma diagnosis, or asthma diagnosis in childhood
 	
Lung function
• Variable expiratory airflow limitation
• Persistent airflow limitation may be present
	History
	• Symptoms intermittent to episodic
	  – May have started before or after age 40
	• May have a history of smoking and/or other toxic exposures, or history of low birth weight or respiratory illness such as tuberculosis
	• Any of asthma features at left (e.g., common triggers: symptoms improve spontaneously or with bronchodilators or ICS; current asthma diagnosis or asthma diagnosis in childhood)
	
	Lung function
	• Persistent expiratory airflow limitation
	• With or without bronchodilator reversbility
		History
		• Dyspnea persistent (most days)
		  – Onset after age 40 years
		  – Limitation of physical activity
		  – May have been preceded by cough/sputum
		  – Bronchodilator provides only limited relief
		• History of smoking and/or other toxic exposure, or history of low birth weight or respiratory illness such as tuberculosis
		• No past current diagnosis of asthma
		
		Lung function
		• Persistent expiratory airflow limitation
		• With or without bronchodilator reversbility

Initial pharmacological treatment (as well as treating comorbidities and risk factors.)		

• ICS-containing treatment is essential to reduce risk of severe exacerbations and death.
  – As-needed low dose ICS-formoterol may be used as reliever.
• Do Not Give LABA and/or LAMA without ICS
• Avoid maintenance OCS
	• ICS-containing treatment is essential to reduce risk of severe exacerbations and death.
	• Add-on LABA and/or LAMA usually also needed
	• Additional COPD treatment as par GOLD
	• Do Not Give LABA and/or LAMA without ICS
	• Avoid maintenance OCS
		• Treat as COPD (see GOLD report)
		  – Initially LAMA and/or LABA
		  – Add ICS as per GOLD for patients with hospitalizations, ≥2 exacerbations/year requiring OCS, or blood eosinophils ≥300/μL
		• Avoid high dose ICS, avoid maintenance OCS
		• Reliever containing ICS is not recommended

Review patient after 2–3 months. Refer for expert advice if diagnostic uncertainty or inadequate response		

(COPD: chronic obstructive pulmonary disease; ICS: inhaled corticosteroid; LABA: long-acting β-agonist; LAMA: long-acting muscarinic antagonist; OCS: oral corticosteroid)

FIG. 4: Differentiating asthma, COPD, and asthma + COPD.

ROLE OF TRAINED LAY HEALTHWORKERS

Asthma outcomes can be improved with interventions by trained lay health workers, as well as by trained nurses and pharmacists.

ACUTE ASTHMA

References to "high flow oxygen" in previous GINA reports have been corrected to "high concentration oxygen".

ASTHMA IN PREGNANCY

A review of guidelines for asthma in pregnancy highlighted the need for more clinical trials, and for clarity in recommendations, as per GINA.

REFERENCES

1. Global strategy for asthma management and prevention. Global Initiative for Asthma (GINA); 2020 update. [online] Available from: https://ginasthma.org/gina-reports/ (Last accessed August, 2021).
2. Beasley R, Holliday M, Reddel HK, Braithwaite I, Ebmeier S, Hancox RJ, et al. Controlled Trial of Budesonide–Formoterol as Needed for Mild Asthma (Novel START Study Team): 52-week, randomized, open-label, parallel-group, controlled trial involving adults with mild asthma. N Engl J Med. 2019;380(21):2020-30.
3. Hardy J, Baggott C, Fingleton J, Reddel HK, Hancox RJ, Harwood M, et al. Budesonide-formoterol reliever therapy versus maintenance budesonide plus terbutaline reliever therapy in adults with mild to moderate asthma (PRACTICAL): a 52-week, open-label, multicentre, superiority, randomised controlled trial. Lancet. 2019;394(10202):919-28.
4. Bateman ED, Reddel HK, O'Byrne PM, Barnes PJ, Zhong N, Keen C, et al. As-needed budesonide-formoterol versus maintenance budesonide in mild asthma. N Engl J Med. 2018;378(20):1877-87.
5. Achakulwisut P, Brauer M, Hystad P, Anenberg SC. Global, national, and urban burdens of paediatric asthma incidence attributable to ambient NO2 pollution: estimates from global datasets. Lancet Planet Health. 2019;3(4):e166-78.
6. Kneale D, Harris K, McDonald VM, Thomas J, Grigg J. Effectiveness of school-based self-management interventions for asthma among children and adolescents: findings from a Cochrane systematic review and meta-analysis. Thorax. 2019:74(5):432-8.
7. Gupta A, Ikeda M, Geng B, Azmi J, Price RG, Bradford ES, et al. Long-term safety and pharmacodynamics of mepolizumab in children with severe asthma with an eosinophilic phenotype. J Allergy Clin Immunol. 2019;144(5):1336-42.e7.
8. Kendzerska T, Aaron SD, To T, Licskai C, Stanbrook M, Vozoris NT, et al. Effectiveness and safety of inhaled corticosteroids in older individuals with chronic obstructive pulmonary disease and/or asthma. A population study. Ann Am Thorac Soc. 2019;16(10):1252-62.

12 Heart Rate an Independent Risk Factor and the Proficient Study

Jagdish Hiremath

INTRODUCTION

Heart rate (HR) is an important clinical index and a relevant cardiovascular risk marker. An elevated resting HR has been found to be an independent risk factor of all cause, noncardiovascular, and cardiovascular mortality in various clinical studies. Thus, along with the traditional risk factors and other potentially confounding demographic and physiological variables such as age, gender, physical, or cardiorespiratory fitness levels, etc., resting HR is a potential marker of risk in cardiovascular patients.[1]

Heart rate is not only a risk factor for cardiovascular events, hypertension, coronary heart disease, and heart failure but it is associated with the entire cardiovascular continuum.[2]

The parasympathetic nervous system and the sympathetic nervous system is responsible for 80% and 20% of resting HR, respectively. Both parasympathetic and sympathetic nervous systems make an equal contribution at close to 140 beats/min (bpm), after which the ratio changes quickly to a more sympathetically dominant system. The sympathetic nervous system has a significantly higher influence in pathological situations that provoke hemodynamic changes, arrhythmias, and metabolic abnormalities which further induces hypertension, heart failure, atherosclerosis, insulin resistance, lipid abnormalities, obesity, and increases cardiovascular and noncardiovascular mortality. It is also associated with the imbalance in the renin–angiotensin–aldosterone system (RAAS) system, thus, inducing release of angiotensin II and additional negative effect on cardiovascular system.[3]

Resting HR has been associated with hypertension, ischemic heart disease, heart failure, and stroke. Thus, the simple measure of this vital sign during the course of the disease should be a warning signal and should lead to treatment and follow-up intensification in order to improve outcomes.

HEART RATE AS A TREATMENT TARGET IN HEART FAILURE AND STABLE ANGINA

The duration of diastole is shortened due to greater myocardial oxygen consumption and decreased myocardial perfusion which in turn is a result of a higher HR. Increased HR also activates an inflammatory endothelial cell response. Thus, increase in high HR leads to the underlying mechanism of heart failure.[4]

Myocardial oxygen demand and coronary blood flow both are a function of HR. High heart decreases supply and increases demand rate leading to an imbalance which results into myocardial ischemia and subsequent angina.[5]

Both for chronic coronary syndrome and heart failure one aims at 60 + 65 bpm.

ROLE OF IVABRADINE IN HEART RATE REDUCTION

Ivabradine is a heart-rate-lowering drug. It acts by selectively and specifically inhibiting the cardiac pacemaker current (I_f) that controls the spontaneous diastolic depolarization in the sinoatrial (SA) node and, hence, regulates the HR. The molecular channel belongs to the hyperpolarization-activated and cyclic nucleotide-gated (HCN) family. Inhibition of the channel disrupts I_f current flow resulting into prolonged diastolic depolarization, slow firing in the SA node, and ultimately reducing the HR. Thus, ivabradine specifically has effects on the SA node and it has no effect on blood pressure, intracardiac conduction, myocardial contractility, or ventricular repolarization. It has been shown to lessen symptoms and reduce ischemia in patients with stable angina pectoris and systolic heart failure.[6]

LANDMARK CLINICAL STUDIES FOR IVABRADINE

Randomized controlled trials on ivabradine such as the BEAUTIFUL (morBidity-mortality EvAlUaTion of the If inhibitor ivabradine in patients with coronary disease and left-ventricULar dysfunction) and SHIFT (Systolic Heart failure treatment with the If inhibitor ivabradine Trial) considered patients with heart failure and stable coronary artery disease (CAD) have found protective effects of ivabradine mainly for HR ≥ 70 bpm.

BEAUTIFUL: Ivabradine 5–7.5 mg BID was assigned to 5,479 eligible patients who had CAD and a left ventricular ejection fraction (LVEF) of <40%. It was found that the safety of giving ivabradine, even in combination with a beta-blocker, and supports a role for ivabradine in patients who cannot tolerate beta-blocker therapy.[7]

SHIFT: About 6,558 patients with symptomatic heart failure and LVEF of 35% or lower, HR of 70 bpm or higher were assigned to have ivabradine 7.5 mg BID and the results supported the importance of heart-rate reduction with ivabradine for improvement of clinical outcomes in heart failure and confirm the important role of HR in the pathophysiology of this disorder.[8]

PROFICIENT STUDY

Medication adherence is a function of dosing frequency especially in patients with chronic cardiovascular diseases. Heart failure management involves multidrug treatment with different dosage regimens. The primary objective of the PROFICIENT study was to assess the noninferiority of the new ivabradine prolonged-release (PR) once-daily formulation compared with the conventional immediate-release (IR) twice-daily formulation with regard to the efficacy and safety parameters in patients with stable chronic heart failure with systolic dysfunction.

The noninferiority of once-daily PR formulation of ivabradine was established with respect to the twice-daily ivabradine IR, when added to background guideline-based medical treatment, in patients with stable chronic heart failure. The safety profile was comparable between the treatment groups.

A separate Holter subgroup analysis was also undertaken in a small subset of patients from the main sample size and it was found that the change in HR was comparable between the treatment groups. It was measured by 24-hour Holter monitoring (mean 24-h HR, mean awake HR, and mean asleep HR). Once daily ivabradine PR effectively maintained the HR in patients shifted from the ivabradine IR twice-daily regimen, and thus may aid in improving treatment compliance.

CONCLUSION

Lower HR (60-65 bpm) is desired in managing Canadian Cardiovascular Society (CCS) and heart failure. Ivabradine alone or along with beta-blockers serves the purpose effectively. Once a day preparation of ivabradine adds to compliance.

REFERENCES

1. Peer N, Lombard C, Steyn K, Levitt N. Elevated resting heart rate is associated with several cardiovascular disease risk factors in urban-dwelling black South Africans. Sci Rep. 2020;10(1):1-8.
2. Nikolovska Vukadinović N, Vukadinović D, Borer J, Cowie M, Komajda M, Lainscak M, et al. Heart rate and its reduction in chronic heart failure and beyond. Eur J Heart Fail. 2017;19(10):1230-41.
3. Tadic M, Cuspidi C, Grassi G. Heart rate as a predictor of cardiovascular risk. Eur J Clin Invest. 2018;48(3).
4. Dobre D, Borer JS, Fox K, Swedberg K, Adams KF, Cleland JG, et al. Heart rate: a prognostic factor and therapeutic target in chronic heart failure. The distinct roles of drugs with heart rate-lowering properties. Eur J Heart Fail. 2014;16(1):76-85.
5. Custodis F, Reil JC, Laufs U, Böhm M. Heart rate: a global target for cardiovascular disease and therapy along the cardiovascular disease continuum. J Cardiol. 2013;62(3):183-7.
6. Tse S, Mazzola N. Ivabradine (Corlanor) for heart failure: the first selective and specific IF inhibitor. P T. 2015;40(12):810-4.
7. Fox K, Ford I, Steg PG, Tendera M, Ferrari R, Beautiful Investigators. Ivabradine for patients with stable coronary artery disease and left-ventricular systolic dysfunction (BEAUTIFUL): a randomised, double-blind, placebo-controlled trial. Lancet. 2008;372(9641):807-16.
8. Swedberg K, Komajda M, Böhm M, Borer JS, Ford I, Dubost-Brama A, et al. Ivabradine and outcomes in chronic heart failure (SHIFT): a randomized placebo-controlled study. Lancet. 2010;376(9744):875-85.

13

Hypertensive Emergencies

Amit A Saraf, Bitukaur Sodhi

INTRODUCTION
Globally, an estimated 26% of the world's population (972 million people) has hypertension and the prevalence is expected to increase to 29% by 2025, driven largely by increases in economically developing nations.[1] Hypertension is a growing problem in India, significantly burdening the health system. According to data from the Global Burden of Disease (GBD) study of 2016, hypertension led to 1.63 million deaths in India in the year 2016 alone.[2] GBD data also showed that over half of the deaths due to ischemic heart disease (54.2%), stroke (56.2%), and chronic kidney disease (54.5%) were attributable to high systolic blood pressure (SBP).[3] India has also been experiencing an increase in the prevalence of hypertension.[4] A cross-sectional, population-based study on a large nationally representative sample of 1.3 million individuals carried out between 2012 and 2014 revealed that the crude prevalence of hypertension in India was 25.3%.[5]

DEFINITION
In 2017, the American College of Cardiology (ACC) and the American Heart Association (AHA) guideline for the prevention, detection, evaluation, and management of high blood pressure (BP) in adults defined hypertension as a SBP ≥ 130 mm Hg and a diastolic blood pressure (DBP) ≥ 80 mm Hg.

Hypertensive (HT) emergencies are conditions where elevated BP (typically ≥ 180/120 mm Hg) represents acute threat to vital organs and patient survival with progressive end organ damage. The common presentations include dyspnea, chest pain, headache, and neurological deficit.[6]

The syndrome was first described by Volhard and Fahr in 1914 and was characterized by severe accelerated hypertension accompanied by evidence of renal disease and by signs of vascular injury to the heart, retina, brain, and kidney and by a rapidly fatal course ending in heart attack, renal failure, or stroke.[7]

ETIOLOGY
It has been seen that atleast 1% of HTs (either essential hypertension or secondary to an underlying cause) will present with HT crisis in their lifetime.

The most common cause of HT crisis in a known HT is noncompliance to medication. This fact highlights the importance of patient education and counseling in prevention of this catastrophe.

Sometimes the diagnosis of hypertension is made in the emergency room when the patient has presented as HT crisis. The presence of de novo malignant hypertension almost always indicates an underlying secondary cause of hypertension and should prompt further work up poststabilization.

Secondary causes of hypertension include:
- Renal—parenchymal disease, renal cysts (including polycystic kidney disease), renal tumors (including renin secreting tumors), and obstructive uropathy
- Renovascular—arteriosclerotic and fibromuscular dysplasia
- Adrenal—primary hyperaldosteronism, Cushing's syndrome, 17 α-hydroxylase deficiency, 11 β-hydroxylase deficiency, 11-hydroxysteroid dehydrogenase deficiency, and pheochromocytoma
- Aortic coarctation
- Obstructive sleep apnea
- Pre-eclampsia/eclampsia
- Neurogenic—psychogenic, diencephalic syndrome, familial dysautonomia, polyneuritis (acute porphyria and lead poisoning), acute increased intracranial pressure, and acute spinal cord section
- Endocrine—hypothyroidism, hyperthyroidism, hypercalcemia, and acromegaly
- Medications—high dose estrogens, adrenal steroids, decongestants, appetite suppressants, cyclosporine, tricyclic antidepressants, monoamine oxidase inhibitors, erythropoietin, cocaine, nonsteroidal anti-inflammatory drugs (NSAIDs), and phencyclidine
- Mendelian forms of hypertension

CLINICAL PRESENTATION

The clinical presentation varies from patient to patient and is related to the particular end organ dysfunction. Common presentations include headache, vomiting, giddiness, dyspnea, loss of consciousness, chest pain, blurring of vision, and weakness of limbs[8] along with extremely elevated BP.

The clinical manifestations as per the involved system are: Central nervous system—dizziness, nausea, vomiting, weakness, HT encephalopathy, intracranial hemorrhage (common sites are basal ganglia especially putamen, thalamus, pons, and cerebellum), subarachnoid hemorrhage, and ischemic stroke.
- Ophthalmological manifestations—ocular hemorrhage blurred vision, loss of sight, exudates, or papilledema on funduscopic examination.
- Cardiovascular manifestations—angina, acute coronary syndrome, left ventricular failure, pulmonary embolism, aortic dissection, and cardiogenic shock.

- Renal manifestations—hematuria, proteinuria, pyelonephritis, elevated serum creatinine and blood urea nitrogen (BUN), and acute renal failure.

PATHOPHYSIOLOGY

Despite of hypertension being around since ages the exact pathophysiology behind it continues to be an enigma. It has been postulated that interplay between various factors is responsible for the development of this disease.

The pathophysiology of hypertension involves the impairment of renal pressure natriuresis, the feedback system in which high BP induces an increase in sodium and water excretion by the kidney that leads to a reduction of the BP. Pressure natriuresis can result from impaired renal function, inappropriate activation of hormones that regulate salt and water excretion by the kidney (such as those in the renin–angiotensin–aldosterone system), or excessive activation of the sympathetic nervous system (**Flowchart 1**).

Genetic influences, obesity, environmental factors, inflammation and immune response alterations, and arterial stiffness are also believed to be playing a crucial role in the development of essential hypertension.

The pathologic consequences of hypertension are varied. Increased pressure exerts stress on the heart and in order to overcome this stress structural and functional adaptations occur in the heart resulting in concentric hypertrophy of the left ventricle. This puts the patient at an increased risk for coronary heart disease, congestive heart failure, stroke, and sudden death.

Hypertension is the strongest risk factor for stroke, also associated with deposition of beta amyloid in the brain and causing dementia. Hypertension exerts its ill effects on the kidneys as well causing glomerular injury, loss of autoregulation of renal blood flow, kick starting a vicious cycle of repeated injury due to increased pressure being transmitted to the glomerulus, hyperfiltration, ultimately progressing to glomerulosclerosis, eventually involving the renal tubules as well, resulting in their atrophy.

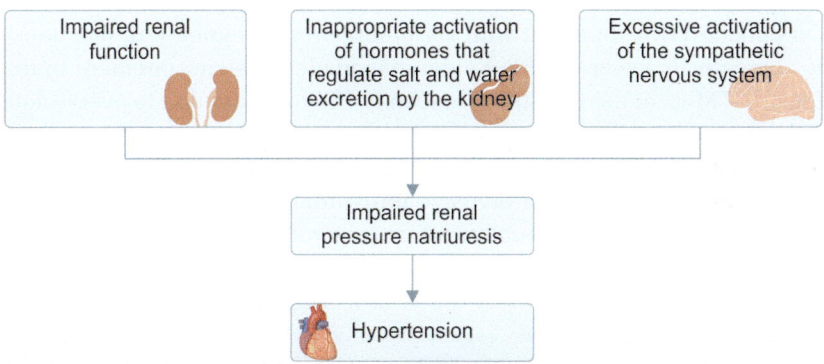

FLOWCHART 1: Pathophysiology of BP surge.

Source: Fuster V, Harrington RA, Narula J, Eapen ZJ. Hurst's the heart, 14th Edition. McGraw-Hill Education; 2017.

In a known HT, the development of HT crisis is most often due to noncompliance to therapy.

It is postulated that sudden increase in the systemic vascular resistance coupled with the failure of autoregulating mechanisms is the first step in the process. The high pressure is responsible for causing endothelial injury and activating the clotting cascade, fibrinoid necrosis of arterioles, and further release of vasoconstrictors augmenting the already elevated BP. If allowed to continue unchecked the cycle of destruction propagates and could lead to death. Hence, recognizing HT emergency is crucial!

MANAGEMENT

History, Physical Examination and Investigations

A detailed history enquiring about the onset and duration of hypertension, history of similar episode in the past, adherence to anti-HT medications, drug history, history of recreational drug use, alcohol use, and any alternative medications being taken.

A thorough physical examination with more emphasis on the cardiovascular and the nervous system. Measuring BP in both arms (a difference in BP of >20 mm Hg should raise concern for aortic dissection), cardiac and lung auscultation, assessment of mental status, and any focal neurological deficit.

Examination of the fundus to look for striate (flame-shaped) hemorrhage and cotton-wool (soft exudates) spots with or without papilledema. It closely parallels the development of severe arteriolar damage (fibrinoid necrosis and proliferative endarteritis) in malignant hypertension.

All the basic laboratory tests, electrocardiogram, chest X-ray, and urine analysis to look for potential secondary causes of hypertension and to determine target organ damage.

Treatment

On encountering a patient with HT emergency, the knee-jerk reaction is to aggressively lower the BP. Kaplan has made a classic statement in this regard—"Most of the catastrophes seen in HT crises are due to overzealous reduction in BP and not because of the elevated BP itself."[9] This is because in a HT, the dynamics of autoregulation of cerebral blood flow are altered when compared to a normotensive individual. So, rapid lowering of BP in these patients could actually end up precipitating cerebral ischemia or infarction as a consequence of decreased cerebral blood flow. In addition to this, the renal and coronary blood flow might also decrease following aggressive reduction.

The initial goal of therapy is to reduce mean arterial pressure by no >25% within minutes to 2 hours or to a BP in the range of 160/100–110 mm Hg. The exceptions are:
- Acute phase of ischemic stroke—BP not lowered unless it is ≥185/110 mm Hg in reperfusion candidates or ≥220/120 mm Hg otherwise.

- Acute aortic dissection—SBP is rapidly reduced to 100/120 mm Hg to be attained in 20 minutes.[10]

The following table gives a list of the preferred drug in selected hypertensive emergencies (**Table 1**).

Parenteral preparations of anti-HTs are used for atleast the first 24 hours, post which shifts to oral anti-HTs can be considered.

ACUTE AORTIC DISSECTION

In this particular emergency, a rapid reduction in the blood pressure is required.
- Drug of choice—intravenous esmolol, a cardioselective β_1 adrenergic receptor blocker
- Dose—the loading dose is 500–1,000 µg/kg/min administered over 1 minute followed by a 50 µg/kg/min infusion rate. The maximum infusion rate is 200 µg.
- Target BP—SBP of <120 mm Hg

HYPERTENSIVE EMERGENCY WITH ACUTE PULMONARY EDEMA

- Drugs of choice—intravenous nitroglycerin (a vasodilator belonging to the class of nitrates), clevidipine (selective arteriolar vasodilator, a third generation dihydropyridine calcium channel blocker), or nitroprusside (a potent arterial and venodilator that decreases preload as well as afterload).
- Dose—initial infusion rate of intravenous nitroglycerin is 5 µg/min. The maximum infusion rate is 20 µg/min.

The initial infusion rate of intravenous sodium nitroprusside is 0.3–0.5 µg/kg/min. The maximum infusion rate is 10 µg/kg/min.

The initial infusion rate of intravenous clevidipine is 1–2 mg/h. The maximum infusion rate is 32 mg/h.

TABLE 1: Drugs in selected hypertensive emergencies.	
Emergencies	**Preferred drugs**
Hypertensive encephalopathy	Nitroprusside, nicardipine, and labetalol
Stroke	Nicardipine, labetalol, and nitroprusside
Myocardial infarction/unstable angina	Nitroglycerin, nicardipine, labetalol, and esmolol
Acute left ventricular failure	Nitroglycerin, enalaprilat, and loop diuretics
Aortic dissection	Nitroprusside, labetalol, and esmolol
Adrenergic crisis	Phentolamine and nitroprusside
Postoperative hypertension	Nitroglycerin, nitroprusside, labetalol, and nicardipine
Pre-eclampsia/eclampsia of pregnancy	Hydralazine, labetalol, and nicardipine

Target BP—20-25% reduction in the first hour and then gradually to 160/100 mm Hg within the next 2-6 hour, and then cautiously to normal over the next 24-48 hour.

HYPERTENSIVE EMERGENCY AND ACUTE RENAL FAILURE

- Drugs of choice—intravenous fenoldopam (dopamine receptor agonist), clevidipine, and nicardipine (second-generation dihydropyridine calcium channel blocker with high vascular selectivity and strong cerebral and systemic vasodilatory activity)
- Dose—the initial infusion rate of intravenous fenoldopam is 0.1-0.3 µg/kg/min. The maximum infusion rate is 1.6 µg/kg/min.

The initial infusion rate of intravenous nicardipine is 5 mg/h. The maximum infusion rate is 30 mg/h.

HYPERTENSIVE EMERGENCY CAUSED BY PHEOCHROMOCYTOMA OR A HYPERADRENERGIC STATE

Drugs responsible for this include cocaine, amphetamines, phencyclidine, or monoamine oxidase inhibitor. Abrupt cessation of clonidine or other sympatholytic drugs could also be the precipitating factor.

- Drugs of choice—intravenous clevidipine, nicardipine, or phentolamine (alpha-adrenergic antagonist).
- Dose—the initial dose of phentolamine is an intravenous bolus dose of 5 mg. Additional bolus doses of 5 mg should be administered intravenously every 10 minutes as needed to reduce the blood pressure to the target level.

HYPERTENSIVE EMERGENCY ASSOCIATED WITH A HIGH PLASMA RENIN STATE

- Drug of choice—intravenous enalaprilat (angiotensin converting enzyme inhibitor).
- Dose—the initial dose of enalaprilat administered intravenously is 1.25 mg over 5 minutes. Additional doses of intravenous enalaprilat may be given up to 5 mg every 6 hour as needed to reach the blood pressure target level.

CONCLUSION

Hypertensive emergency is an acute, life threatening manifestation of uncontrolled or hitherto undiagnosed hypertension associated with high mortality and morbidity. Easy availability of oral and parenteral formulations of anti-HTs has proven lifesaving in the crisis but as the old adage goes—prevention is better than cure, lifestyle interventions, and strict compliance to medications can to an extent help in preventing the occurrence of this catastrophe!

REFERENCES

1. Kearney PM, Whelton M, Reynolds K, Muntner P, Whelton PK, He J. Global burden of hypertension: analysis of worldwide data. Lancet. 2005;365(9455):217-23.
2. Gakidou E, Afshin A, Abajobir AA, Abate KH, Abbafati C, Abbas KM, et al. Global, regional, and national comparative risk assessment of 84 behavioural, environmental and occupational, and metabolic risks or clusters of risks, 1990-2016: A systematic analysis for the Global Burden of Disease study 2016. Lancet. 2017;390(10100):1345-422.
3. Institute for Health Metrics and Evaluation (IHME). (2017). GBD Compare Data Visualization.[online] Available from: https://vizhub.healthdata.org/gbd-compare/# (Last accessed August, 2021).
4. Gupta R, Gaur K, S Ram CV. Emerging trends in hypertension epidemiology in India. J Hum Hypertens. 2019;33(8):575-87.
5. Geldsetzer P, Manne-Goehler J, Theilmann M, Davies JI, Awasthi A, Vollmer S, et al. Diabetes and hypertension in India: A nationally representative study of 1.3 million adults. JAMA Intern Med. 2018;178:363-72.
6. Karnik ND, Padwal NJ. The Crisis in Hypertension. J Assoc Physicians India. 2017;65(6):11-3.
7. Volhard F, Fahr T. Die brightsche Nierenkrankheit: Klinik, Pathologie und Atlas. Berlin: Springer; 1914.
8. Varun MS, Gangaram U, Nagabushana MV, Siddappa HG, Soren B. Clinical study of hypertensive crisis at a tertiary care hospital of South India. Int J Adv Med. 2018;5(5):1168-71.
9. Kaplan NM, Victor RG, Flynn JT. Hypertensive emergencies. In: Kaplan NM, Victor RG (Eds). Kaplan's Clinical Hypertension, 11th Edition. Philadelphia: Lippincott Williams and Wilkins; 2015. pp. 263-75.
10. Jameson JL, Fauci AS, Kasper DL, Hauser SL, Longo DL, Loscalzo J. Harrison's Principles of Internal Medicine, 20th edition. New York, NY: McGraw-Hill; 2018.

14. Hyponatremia in the Intensive Care Unit: Step Wise Approach to Diagnosis and Management

Niwrutti Hase, Aniket Hase

INTRODUCTION
- Hyponatremia is defined as a serum or plasma sodium <135 mEq/L (normal serum sodium is 135-145 mEq/L).
- Hyponatremia is common electrolyte disorder seen in critical care settings.
- It occurs in 30-40% of intensive care unit (ICU) patients.
- Acute hyponatremia is defined as a fall in serum sodium over a period of <48 hours.
- Studies have shown hyponatremia patients had longer ICU stay, mechanical ventilation days, and higher mortality than patients having normal serum sodium level.
- Hyponatremia can present with life threatening neurological complications. This is medical emergency.
- Judicious and prompt treatment is indicated. Over correction can results in dreaded complication of osmotic demyelination (OSD) leading to worsening of neurological deficit.
- Osmotic demyelination can be prevented following certain rules of correction and relowering of plasma sodium by infusing hypotonic fluid and judicious use of desmopressin.
- Hyponatremia has multiple pathophysiological mechanisms which demands careful multistep diagnostic approach to determine the cause and appropriate treatment.
- Hyponatremia does not mean salt capsules and vaptans. Treatment has to be individualized according to underlying pathophysiologic mechanisms.
- Dysnatremias hyponatremias or hypernatremia's are water regulation disorders.
- In absence of renal failure if water intake exceeds the capacity of kidney to excrete the maximum water results in hyponatremia.
- Hyponatremia suggests there is excess of free water in body relative to sodium. Hypernatremia suggests loss of free water and there is free water deficit.
- Treatment of hypervolemic and euvolemic hyponatremia, we have got now new weapon—vaptans—demands judicious use.
- *Aim of this article:* A case based stepwise approach to diagnosis and treatment of hyponatremias in ICU settings.

A CASE
- 45-year-old male Mr B P (Referred to nephrology: To rule out uremia)
- Diagnosed to have tuberculosis pleural effusion
- Started on antituberculous treatment (ATT) 4 days back
- History of anorexia nausea, and vomiting
- Abnormal behavior
- Hiccups—intractable
- Imbalance while walking
- Decreased urine output

On Physical Examination
Patient conscious but not oriented. He was rowdy. His pulse was 100/min with BP: 100/70 mm Hg. There was jaundice no or on anemia or no edema feet or face. He had flaps (asterixis). No signs of dehydration. Liver spleen not palpable, and no focal neurological deficit. Plantar flexor. Other systems were unremarkable except right-sided pleural effusion.

Investigations
Hemoglobin (Hb): 13 g/dL, packed cell volume (PCV): 40.5, mean corpuscular volume (MCV): 90 fL, White blood cell (WBC): 9,800/mm^3, N68, L20, E04, M08. PLC: 3.4 L.

Urine albumin: Trace and no active sediments.

Blood urea nitrogen (BUN): 8.0 mg/dL, SCr: 0.7 mg/dL, Serum uric acid: 3.0 mg/dL. serum Na: 109 mEq/L, Potassium: 5.8 mEq/L, Cl: 89, HCO$_3$: 18 mEq/L.

Alanine transaminase/aspartate transaminase (ALT/AST): 17/32, serum proteins: T: 6.8, albumin: 4.2 g/dL.

Patient has symptomatic severe hyponatremia mild hyperkalemia. He is euvolemic and has normal renal functions. What are the steps in diagnosis and management?
- Investigations to be ordered
- Serum osmolality: 245 mOsm/kg
- Urine osmolality: 570 mOsm/kg
- Urinary sodium: 56 mmol/L
- Urinary potassium: 30 mmol/L

Step 1: Look at Osmolality
Sodium is the main extracellular cation. The main function of serum sodium is maintenance of extracellular osmolality. The measurement of serum osmolality is the first step in evaluation of hyponatremia. The normal serum osmolality is 285–295 mOsm/kg H$_2$O. Low serum osmolality suggests true hyponatremia. If osmolality is normal, it is isotonic or pseudohyponatremia which is caused by severe elevation of lipids or plasma proteins. This is detected only by flame photometer which measures the sodium concentration in whole plasma and assumes that the plasma water is 93%

of the plasma. Marked increase in lipids or proteins dilutes the serum sodium concentration and flame photometry gives falsely low sodium. Sodium concentration measured by ion selective electrode which measure the concentration in the aqueous portion of plasma gives more accurate reading, avoiding these pseudo-readings. Pseudohyponatremia does not require any treatment.

Hypertonic hyponatremia: Serum osmolality is higher than 295 mOsm/kg H_2O. The common causes are hyperglycemia and mannitol infusion. An increase in extracellular osmolality because of these osmotically active particles produces shift of water from intravascular compartment to extracellular fluid (ECF) which dilutes the sodium in plasma and causes low sodium. For every 100 mg/dL that the glucose is above 100 mg/dL, the sodium falls by 1.6 mEq/L.

Our patient has osmolality 245, low osmolality suggests it is true hyponatremia: Hypotonic hyponatremia

Step 2: *Get urinary osmolality done: Decide antidiuretic hormone (ADH)-dependent or ADH-independent hyponatremia.*
- *Urine osmolality <100:* Very dilute urine. There is no ADH in circulation. Hyponatremia is independent of ADH.
- *Causes:* Primary polydipsia, low solute intake (tea and toast diet,) and Beer potomania.
- *Urine osmolality >100:* This will suggest ADH-dependent hyponatremia.

Step 3: *Once, it is diagnosed as ADH-dependent true hyponatremia, step 3 will be assessment of the volume status.*
- Hypovolemia with hyponatremia
   - Renal losses (urinary sodium >20 mEq/L)
      - Diuretics
      - Salt losing nephropathy
      - Postobstructive diuresis
      - Diuretic phase of acute tubular necrosis
      - Osmotic diuretics
      - Mineralocorticoid deficiency
      - Renal tubular acidosis (RTA) bicarbonaturia and metabolic alkalosis
   - Extra renal losses (urinary sodium <20 mEq/L)
      - Diarrhea, vomiting, burns, and third spacing of fluids

Signs of hypovolemia: Decreased weight, tachycardia, postural hypotension, decreased skin turgor, dry mucous membranes, low jugular venous pressure, and slow capillary refill. Low central venous pressure (CVP), pulmonary capillary wedge, increased blood urea nitrogen (BUN): Creatinine ratio, hemoglobin, hematocrit, uric acid, and specific gravity on urinalysis.
- Hypervolemia with hyponatremia (hyponatremia with edema)
   - Total body water is increased as compare to sodium
   - Urine sodium >20 mEq/L: Acute/chronic renal failure
   - Urine sodium <20 mEq/L: Nephrotic syndrome, cardiac failure, and cirrhosis of liver

- Euvolemic hyponatremia (hyponatremia without edema or dehydration)
  - Urinary sodium 20-40 mEq/L: Give infusion of 0.9% saline over 24 hours if serum sodium increases by 5-6 mEq/L will suggest hypovolemia. If serum sodium decreases by 5 mEq/L suggests syndrome of inappropriate antidiuretic hormone secretion (SIADH) or reset osmostat.
  - Urinary sodium >40 mEq/L: Euvolemic hyponatremia
  - *Causes:* Glucocorticoid deficiency, hypothyroidism, physical and emotional stress, drugs, and SIADH.

Diagnostic criteria for SIADH: Up to 60% of all euvolemic hyponatremias are SIADH.

Essential criteria:
- Hyponatremia: Serum sodium <135 mEq/L
- Plasma osmolality <275 mOsm/kg H_2O
- Euvolemia
- Urinary osmolality >200 mOsm/kg H_2O
- Urinary sodium >20 mEq/L
- Normal renal, cardiac, hepatic, adrenal, pituitary, and thyroid function
- No history of antidiuretic drugs
- No emotional or physical stress
- Normal arterial blood gas (ABG) and potassium handling

Supplemental features:
- Uric acid < 4
- Blood urea nitrogen (BUN) <10
- Failure to correct hypoNa after NS infusion
- Correction of hypoNa after fluid restriction
- Fractional urea excretion >55%
- Fractional uric acid excretion >12%
- Increased serum ADH level

Once the diagnosis of SIADH is done next step will be to determine the cause (**Box 1**).

SYMPTOMS OF HYPONATREMIA

Symptoms of hyponatremia is due to osmotic shift of water from hypotonic ECF to relative hypertonic intracellular compartment (ICF) resulting cellular swelling (edema). Life threatening edema is brain edema responsible for neurologic symptoms and signs. Symptoms depend upon rapidity with which serum is reduced and level of serum sodium. Within 24-48 hours brain cell adapt to hyponatremia by lowering intracellular osmolality. Spectrum of symptoms can range from no symptoms to life threatening seizures coma due to uncal and cerebellar herniation (**Table 1**).

Analysis of case: Patient presented with nausea, vomiting, hiccup, altered sensorium had flaps, all symptoms and signs are attributed to hyponatremia. Hyponatremia with low osmolality suggests true hyponatremia. Urinary

> **Box 1: Causes of syndrome of inappropriate secretion of antidiuretic hormone (SIADH).**
>
> *Ectopic production of antidiuretic hormone (ADH) by neoplastic tumor:*
> - Lung carcinoma (small cell carcinoma)
> - Pancreatic carcinoma
> - Stomach carcinoma
> - Lymphoma
> - Thymoma
> - Duodenum carcinoma
> - Mesothelioma
> - Prostate cancer
> - Ewing's Sarcoma
>
> *Central nervous system (CNS) disorders:*
> - Stroke
> - Meningitis
> - Encephalitis
> - Head injury
> - Subdural hematoma
> - Brain tumor
> - Subarachnoid hemorrhage—cerebral salt wasting
> - Hydrocephalus
> - Guillain–Barré syndrome
> - Acute intermittent porphyria
> - CNS lupus
>
> *Pulmonary disorders:*
> - Pneumonias, lung abscesses, bronchiectasis, tuberculosis, and legionella
> - Cystic fibrosis
> - Acute asthma
>
> *Drugs:*
> - Tricyclic antidepressants
> - Selective serotonin reuptake inhibitors
> - Carbamazepine
> - Valproate
> - Oxycarbamazepine
> - Vincristine
> - Vinblastine
> - Cyclophosphamide
> - Ifosfamide
> - 3,4-methylenedioxymetha-mphetamine (MDMA) (ecstasy)
> - Antipsychotic drug
> - Ciprofloxacin
> - Oxytocin
> - Arginine vasopressin (AVP) analogs
> - Narcotics
> - Nicotine
> - Amiodarone
>
> *Miscellaneous:*
> - Human immunodeficiency virus-acquired immunodeficiency syndrome (HIV-AIDS)
> - Pain, stress, acute injury, postsurgery-nonosmotic-induced ADH may persist for 2–5 days
> - Idiopathic in elderly
> - Endurance exercise

osmolality 570 suggests ADH-dependent hyponatremia. Patient is euvolemic clinically. Urinary sodium 60, normal renal function suggests possibility of SIADH. As per criteria, thyroid-stimulating hormone (TSH) was normal. Serum cortisol was low. Adrenocorticotropic hormone (ACTH) was high suggesting primary adrenal insufficiency. Computed tomography (CT) abdomen showed adrenal calcification. Other findings suggested adrenal insufficiency are hypercalcemia and metabolic acidosis. Patient was treated with 3% saline as patient had neurological symptoms. Started on replacement doses of prednisolone.

TABLE 1: Signs and symptoms of hyponatremia.

Symptoms	Signs
• Loss appetite and anorexia • Nausea, vomiting, and hiccup • Weakness and lethargy • Muscle cramps • Agitation • Drowsiness • Disorientation • Ataxia • Convulsions and coma • Chronic hyponatremia may be associated with declining cognitive function • Fall and fractures in elderly	• Flapping tremors (asterixis) • Depressed/absent reflexes • Disorientation • Altered sensorium • Hypothermia • Respiratory depression • Cheyne–Stokes respiration • Seizures • Coma

MANAGEMENT OF HYPONATREMIA

Factors need to be considered while planning treatment of hyponatremia.
- The presence or absence of neurological symptoms
- Duration of hypo-osmolality acute < 48 hours or chronic > 48 hours
- The patients volume status: Hypovolemic, hypervolemic, or euvolemic
- The degree of hyponatremia
- Step wise approach in **Box 2**.

CONCLUSION

- Hyponatremia does not mean salt capsules and vaptans individualized therapy is required.
- Hyponatremia cannot be managed without doing serum osmolality, urine osmolality, urine sodium, urine potassium, and serum uric acid.
- Frequent monitoring of serum sodium is required to prevent rapid correction. Treatment should not be worse than disease.
- Keep strict intake of fluids, sodium, and urine output of water and sodium. If there is positive balance of water serum, sodium will be decreased or not increased as expected. Excessive negative balance may result in rapid correction.
- To increase serum sodium infusate, sodium should be greater than sum of urinary sodium and potassium.
- Keep watch on serum potassium. Serum sodium is equal to total body sodium plus total body potassium divided by total body water. Correction of hypokalemia will increase the serum sodium.
- Remember 1 g sodium is equal to 43 mEq of sodium. 1 g of salt gives 17 mEq of sodium.
- Various formulas used in correction are not substitute for frequent monitoring of serum sodium.

> **Box 2: Factors while planning treatment of hyponatremia.**
>
> - *Hyponatremia <125 mEq/L acute duration <48 h:*
>   Neurological symptoms convulsions coma, suspected cerebral herniation treat as emergency: Maintain airway, breathing, and circulation (ABC)
>   - About 3% hypertonic saline 150 mL IV or 1–2 mL/kg over 5–10 min should be administered as soon as possible. If the patient does not improve clinically after the first bolus, repeat a second bolus of hypertonic saline. It is important to stop all fluids after the second bolus to avoid raising the serum sodium any further
>   - Check serum sodium every 2 hourly follow rule of 6—correct by 6 mEq in 6 h and then 6 mEq a day
>   - If 3% saline is not available, use 60 cc of sodium bicarbonate
>   - Start evaluating volume status and determine the underlying cause of hyponatremia
> - *Hypovolemic hyponatremia*:
>   - The priority is to restore adequate circulating volume
>   - Use 0.9% saline or ringer lactate as fluid
>   - As volume depletion get corrected, ADH will get suppressed. Urine volume will increase and urine will be dilute if you do not replace volume there will be chances of rapid correction and OSD
>   - To prevent rapid correction, monitor urine out
>   - Insert foleys catheter if urine output >100 cc/h urine osmolality <100. Consider desmopressin and fluid restriction prevent rapid correction
> - *Hypervolemic hyponatremia*:
>   - Fluid restriction
>   - Salt restriction
>   - Diuretics
>   - Vaptans
> - *Euvolemic hyponatremia*:
>   - Find out the cause
>   - Treat the cause like hypothyroidism and adrenal insufficiency
> - *If SIADH*—Neurological symptoms treat with 3% saline 1 cc/kg/h with monitoring not increase >6 in 6 h than 6 mEq/day
>   - If patient is asymptomatic, restrict the fluid intake
>   - Restrict all the fluid not just water
>   - Aim the fluid restriction 500 mL/day below the 24 h urine out
>   - Encourage high salt and high protein diet
>   - Sum of urine concentration of sodium plus potassium is <1 restrict the water intake 500 mL/day less than urine output. If urine output is 1.5 L/day, restrict all fluids to 1 L/day
>   - If sum of urine concentration of sodium plus potassium is >1, patient may not respond to fluid restriction

Continued

Continued

- Other predictor of failure to fluid restriction will be high urinary osmolality >500, urine output <1500 mL/day. Increase in serum sodium <2 mEq/L/day after fluid restriction for 24–48 h.
- If no response to fluid restriction, other options are demeclocycline 300–600 mg twice per day or tolvaptan 15 mg/day orally. High protein diet oral urea may also help
- Tolvaptan binds to the V2 receptors in renal collecting tubules/ducts. It is vasopressin antagonist
  - Uses:
    - Euvolemic/hypervolemic hypo Na^+
    - Contraindicated in hypovolemia hyponatremia and acute hyponatremia or in patients with S. Na < 115 mmol/L
    - It produces slow aquaresis water diuresis
  - Adverse effects:
    - Thirst and dry mouth
    - Concomitant use of vaptan and potent, CYP3A4 inhibitors such as ketoconazole, itraconazole, clarithromycin, ritonavir, or indinavir are contraindicated
    - Treat the underlying cause of SIADH, if possible

(ADH: antidiuretic hormone; OSD: osmotic demyelination; SIADH: syndrome of inappropriate secretion of antidiuretic hormone)

RECOMMENDED READINGS

1. Palmer BF. Hyponatremia in the intensive care unit. Semin Nephrol. 2009;29(3): 257-70.
2. Saab G. Disorder of Water balance. In: Cheng S, Vijayan A (eds). Nephrology Subspeciality Consult, 3rd edition. Philadelphia: Wolter Kluwer; 2014. pp. 39-49.
3. Helman A. Tips to Assess Rapid Onset of Hyponatremia to Prevent Overcorrection and Diagnose Underlying Cause. ACEP Now. 2017;36(3).
4. Spasovski G, Vanholder R, Allolio B, Annane D, Ball S, Bichet D, et al. Clinical practice guideline on diagnosis and treatment of hyponatraemia. Nephrol Dial Transplant. 2014;29(Suppl 2):i1-i39.
5. Faubel S, Topf J. The Fluid, Electrolyte & Acid-Base Companion. San Diego, CA: Alert and Oriented Pub; 1999.

15 Importance of Influenza Vaccination in Adult Population

Leong Hoe Nam

INTRODUCTION

There is a heavy burden of influenza on world. Every year, an estimated 20-30% of the children and 5-10% of adults are infected. This leads to 3-5 million cases of severe diseases and 650,000 deaths. Yet, all these unnecessary morbidity and mortality may be preventable.

Influenza has caused global pandemics (**Table 1**).

It is with certainty that there will be yet another influenza pandemic. What is unknown is when and how many deaths it can cause. Like the recent H1N1 swine flu, it will appear unexpectedly from an unexpected country and host.

Vaccines have been developed to prevent influenza vaccine. First there was a monovalent vaccine directed against influenza A. Subsequently, there more strains were included and there are now up to four strains of influenza in each vaccine. Two from influenza A (H1N1 and H3N2 strains), and two from influenza B (Victoria and Yamagata strains). The change from 3 to 4 valent influenza vaccine occurred only recently, when the influenza B strain diverged to form the two distinct Victoria and Yamagata strains in the 1980s. Though both are influenza B, they do not offer cross protection, and are genetic and phylogenetically distinct. The previous three valent influenza vaccine provide the required cover for the annual vaccination. Epidemiological studies from North America, Europe, and Australia showed that World Health Organization (WHO) recommendations predicted the right circulating influenza B strain only half the time. This lowers the influenza vaccine overall efficacy.

TABLE 1: Flu pandemic.				
Year	1918	1957	1968	2009
Type of influenza	H1N1 Spanish flu	H2N2 Asian flu	H3N2 Hong Kong flu	H1N1 Swine flu
Deaths	50–100 million	2 million	1 million	200,000 million
Cause	Direct transmission from birds to humans	Genetic RNA reassortment between animal and human viruses can produce a new strain. This can occur when two different influenza viruses infect the same host		

Influenza seasons are unique to locations. Though north of the equator, New Delhi and Dhaka peak months of influenza transmission occurs in July to August. Knowledge of this allows more directed and timed vaccination strategies. Countries in the South East Asia, e.g., Malaysia, Singapore, and Indonesia have influenza transmission all year round. Bangkok and Vientiane have it in August to September each year.

The burden of influenza is greater in individuals with pre-existing chronic diseases. Diabetes mellitus, lung diseases, stroke, cancer, and heart diseases represent the five major noncommunicable diseases worldwide. They account for 63% of all deaths. When influenza infects individuals with pre-existing chronic diseases, the death rate rises.

Diabetes mellitus has a five times increased risk of hospitalization for influenza, 25× increased risk of pneumonia and 30-90× increased risk of death. The risk increases during a pandemic year. This results in excess 13-60 deaths per 10,000 in those aged 65 years and above

The risk of heart attack is five times more likely in the 3 days following the diagnosis of systematic respiratory infection. Most of these were non-ST elevation myocardial infarction. Risk of stroke is three times higher after an influenza infection. Case fatality in individuals with chronic obstructive airway diseases rises from 0.01% to 30% after an infection with influenza A.

Even if the individual survives the initial insult of the respiratory infection, individuals previously admitted to the intensive care for pneumonia have poorer quality of life as measured by mobility, self-care, daily activities of living, pain, and depression. An additional 10% die after the first month of hospitalization from other complications.

Vaccines have been proven to work effectively in the elderly and individuals with noncommunicable diseases. Case control studies demonstrate a 51% reduction in odds ratio of developing a myocardial infarction after influenza vaccination. In several postmyocardial infarction studies, influenza vaccination reduced subsequent cardiovascular events. The Thai study by Arintaya Phrommintikul et al. published in European Heart Journal in 2011 showed a reduction in a major cardiovascular event by 30% and cardiovascular death by 61% (**Fig. 1**).

In chronic obstructive pulmonary disease (COPD) patients, risk reduction of acute respiratory illness is greater in those with more severe diseases. With relative reduction in from unity to 0.4-0.25.

Vaccine efficacy has been shown in the community-dwelling elderly with risk reduction of 27% for hospitalization and 48% for death.

Amongst the adults, pregnant women are at higher risk of hospitalization and pneumonia from influenza. With vaccination of the pregnant mother at their second to third trimester, we see children born to vaccinated mothers have lower risk of acquiring influenza or influenza-related hospitalization for their first 6 months of life. This benefit is lost after 6 months.

The influenza vaccine is in general well tolerated with a small risk of transient fever, aches, and pains on the site of injection. Only contraindications are in individuals who are known to have allergies to the influenza vaccine

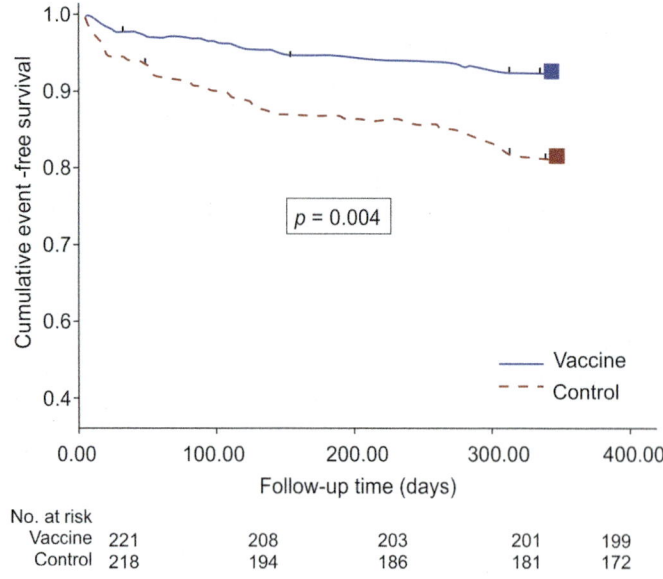

FIG. 1: Kaplan–Meier curves of event-free survival for major adverse cardiovascular events.

Source: Phrommintikul A, Kuanprasert S, Wongcharoen W, Kanjanavanit R, Chaiwarith R, Sukonthasarn A. Influenza vaccination reduces cardiovascular events in patients with acute coronary syndrome. Eur Heart J. 2011;32(14):1730-5.

or its compounds. Most influenza vaccines are made from eggs. Unless an individual has known anaphylactic reaction to egg, individuals with egg allergy may still receive the influenza vaccine safely. Individuals with a history of Guillain–Barré Syndrome (acute GBS) is not recommended to have the vaccine. There is a rare 1 in 1,000,000 chance of developing GBS with influenza vaccine. This is however, still much lower than the estimated 2 in 1,000,000 chance of acute GBS with acute wild type influenza infection.

Eventually, the doctor is the most important determinant in convincing the individual to receive the vaccine. The responsibility of getting the patient vaccinated falls on our hands as their physicians. Getting one vaccinated is saving one life.

REFERENCES

1. Grau AJ, Fischer B, Barth C, Ling P, Lichy C, Buggle F. Influenza vaccination is associated with a reduced risk of stroke. Stroke. 2005;36(7):1501-6.
2. Phrommintikul A, Kuanprasert S, Wongcharoen W, Kanjanavanit R, Chaiwarith R, Sukonthasarn A. Influenza vaccination reduces cardiovascular events in patients with acute coronary syndrome. Eur Heart J. 2011;32(14):1730-5.
3. McMillan M, Kralik D, Porritt K, Marshall HS. Influenza vaccination during pregnancy: a systematic review of effectiveness and safety. JBI Database of Systematic Reviews and Implementation Reports. 2014;12(6):251-381.

16
Interpreting the Link Between Hyperuricemia and Cardiometabolic Disorders and Management

Ayan Kumar Dey, Alan F Almeida

INTRODUCTION

Uric acid (UA), an end product of purine metabolism, has been an enigma to clinicians, epidemiologists, and research scientists alike. Inability of the human body to generate allantoin due to the unexpressed uricase gene means that UA is maintained at the theoretical limit of solubility in the serum (6.8 mg/dL).

Uric acid is known to have antioxidant activity suggesting that hyperuricemia might be the body's protective response to oxidative stress. Nevertheless, newer studies show an association of hyperuricemia with cardiometabolic disorders like hypertension, insulin resistance, metabolic syndrome (MetS), nonalcoholic fatty liver disease (NAFLD), renal failure, and all-cause mortality.

In an Indian population of diabetics and hypertensives, the overall prevalence of hyperuricemia was about 25% with higher prevalence in males (27.5%) as compared to females (22.3%). The growing burden of hyperuricemia parallels rising cardiometabolic disorders. Understanding this relationship has clinical implications in reducing UA levels in such disorders.

HYPERURICEMIA AND ITS CLINICAL IMPLICATION

Evolutionary researchers have long debated the need for mammals to have a repressed uricase gene. Studies looking for UA beyond just an inert weak organic acid, showed that UA was indeed a powerful antioxidant in the extracellular milieu, scavenging oxygen radicals, chelating transition metals to reduce, for instance, iron ion-mediated oxidation. It prevented lipid and protein peroxidation, protected low-density lipoprotein (LDL) from oxidation and inactivated cofactors necessary for nitric oxide (NO) synthase. Together, these were thought to have protective effects on aging, atherosclerosis, and cancer.

Paradoxically, in vitro and cellular studies have also shown UA to have pro-oxidant effects, based on its chemical microenvironment. It oxidizes already oxidized LDLs containing lipid peroxidation products which result in plaque formation and atherosclerosis. Urate can react directly with NO under aerobic conditions to generate unstable nitrosated products. Reduced

NO bioavailability has been associated with endothelial dysfunction, hypertension, and insulin resistance. UA can impair acetylcholine-induced forearm vasodilation, thereby diminishing vascular compliance. Adipogenic differentiation of precursor cells can generate reactive oxygen species in the environment of hyperuricemia which in turn leads to inflammation and insulin resistance in the obese.

Thus, there remains a complex relationship between hyperuricemia and its pro-oxidant versus antioxidant role in human physiology.

CAUSE OF HYPERURICEMIA AND ITS CLINICAL RELEVANCE

Hyperuricemia has two distinct pathophysiologies related to overproduction or under-excretion/increased reabsorption.

The kidney excretes up to 70% of UA with the rest being handled in the gastrointestinal tract. Humans predominantly reabsorb urate from proximal tubules. Urate transporter 1 (URAT1), the major organic anion transporter linked to reabsorption, has an increased expression in obesity and insulin resistance (in animal studies). Polymorphisms in URAT1 have shown association with hypertension and MetS. Genome wide association studies have established association of loci in urate transporter genes such as *SLC2A9, ABCG2,* and *GLUT9* with diabetes mellitus in an Indian population too.

Alternatively, hyperuricemia can result with increased oxidative stress that accompanies the activation of xanthine oxidoreductase (XOR) leading to higher conversion to xanthine oxidase (XO), increased levels of which are a rich source of oxygen radical species. This causes deleterious effects on vascular smooth muscles and alters neurohormonal responses. XOR can generate superoxides via NADH oxidase activity having direct action on endothelial function, hypertension, and heart failure (HF). Indian studies have shown a direct correlation between flow-mediated vasodilatation and hyperuricemia, suggesting significant endothelial dysfunction even with asymptomatic hyperuricemia.

Understanding these pathways has therapeutic implications. While increased reabsorption could be managed with uricosuric agents, XOR pathway-induced hyperuricemia could be treated with XO inhibitors. Whether this theoretical basis translates into clinically meaningful difference will be discussed further.

HYPERURICEMIA AND ITS RELATION TO CARDIOMETABOLIC DISORDERS

Cardiometabolic disorders represent a consortium of inter-related risk factors such as hypertension, elevated blood sugars, obesity, NAFLD, HF, and raised triglycerides. Whether its association with hyperuricemia is causative, coincidental, or merely a response to underlying oxidative stress is a fiercely debated topic.

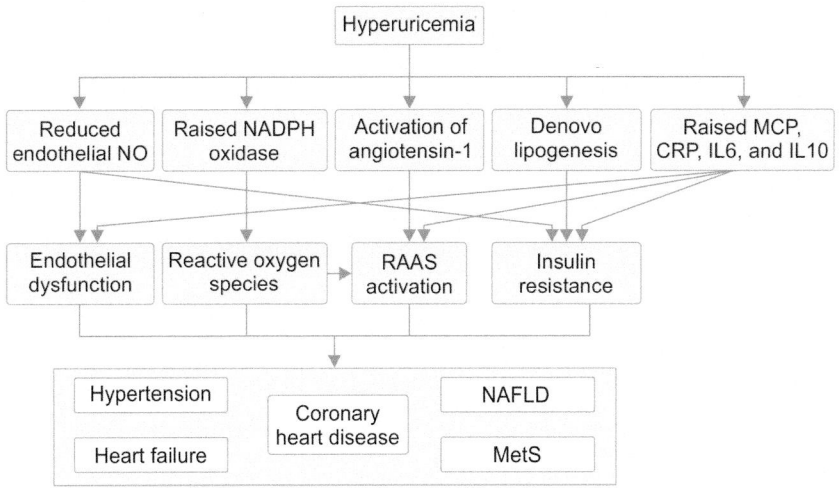

FIG.1: Hyperuricemia effects: Complex interplay.

(CRP: C-reactive protein; IL: interleukin; MCP: monocyte chemoattractant protein; MetS: metabolic syndrome; NAFLD: non-alcoholic fatty liver disease; NO: nitric oxide; RAAS: renin–angiotensin–aldosterone system)

Studies like PAMELA (Pressioni Arteriose Monitorate E Loro Associazioni) have shown causative effects of hyperuricemia with development of hypertension. Risk increases (1.29-fold for males and 1.57-fold for females) have been noted. This remains true for cardiovascular disorders (CVD) including subclinical atherosclerosis. Recent meta-analyses reported that for every 1 mg/dL increase in UA levels, the risk rose for incident hypertension by 13%, overall coronary heart disease by 20%, coronary artery calcification by 31%, and HF by up to 19%. Trials, like ERIKA, showed a direct correlation of hyperuricemia with cardiovascular and all-cause mortalities. Several longitudinal studies have found that hyperuricemia not only acts as a risk factor for HF incidence, but is also associated with severity of the disease and poorer prognosis.

Raised UA, historically a part of the MetS, was earlier thought to be a secondary effect of hyperinsulinemia causing lower renal excretion of UA by tubular reabsorption. However, recent epidemiologic studies have shown that it often precedes insulin resistance and that serum UA is an independent risk factor for the development of MetS. Studies like ROTTERDAM have shown significant associations with prediabetes, while prospective cohort studies demonstrated up to a 75% higher chance of developing diabetes mellitus with persistent hyperuricemia.

Chronic kidney disease (CKD) remains an important arm of the cardiometabolic disorder contributing to accelerated atherosclerosis, predisposing to malnutrition, and potentiating chronic inflammation. Hyperuricemia has been found to be an independent risk factor for renal dysfunction in the normal population and in patients with hypertension, diabetes, and CKD. Higher quartiles of UA conferred a 2.14-fold risk of developing endstage renal disease. UA levels also predicted estimated glomerular filtration rate (eGFR) decline. This remained true even for renal transplant recipients.

Large database studies like preventive cardiology information system (PreCIS) documented that each 1 mg/dL increment in UA levels correlated with up to 39% increase in the risk of death in patients with high risk of CVD. Concordance index analyses confirmed improved predictive accuracy of hyperuricemia in models that included Framingham Heart Study Score factors and MetS components.

These studies indicate a growing consensus of hyperuricemia contributing to cardiometabolic disorders. This leads us to the question: Will treating hyperuricemia improve these cardiometabolic disorders?

MANAGING HYPERURICEMIA

The various urate lowering therapies (ULT) are outlined in **Figure 2**.

XANTHINE OXIDASE INHIBITORS

Xanthine oxidase inhibitors (XOi), the cornerstone of management of hyperuricemia and gout; have shown beneficial effects on cardiovascular outcomes (CVO). In experimental models, allopurinol attenuated hypertension and reduced the risks of strokes and myocardial infarctions. Blood pressure (BP) and UA-independent effects on the vasculature were noted, including regression of left ventricular hypertrophy and improved endothelial function. Allopurinol use in MetS has shown improved proinflammatory endocrine imbalance with decreased macrophage infiltration in adipose tissues and decreased insulin resistance in animal studies.

Febuxostat has similarly shown beneficial effects on CVO with initial studies suggesting a role in retarding CKD progression. Topiroxostat, the

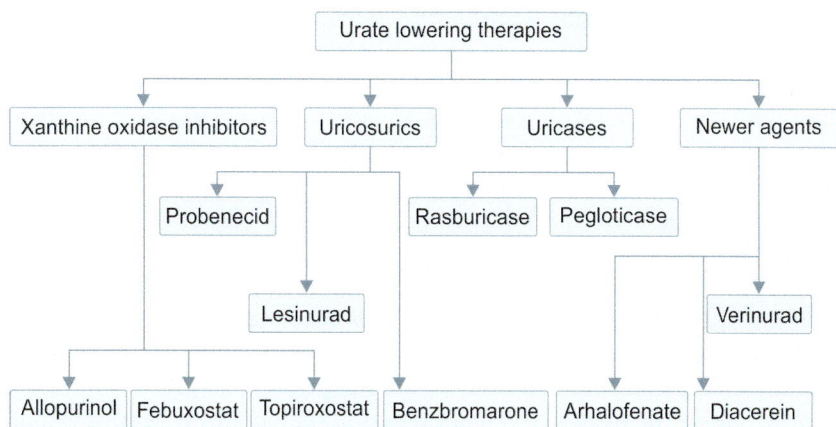

FIG 2: Urate lowering therapies.

TABLE 1: Xanthine oxidase inhibitors trials.

Medications	Favorable Trials	Negative Association Trials
Allopurinol	Agarwal et al. Journal of Clinical Hypertension. 2013: Allopurinol associated with small but significant drop in BP in hypertensive patients	CKD-FIX trial: NEJM 2020: no effect on eGFR decline with Allopurinol in CKD stage 3 or 4 and macroalbuminuria
	Liu et al. Clinical Endocrinology. 2015: Allopurinol treatment improved renal function in type 2 diabetics and asymptomatic hyperuricemia over 3 years	PERL study NEJM 2020: no evidence of clinically meaningful benefits of serum urate reduction with allopurinol on kidney outcomes among patients with type 1 diabetes and early-to-moderate diabetic kidney disease
	Takir et al. J Investig Med. 2015: Lowering Uric Acid With Allopurinol Improved Insulin Resistance and Systemic Inflammation in Asymptomatic Hyperuricemia	Kostka-Jeziorny et al. Blood Press. 2011: Allopurinol does not produce additional antihypertensive effects in patients with treated arterial hypertension
	Li et al. Br J Clin Pharmacol. 2011: Higher doses of allopurinol associated with better control of urate and lower risks of both cardiovascular events and mortality	EXACT HF study. Circulation. 2015: In high-risk HF patients with reduced ejection fraction and elevated uric acid levels, xanthine oxidase inhibition with allopurinol failed to improve clinical status, exercise capacity, quality of life, or left ventricular ejection fraction at 24 weeks
	Singh et al. BMC Cardiovasc Disord. 2017: Current allopurinol use protected against the occurrence of acute cardiovascular events in patients with gout and diabetes	
	Kasper et al. American Journal of Medicine. 2016: Allopurinol treatment is associated with a decreased cardiovascular risk among hyperuricemic patients	
	MacIsaac et al. Hypertension. 2016: Allopurinol use is associated with lower rates of stroke and cardiac events in older adults with hypertension, particularly at higher doses	

Continued

Continued

Medications	Favorable Trials	Negative Association Trials
Febuxostat	Ito et al. Intern Med. 2016: Renoprotective effect with Febuxostat, more in nondiabetics than diabetics. Retrospective observational study of 160 patients	FEATHER trial. Am J Kidney Dis. 2018: Compared to placebo, febuxostat did not mitigate the decline in kidney function among patients with stage 3 CKD and asymptomatic hyperuricemia
	FREED study: Febuxostat significantly decreased serum uric acid levels, and was associated with reduction of cerebral, cardiovascular, and renal events in patients aged 65 years or older	CARES study. N Engl J Med. 2018: In patients with gout and major cardiovascular coexisting conditions, febuxostat was noninferior to allopurinol with respect to rates of adverse cardiovascular events. All-cause mortality and cardiovascular mortality were higher with febuxostat than with allopurinol
	FAST trial. Lancet. 2020: Febuxostat was noninferior to allopurinol therapy with respect to the primary cardiovascular endpoint, and its long-term use was not associated with an increased risk of death or serious adverse events compared with allopurinol	
Topiroxostat	UPWARD study. Clin Exp Nephrol. 2018: Topiroxostat provides strict control of the serum uric acid level preventing decline of eGFR in patients with diabetic nephropathy, but no effect on proteinuria	TROFEO trial sub-analysis. Ann Thorac Cardiovasc Surg. 2020: Febuxostat had stronger renoprotective and antioxidant effects than topiroxostat in patients with hyperuricemia and CKD. Significantly higher uric acid levels with topiroxostat
	ETUDE study. Nephrology. 2018: Topiroxostat 160 mg daily-reduced albuminuria in 80 patients with diabetic nephropathy	

newest XOi, in the ETUDE and UPWARD trials, confirmed the positive impact on renal function in patients with overt diabetic nephropathy.

In **Table 1**, various trials and negative association trials are summarized.

However, there are trials which have failed to replicate this association like OPT-CHF which did not find clinical improvements with oxypurinol in moderate-to-severe systolic HF patients. Data from the EXACT-HF study showed no improvement in left ventricular ejection fraction (LVEF) with allopurinol in high-risk HF patients.

With regards to CKD progression, two seminal studies CKD-FIX (Controlled Trial of Slowing of Kidney Disease Progression from the Inhibition of Xanthine Oxidase) and PERL (Preventing Early Renal Loss in Diabetes trial) have conclusively proven that reducing hyperuricemia with allopurinol does not result in slowing the rate of CKD. It was postulated that circulating UA may not be playing a causal role in CKD progression. Trials like FEATHER have failed to show any effect of febuxostat on GFR decline. Moreover, CARES had suggested increased cardiovascular adverse outcomes and mortality with febuxostat, which was later refuted in a follow-up large prospective trial called FAST.

URICOSURICS

This class of drugs promotes UA excretion via inhibition of reabsorption by urate channels in the kidneys. Drugs like probenecid and benzbromarone were the prototype URAT1 inhibitors which showed some effect on CVO initially. However, due to significant drug interactions, safety profile issues and newer ULTs, these drugs are limited in their clinical use. Interesting to note is the renewed interest of probenecid as a positive inotropic and lusitropic agent with newer studies being conducted to see its benefit in HF.

LESINURAD

This novel uricosuric agent inhibits URAT1 and possibly OAT4, thereby augmenting its efficacy. Pivotal phase 3 trials like CLEAR 1 and 2 showed robust decreases in UA levels with lesinurad, albeit with significant renal dysfunction due to urate nephropathy. CRYSTAL trial showed lesinurad to have a good add-on effect to febuxostat in lowering UA levels in gout. Its use remains currently restricted as add-on therapy for hyperuricemia refractory to XOi. Its role in cardiometabolic disorders remains to be explored.

URICASES

Rasburicase and Pegloticase are extremely potent uricases which degrade UA into the more water soluble allantoin. These are generally third-line treatment options and restricted in their use to management of tumor lysis syndrome. Their role in mitigating long-term cardiometabolic outcomes will need logistical and financial obstacles to be overcome.

NEWER AGENTS

A growing understanding of urate transporters in the kidney has enabled potential targets for newer drugs. Uricosuric agents like arhalofenate, diacerein, tranilast, levotofisopam and verinurad are being evaluated in phase 2 trials. It will be interesting to see their long-term effects in cardiometabolic disorders.

CONCLUSION

There is a growing consensus that hyperuricemia may have causal association with cardiometabolic disorders. However, while numerous studies associate hyperuricemia with cardiometabolic disorders, few large-scale studies show conclusive evidence of lowering UA levels and hard-end-point outcomes.

Dietary adjustments and lifestyle modifications remain the cornerstone of holistic management of cardiometabolic disorders. Perhaps, ULT might be better as an add-on therapy to BP management, weight loss, better lipid profiles, and controlled sugars.

More long-term data on benefits of lowering UA on hard end-points in CVD such as death, myocardial infarction, and stroke is needed. Newer agents with targeted approaches might bring a fresher perspective and better understanding of this long-standing enigma.

SUGGESTED READINGS

1. Patel H, Shah D. Hyperuricemia prevalence in Indian subjects with underlying comorbidities of hypertension and/or type 2 diabetes: a retrospective study from subjects attending hyperuricemia screening camps. Int J Res Med Sci. 2020;8(3):794.
2. Borghi C, Domienik-Karłowicz J, Tykarski A, Widecka K, Filipiak K, Jaguszewski M, et al. Expert consensus for the diagnosis and treatment of patients with hyperuricemia and high cardiovascular risk: 2021 update. Cardiol J. 2021;28(1):1-14.
3. Benn CL, Dua P, Gurrell R, Loudon P, Pike A, Storer RI, et al. Physiology of Hyperuricemia and Urate-Lowering Treatments. Front Med. 2018;5:160.
4. Shukla V, Fatima J, Varshney AR, Joshi P, Kugashiya R. Study of Endothelial Dysfunction by Flow Mediated Vasodilation in Individuals with Asymptomatic Hyperuricemia. J Assoc Physicians India. 2021;69(2):39-42.
5. Johnson RJ, Bakris GL, Borghi C, Chonchol MB, Feldman D, Lanaspa MA, et al. Hyperuricemia, Acute and Chronic Kidney Disease, Hypertension, and Cardiovascular Disease: Report of a Scientific Workshop Organized by the National Kidney Foundation. Am J Kidney Dis. 2018;71(6):851-65.
6. Brucato A, Cianci F, Carnovale C. Management of hyperuricemia in asymptomatic patients: A critical appraisal. European J Int Med. 2020;74:8-17.
7. Doria A, Galecki AT, Spino C, Pop-Busui R, Cherney DZ, Lingvay I, et al. Serum Urate Lowering with Allopurinol and Kidney Function in Type 1 Diabetes. N Engl J Med. 2020;382(26):2493-503.
8. Badve SV, Pascoe EM, Tiku A, Boudville N, Brown FG, Cass A, et al. Effects of Allopurinol on the Progression of Chronic Kidney Disease. N Engl J Med. 2020;382(26):2504-13.
9. Chang CC, Wu CH, Liu LK, Chou RH, Kuo CS, Huang PH, et al. Association between serum uric acid and cardiovascular risk in nonhypertensive and nondiabetic individuals: The Taiwan I-Lan Longitudinal Aging Study. Sci Rep. 2018;8(1):5234.
10. Remedios C, Shah M, Bhasker AG, Lakdawala M. Hyperuricemia: a Reality in the Indian Obese. Obes Surg. 2012;22(6):945-8.

17. Masked Hypertension: How Worrisome?

SB Gupta

INTRODUCTION

Masked hypertension is an emerging clinical entity with increased cardiovascular risk, however, not so well documented and with under-recognized prevalence. Need to identify early to reduce cardiovascular morbidity and mortality is important.

With the advent of ambulatory blood pressure monitoring (ABPM) and concept of home blood pressure (BP) monitoring, beyond normal BP, and sustained hypertension. Two additional entities have been documented (**Fig. 1**):
1. White-coat hypertension (WCH)
2. Masked hypertension (MH)

White-coat hypertension is an entity where the office (clinic) BP is high and out-of-office (home) BP is normal and the reverse where out-of-office BP is high and office BP is normal is masked hypertension (MH).

By definition, masked hypertension is a condition where clinic or office BP is normal (<140/90 mm Hg), but out-of-office or home BP is elevated (ambulatory daytime BP or home BP > 130/85 mm Hg).

Home- or self-monitoring of BP (SBPM) is a convenient method to measure out-of-office BP, however, ABPM is the gold standard.

Further, HBPM (or SBPM) is taken during daytime and always in resting state, while ABPM gives the readings for the night-time also. And, there is

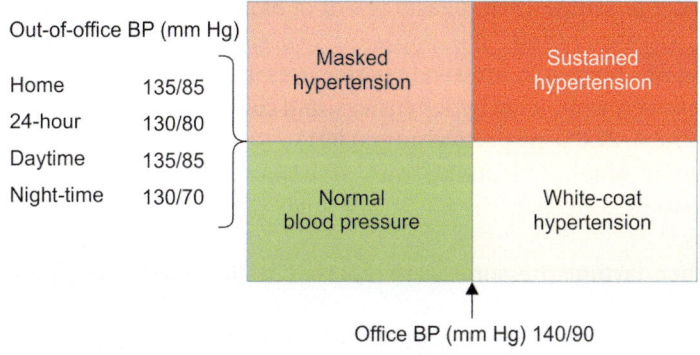

FIG. 1: Hypertension subsets.

growing evidence that an elevated night-time, BP may be the better predictor of risk.[1,2]

Primary objective is to identify patients in the population who are not receiving treatment and are having masked hypertension and also the patients who are being treated for hypertension, but not adequately, masked uncontrolled hypertension (MUCH).

Prevalence

The Ohasama study reported the prevalence of MH as 10.4%.[3] The PAMELA (Pressioni Arteriose Monitorate E Loro Associazioni) study found MH in 9% of their subjects.[4] Salenta et al. reported 23% MH in their normal volunteers.[5] Differences could be attributed to different cut-off values for the BP.

The 11-country IDACO (International Database on Ambulatory Blood Pressure in Relation to Cardiovascular Outcomes) on 1,168 untreated patients of middle age and elderly patients with mean age of 64 years having isolated systolic hypertension, using daytime ABPM reported 314 (26.9%) had sustained hypertension, 334 (28.5%) had WCH and 520 (44.5%) had MH.[6] In another 11-country, IDACO report showed the prevalence of MH in untreated nondiabetic patients as 18.8% and in the treated nondiabetic patients as 30.5%. In contrast, the prevalence of MH in untreated diabetic patients and treated diabetic patients was 29.3% and 42.5%, respectively.[7]

Masked hypertension has also been reported in children. Lurbe et al. reported 45 children (7.6%) having MH in a cohort of 592 children with mean age 10.2 years.[8] In another study of 85 children, 9.4% children had MH. Children having MH had significantly higher left ventricular mass as compared to normotensive children.[9]

CAUSES

Certain factors may selectively lead to higher ambulatory BP, especially lifestyle factors like smoking, alcohol, physical activity, and stress.

Liu et al. found a nonsignificant higher tendency of smokers in masked hypertensives (23% vs. 16%).[10] The Second Australian National Blood Pressure Study[11] also showed that masked hypertension was more in smokers. The SHEAF (Self measurement of blood pressure at Home in the Elderly, Assessment and Follow-up) study,[12] in elderly hypertensives reported smoking was highest in masked hypertensives as compared to uncontrolled hypertensives, white-coat hypertensives, and controlled hypertensives (35%, 34.4%, 23.6%, 27.6%, respectively; $p < 0.001$).

Regular alcohol drinking was associated with masked morning hypertension as detected by SBPM in a study of one Japanese hypertensive patients.[13]

Higher daytime pressures were reported in the subjects who were more physically active.[14]

Further, SHEAF study reported that masked hypertensives was more common in males and in patients who have diabetes or with history of stroke or coronary artery disease.[15]

Shortened sleep time, obstructive sleep apnea, and sedentary obese individuals predispose to masked hypertension.

PROGRESSION

Masked hypertension is thought to be a precursor of sustained hypertension. 5-year Quebec population study with baseline MH, one-third progressed to sustained hypertension, one-third regressed to normotension, and one-third remained masked hypertension.[16]

Masked Hypertension and Target Organ Damage

Higher left ventricular mass, more carotid atherosclerosis were reported masked hypertensives as compared to true normotensives and were almost same as in true hypertensives. The left ventricular mass index (LVMI) was 73 g/m^2, 86 g/m^2, and 90 g/m^2 in true normotensives, masked hypertensives, and true hypertensives, respectively. 15% of true hypertensives and 28% of both masked and true hypertensives showed carotid plaques.[10] The PAMELA study[4] also reported higher LVMI in masked hypertensives (91 g/m^2) as compared to true normotensives (79 g/m^2) and almost similar to true hypertensives (94 g/m^2). Higher carotid intima-media thickness (IMT) and higher pulse wave velocity were reported in masked hypertensives than in normotensive subjects in a Japanese study.[17]

Cardiovascular mortality and stroke morbidity were higher in both masked and sustained hypertensives as compared to normotensive subjects, as reported by Ohkubo et al. in the Ohasama study.[18] Björklund et al. also reported in 578 untreated 70-year old men that isolated ambulatory MH are a predictor of cardiovascular morbidity.[19] Higher prevalence of cardiovascular and all-cause mortality were reported in subjects with masked hypertension in comparison to subjects with normal office and 24-h BP in the PAMELA study by Mancia et al.[20]

Masked Uncontrolled Hypertension

Masked hypertension in treated patients is entirely different. Here, clinic readings give us a false impression that BP is adequately under control, however, this is not the case as home BP is higher. It is important to know the prevalence of MUCH and its impact on prognosis.

The SHEAF study[12] reported the prevalence of MUCH as 9.4%, while the J-HOME study[21] reported 19%. Pierdomenico et al. reported masked hypertension (daytime pressure <135/85 mm Hg) in one-third patients in whom clinic pressure was under control (<140/90 mm Hg).[22]

In the SHEAF study,[12] the hazard ratio (HR) was 2.06 for cardiovascular events in patients with MUCH as compared to patients whose BP was well controlled both at clinic and at home. Pierdomenico et al. reported the higher event rates of fatal and nonfatal cardiovascular events in MUCH group in comparison to patients with controlled hypertension, 100 patient-years as 2.42 in MUCH group and 0.87 in controlled hypertension group.[22]

The Ohasama study[18] also reported increased HR for cardiovascular disease mortality/stroke morbidity in treated MH patients.

Treatment of Masked Hypertension and Regression of Target Organ Damage

A prospective study of 80 nondiabetic hypertensive patients on antihypertensive treatment and achieved BP control both in clinic and on ABPM with mean follow-up of 30 months, showed regression in LVMI (117 ± 23 g/m^2 at baseline, 95 ± 22 g/m^2 at follow-up, $p < 0.01$), prevalence of LVH with concentric remodeling (46% at baseline, 34.4% at follow-up, $p =$ NS), or microalbuminuria (3.9% at baseline, 3.9% at follow-up, $p < 0.05$).[23]

CONCLUSION

It is quite clear that MH is worrisome and should be taken seriously and always to be kept in mind for investigation. There are substantial number of people in general population who are undiagnosed and, hence, not treated and are the candidates for increased cardiovascular risk, needs to be recognized and treated adequately. Further in the treated group also, we shall identify MUCH and offer to control their BP in out-of-office settings.

Home- or self-monitoring of BP is the most convenient and cost-effective method to identify and for follow-up purposes and ABPM may be used initially to firmly diagnose the condition and later, if required in doubtful cases.

Patients whose BP at clinic in high-normal range, smokers, and/or with risk factors like diabetes or chronic kidney disease shall always in close watch.

REFERENCES

1. Kikuya M, Ohkubo T, Asayama K, Metoki H, Obara T, Saito S, et al. Ambulatory blood pressure and 10-year risk of cardiovascular and noncardiovascular mortality: the Ohasama study. Hypertension. 2005;45(2):240-5.
2. Hoshide S, Ishikawa J, Eguchi K, Ojima T, Shimada K, Kario K. Masked nocturnal hypertension and target organ damage in hypertensives with well controlled self-measured home blood pressure. Hypertens Res. 2007;30(2):143-9.
3. Imai Y, Tsuji I, Nagai K, Sakuma M, Ohkubo T, Watanabe N, et al. Ambulatory blood pressure monitoring in evaluating the prevalence of hypertension in adults in Ohasama, a rural Japanese community. Hypertens Res. 1996;19(3):207-12.
4. Sega R, Trocino G, Lanzarotti A, Carugo S, Cesana G, Schiavina R, et al. Alterations of cardiac structure in patients with isolated office, ambulatory, or home hypertension: data from the general population (Pressione Arteriose Monitorate e Loro Associazioni (PAMELA) Study). Circulation. 2001;104(12):1385-92.
5. Selenta C, Hogan BE, Linden W. How often do office blood pressure measurements fail to identify true hypertension? An exploration of white-coat normotension. Arch Fam Med. 2000;9:533-40.
6. Franklin SS, Thijs L, Hansen TW, Li Y, Boggia J, Kikuya M, et al. Significance of white-coat hypertension in older persons with isolated systolic hypertension: a meta-analysis using the International Database on Ambulatory Blood Pressure in Relation to Cardiovascular Outcomes population. Hypertension. 2012;59(3):564-71.
7. Franklin SS, Thijs L, Li Y, Hansen TW, Boggia J, Liu Y, et al. Masked hypertension in diabetes mellitus: treatment implications for clinical practice. Hypertension. 2013;61(5):964-71.

8. Lurbe E, Torro I, Alvarez V, Nawrot T, Paya R, Redon J, et al. Prevalence, persistence, and clinical significance of masked hypertension in youth. Hypertension. 2005;45(4):493-8.
9. Stabouli S, Kotsis V, Toumanidis S, Papamichael C, Constantopoulos A, Zakopoulos N. White-coat and masked hypertension in children: association with target-organ damage. Pediatr Nephrol. 2005;20(8):1151-5.
10. Liu JE, Roman MJ, Pini R, Schwartz JE, Pickering TG, Devereux RB. Cardiac and arterial target organ damage in adults with elevated ambulatory and normal office blood pressure. Ann Intern Med. 1999;131(8):564-72.
11. Wing LM, Brown MA, Berlin LJ, Ryan P, Reid CM; ANBP2 Management Committee and Investigators. 'Reverse white-coat hypertension' in older hypertensives. J Hypertens. 2002;20(4):639-44.
12. Bobrie G, Chatellier G, Genes N, Clerson P, Vaur L, Vaisse B, et al. Cardiovascular prognosis of "masked hypertension" detected by blood pressure self-measurement in elderly treated hypertensive patients. JAMA. 2004;291(11):1342-9.
13. Ishikawa J, Kario K, Eguchi K, Morinari M, Hoshide S, Ishikawa S, et al. Regular alcohol drinking is a determinant of masked morning hypertension detected by home blood pressure monitoring in medicated hypertensive patients with well controlled clinic blood pressure: the Jichi Morning Hypertension Research (J-MORE) study. Hypertens Res. 2006;29(9):679-86.
14. Leary AC, Donnan PT, MacDonald TM, Murphy MB. The influence of physical activity on the variability of ambulatory blood pressure. Am J Hypertens. 2000;13(10):1067-73.
15. Bobrie G, Genes N, Vaur L, Clerson P, Vaisse B, Mallion JM, et al. Is "isolated home" hypertension as opposed to "isolated office" hypertension a sign of greater cardiovascular risk? Arch Intern Med. 2001;161(18):2205-11.
16. Trudel X, Milot A, Brisson C. Persistence and progression of masked hypertension: a 5-year prospective study. Int J Hypertens. 2013;2013:836387.
17. Matsui Y, Eguchi K, Ishikawa J, Hoshide S, Shimada K, Kario K. Subclinical arterial damage in untreated masked hypertensive subjects detected by home blood pressure measurement. Am J Hypertens. 2007;20(4):385-91.
18. Ohkubo T, Kikuya M, Metoki H, Asayama K, Obara T, Hashimoto J, et al. Prognosis of "masked" hypertension and "white-coat" hypertension detected by 24-h ambulatory blood pressure monitoring 10-year follow-up from the Ohasama study. J Am Coll Cardiol. 2005;46(3):508-15.
19. Björklund K, Lind L, Zethelius B, Andrén B, Lithell H. Isolated ambulatory hypertension predicts cardiovascular morbidity in elderly men. Circulation. 2003;107(9):1297-302.
20. Mancia G, Facchetti R, Bombelli M, Grassi G, Sega R. Long-term risk of mortality associated with selective and combined elevation in office, home, and ambulatory blood pressure. Hypertension. 2006;47:846-53.
21. Obara T, Ohkubo T, Kikuya M, Asayama K, Metoki H, Inoue R, et al. Prevalence of masked uncontrolled and treated white-coat hypertension defined according to the average of morning and evening home blood pressure value: from the Japan Home versus Office Measurement Evaluation Study. Blood Press Monit. 2005;10(6):311-6.
22. Pierdomenico SD, Lapenna D, Bucci A, Di Tommaso R, Di Mascio R, Manente BM, et al. Cardiovascular outcome in treated hypertensive patients with responder, masked, false resistant, and true resistant hypertension. Am J Hypertens. 2005;18(11):1422-8.
23. Cuspidi C, Meani S, Fusi V, Valerio C, Catini E, Magrini F, et al. Isolated ambulatory hypertension and changes in target organ damage in treated hypertensive patients. J Hum Hypertens. 2005;19(6):471-7.

18. Myelodysplastic Syndrome: What a Physician Should Know?

Dipanjan Haldar

INTRODUCTION

Myelodysplastic syndrome (MDS) encompasses of a heterogeneous group of clonal disorders characterized by ineffective erythropoiesis and bone marrow failure. The manifestations in MDS are quite varied and may range from mild anemia to life threatening pancytopenia and risk of transformation to acute myeloid leukemia (AML).

In this mini review, the clinical presentation, investigations to confirm the diagnosis, risk stratification, and approach to treatment are discussed.

CASE

- 84-year-old male-presented with new-onset decreased exercise tolerance, fatigue, and dizziness of 2 months duration. Physical examination did not show any hepatosplenomegaly.
- His complete blood count showed hemoglobin of 5.1 g/dL, white blood cell count of $3.5 \times 10^3/\mu L$, and Plt 110,000/µL. The mean corpuscular volume was 127 fL. Differential count showed 55% neutrophils, 32% lymphocytes, 12% monocytes, and 1% eosinophil.
- After ruling out nutritional deficiencies, bone marrow aspiration and biopsy was done which showed significant dyserythropoiesis, no ring sideroblasts, blast count of 3%, and loss of chromosome-Y on karyotyping.
- He was diagnosed as MDS—single lineage dysplasia, revised International Prognostic Scoring System (IPSS-R) low risk and started on injection darbepoetin 500 µ every 3 weeks.
- He became transfusion independent in a month and is asymptomatic at 1 year follow-up.

Approach to Diagnosis[1]

The approach to such a patient starts with exclusion of other common causes of anemia such as nutritional deficiencies, blood loss, and hemolysis. A careful examination of blood smear is mandatory to look for any atypical cells/blasts and evidence of dysplasia. For any unexplained cytopenias involving single or multiple lineages, a bone marrow aspiration and biopsy is recommended along with immunophenotyping, karyotyping as well as fluorescence in situ hybridization (FISH) studies to rule out MDS. A genetic mutation analysis is recommended for all cases specially the ones with equivocal dysplasia on morphology to look for any underlying genetic markers of MDS as some of this genetic markers have prognostic impact as well as specific-targeted therapy. The approach to diagnosis of MDS is summarized in **Figure 1**.

Clinical Features of Myelodysplastic Syndrome

The patients of MDS can have nonspecific presentation. Many patients are asymptomatic and diagnosis is made on finding abnormalities found on routine blood counts (e.g., anemia, neutropenia, and thrombocytopenia). Alternatively, patients can have symptoms or complications resulting from cytopenias (e.g., infection, fatigue, bleeding, and easy bruising).

Patients can present with unexplained anemia which is the most common cytopenia as fatigue, weakness, exercise intolerance, angina, and dizziness. Recurrent infections—bacterial infections, skin infections, fungal, viral, or mycobacterial infection secondary to severe neutropenia can be one of the first manifestations. Patients with severe thrombocytopenia can have recurrent petechiae and/or purpura.

Autoimmune abnormalities such as rheumatoid arthritis, pernicious anemia, psoriasis, and polymyalgia rheumatica can be rare manifestations of MDS.

Classification and Diagnostic Criteria of Myelodysplastic Syndrome[2]

Various classification systems have been proposed for MDS-French American British (FAB) classification, World Health Organization (WHO) 2008 and WHO 2016 classification. Essentially, they are based on number of lineages affected by dysplasia, blast percentage, presence or absence of ringed sideroblasts, presence of 5q deletion abnormality as a defining feature or presence of any other defining clonal cytogenetic abnormalities. The 2008 and 2016 classification of MDS are summarized in **Table 1**.

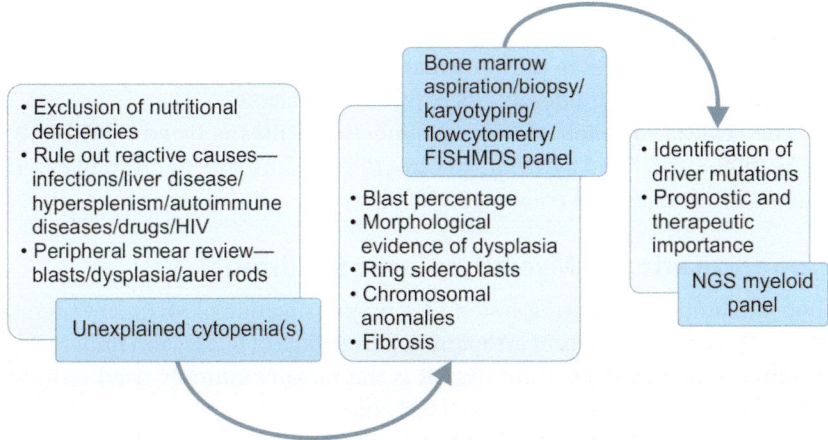

(FISH: fluorescence in situ hybridization; HIV: human immunodeficiency virus; NGS: next-generation sequencing)

FIG. 1: Approach to diagnosis of myelodysplastic syndrome (MDS).

TABLE 1: World Health Organization (WHO) 2008 and WHO 2016 classification of myelodysplastic syndrome (MDS).

2008 WHO classification	2016 WHO classification
Refractory cytopenia with unilineage dysplasia (RCUD) encompassing refractory anemia (RA), refractory neutropenia (RN), and refractory thrombocytopenia (RT)	MDS with single lineage dysplasia (MDS-SLD)
Refractory cytopenia with multilineage dysplasia (RCMD)	MDS with multilineage dysplasia (MDS-MLD)
Refractory anemia with ringed sideroblasts (RARS)	MDS with ring sideroblasts (MDS-RS)
	MDS-RS with single lineage dysplasia (MDS-RS-SLD)
	MDS-RS with multilineage dysplasia (MDS-RS-MLD)
Myelodysplastic syndrome associated with isolated del(5q)	MDS with isolated del(5q)
	MDS with excess blasts (MDS-EB)
Refractory anemia with excess blasts-1 (RAEB-1)	MDS-EB-1
Refractory anemia with excess blasts-2 (RAEB-2)	MDS-EB-2
Myelodysplastic syndrome, unclassified (MDS-U)	MDS, unclassifiable (MDS-U)
	With 1% blood blasts
	With single lineage dysplasia and pancytopenia
	Based on defining cytogenetic abnormality
Refractory cytopenia of childhood	Refractory cytopenia of childhood

The present WHO 2016 classification scheme is based on three factors:
1. Number of cytopenias in the peripheral blood
2. Dysplastic changes in the bone marrow
3. Percentage of ring sideroblasts in the bone marrow

The criteria for each of these diagnostic entities is listed in **Table 2**. Cytopenias are defined as: Hemoglobin <10 g/dL; absolute neutrophil count <1800/mm^3 and platelet count <100,000/mm^3.

Prognostication of Myelodysplastic Syndrome[3]

There are number of scoring systems for prognostication of MDS. In general, they are based on severity of cytopenias, percentage of blasts, and underlying chromosomal anomalies. The IPSS-R is the most commonly used scoring system for MDS. This is summarized in **Table 3**.

The prognosis is remarkably different across risk groups with survival in the very low risk group extending beyond 8 years where as the very high risk group, survival ranges to only few months (**Table 4**).

TABLE 2: Diagnostic criteria for myelodysplastic syndrome (MDS) World Health Organization (WHO) 2016 classification based on peripheral blood and bone marrow findings.

Subtype	Blood	Bone marrow
MDS with single lineage dysplasia (MDS-SLD)	Single or bicytopenia	Dysplasia in ≥10% of one cell line and <5% blasts
MDS with ring sideroblasts (MDS-RS)	Anemia, no blasts	≥15% of erythroid precursors with ring sideroblasts, or ≥5% of ring sideroblasts, and <5% blasts
MDS with multilineage dysplasia (MDS-MLD)	Cytopenia(s), <1 × 10^9/L monocytes	Dysplasia in ≥10% of cells in ≥2 hematopoietic lineages, ±15% ring sideroblasts, and <5% blasts
MDS with excess blasts-1 (MDS-EB-1)	Cytopenia(s), ≤2–4% blasts, <1 × 10^9/L monocytes	Unilineage or multilineage dysplasia, 5–9% blasts, and no auer rods
MDS with excess blasts-2 (MDS-EB-2)	Cytopenia(s), 5–19% blasts, <1 × 10^9/L monocytes	Unilineage or multilineage dysplasia, 10–19% blasts, ±auer rods
MDS with isolated del(5q)	Anemia, platelets normal or increased	Unilineage erythroid dysplasia, isolated del(5q), and <5% blasts
MDS, unclassifiable (MDS-U)	Cytopenia(s), +1% blasts on at least two occasions	Unilineage dysplasia or no dysplasia but characteristic MDS cytogenetics, <5% blasts
Refractory cytopenia of childhood	Cytopenias and <2% blasts	Dysplasia in 1–3 lineages and <5% blasts

TABLE 3: The Revised International Prognostic Scoring System (IPSS-R).

Prognostic variable	Scores						
	0	0.5	1.0	1.5	2.0	3.0	4.0
Cytogenetics#	Very good		Good		Intermediate	Poor	Very poor
Bone marrow blast (%)	≤2		>2 to <5		5–10	>10	
Hb (g/dL)	≥10		8 to <10		<8		
Platelets (cells/μL)	≥100	50 to 100	<50				
Absolute neutrophil count (cell/μL)	≥0.8	<0.8					

Approach to Treatment[4]

Since, MDS is such a heterogeneous group of disorder with such a wide range in clinical severity as well as prognosis, the treatment approach to MDS depends on multiple factors such as—age of the patient, risk stratification of MDS, cellularity of bone marrow, presence of 5q deletion abnormality,

TABLE 4: Revised International Prognostic Scoring System (IPSS-R) impact on survival in myelodysplastic syndrome (MDS).

Risk group	IPSS-R Score	Median survival (years)
Very low	≤1.5	8.8
Low	>1.5 to 3.0	5.3
Intermediate	>3 to 4.5	3.0
High	>4.5 to 6	1.6
Very high	>6	0.8

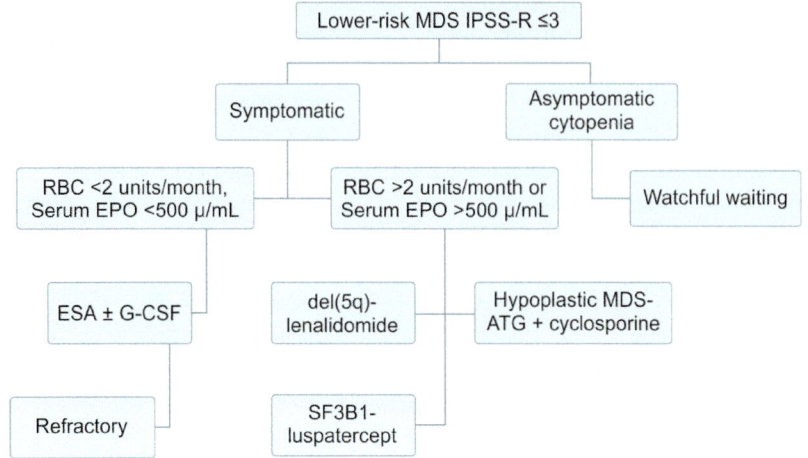

(ATG: antithymocyte globulin; EPO: erythropoietin; ESA: erythropoietin stimulating agents; G-CSF: granulocyte colony stimulating factor; IPSS-R: revised-International Prognostic Scoring System; MDS: myelodysplastic syndrome)

FLOWCHART 1: Treatment scheme for low-risk MDS.

presence of SF3B1 mutation as well as availability of prospective donor for allogenic transplant.

Asymptomatic patients with low-risk MDS are followed by watchful waiting. Erythropoietin stimulating agents (ESAs) with or without granulocyte-colony stimulating factor (G-CSF), lenalidomide for 5q deletion patients, antithymocyte globulin (ATG) plus cyclosporine therapy are all therapeutic options for low-risk MDS patients. Luspatercept is a recently approved molecule that works by binding transforming growth factor-β in MDS with ringed sideroblasts.[5]

Therapeutic option for high-risk MDS patient generally depends on whether the patient is eligible for bone marrow transplant based on age and performance status. Allogenic bone marrow transplant like is the only curative option for high-risk MDS patients and should be pursued in all young and fit patients, if they have suitable donor. On the other hand, patients without suitable donor or patients unfit for allogenic hematopoietic stem cell transplantation (HSCT) are generally treated with hypomethylating agents like azacitidine. The treatment approach to low and high-risk MDS is shown in **Flowcharts 1** and **2**, respectively.

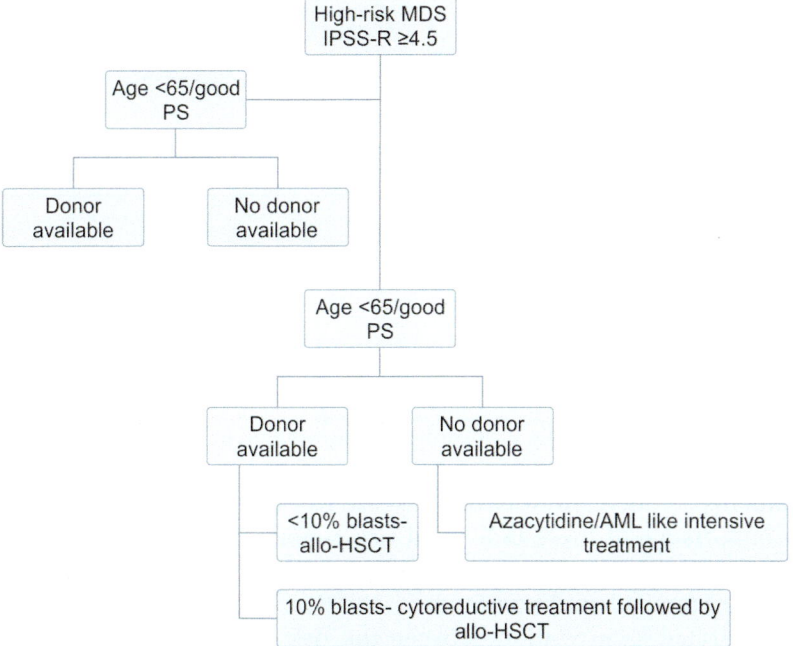

(Allo-HSCT: allogeneic hematopoietic stem cell transplant; AML: acute myeloid leukemia; MDS: myelodysplastic syndrome; PS: performance status)

FLOWCHART 2: Treatment scheme for high-risk MDS.

REFERENCES

1. Hamid GA, Al-Nehmi AW, Shukry SA. (2019). Diagnosis and classification of myelodysplastic syndrome. [online] Available from: https://www.intechopen.com/chapters/64871 (Last accessed August, 2021).
2. Barbui T, Thiele J, Gisslinger H, Kvasnicka HM, Vannucchi AM, Guglielmelli P, et al. The 2016 WHO classification and diagnostic criteria for myeloproliferative neoplasms: document summary and in-depth discussion. Blood Cancer J. 2018;8(15).
3. Greenberg PL, Tuechler H, Schanz J, Sanz G, Garcia-Manero G, Solé F, et al. Revised international prognostic scoring system for myelodysplastic syndromes. Blood. 2012;120(12):2454-65.
4. Hellström-Lindberg E, Tobiasson M, Greenberg P. Myelodysplastic syndromes: moving towards personalized management. Haematologica. 2020;105(7): 1765-79.
5. Markham A. Luspatercept: First Approval. Drugs. 2020;80(1):85-90.

19. Approach to Metabolic Syndrome

L Sreenivasamurthy

INTRODUCTION

The concept of a metabolic syndrome was introduced in the 1920s.[1] Between 1950 and 1975, many of the individual risk factors for later development of atherosclerotic cardiovascular disease (ACVD) were identified,[1] and the importance of these individual risk factors to predict multivariate CVD risk in patients without overt CVD was further substantiated by data from the Framingham Heart Study.[2,3] The Framingham Heart Study also demonstrated a correlation between the risk of CVD and the number risk factors[3] such as obesity, type 2 diabetes mellitus (T2DM), arterial hypertension, and hyperlipidemia. These conditions were often found to cluster together.[4] Later work highlighted the important role of central obesity and hyperinsulinemia,[5,6] and in 1988, Reaven et al. proposed the existence of an insulin resistance syndrome, later renamed metabolic syndrome which recognized insulin resistance as an underlying mechanism for the development of CVD risk factors such as dyslipidemia, T2DM, and arterial hypertension.[7] In addition to overt T2DM and CVD, many other morbid outcomes of the metabolic syndrome have been reported including liver diseases, i.e., nonalcoholic fatty liver disease (NAFLD) and nonalcoholic steatohepatitis,[8,9] malignancies,[10] polycystic ovarian syndrome,[11] sleep apnea,[12] and gall bladder disease.[13] Of great concern is that its prevalence is increasing among children and young adults,[14] particularly in women, in whom it has been associated with increased risk for gestational diabetes, gestational hypertension, and sexual dysfunction.

DEFINITION

In 2005, a harmonization of the definition was published by the International Diabetes Federation and the American Heart Association (AHA)/National Heart, Lung, and Blood Institute, together with the World Heart Federation, International Atherosclerosis Society, and International Association for the Study of Obesity.[15] In a joint statement, the metabolic syndrome was defined by the presence of at least three out of five individual risk factors: elevated waist circumference, dyslipidemia, i.e., elevated triglycerides and decreased high-density lipoprotein (HDL) cholesterol, elevated blood pressure, and elevated fasting glucose (**Table 1**).[16]

TABLE 1: Five individual risk factors with their treatments.

Criterion	Cut-off value	Treatments
Waist circumference	• ≥102 cm (≥40 in) in men • ≥88 cm (≥35 in) in women	N/A
Elevated triglycerides	• ≥150 mg/dL (1.7 mmol/L)	Or on drug treatment for elevated triglycerides
Reduced HDL-C	• <40 mg/dL in men • <50 mg/dL in women	Or on drug treatment for reduced HDL
Elevated blood pressure	• ≥130 mm Hg systolic pressure • ≥85 mm Hg diastolic pressure	Or on antihypertensive treatment in patient with history of hypertension
Elevated fasting glucose	≥100 mg/dL	Or on drug treatment for elevated glucose

(HDL-C: high-density lipoprotein cholesterol)

In addition to the above factors, other comorbidities are also associated with the metabolic syndrome, i.e., the proinflammatory state, prothrombotic state, NAFLD, cholesterol gallstone disease, and reproductive disorders.

EPIDEMIOLOGY

The metabolic syndrome has been recognized to be a common complex entity emerging as a major public health concern and epidemic worldwide. This condition is not a disease as per. The prevalence rate of metabolic syndrome is reported to be approximately 25% in American adults.

The prevalence of the metabolic syndrome has been reported to be rising also in Asian countries such as China, India, and South Korea in addition to the USA and Europe. The metabolic syndrome is important not only in view of its high prevalence worldwide but because of its possible role in prediction of development of T2DM and cardiovascular disease (CVD). NAFLD and cholesterol gallstone disease have been recognized as two major hepatic components of the metabolic syndrome (**Table 2**).

COVID-19 AND METABOLIC SYNDROME

The severe and worse outcomes of coronavirus disease 2019 (COVID-19) have been to be associated with comorbidities such as diabetes, hypertension, and obesity in recent studies suggesting the association of metabolic syndrome and its components with severity of COVID-19.

The potential risks for severe COVID-19 in obesity are due to enhanced expression of angiotensin-converting enzyme 2 (ACE2) receptors in obesity which makes it more likely for the virus to enter into the human body in obese people as compared with nonobese people, which may increase cytokines release and result in exacerbation of COVID-19. The greater expression of ACE2 may also expand the distribution of severe acute respiratory syndrome coronavirus 2 (SARS-CoV-2) in human body inducing severe COVID-19.

TABLE 2: Diagnostic criteria for metabolic syndrome.

	WHO 1998	EGSIR 1999	ATP III 2001	AACE 2003	IDF 2005	AHA/NHLBI 2005	AHA/NHLBI+ IDF 2009
Definition of MetS	Insulin resistance + any other two components	Plasma insulin concentration >75th percentile of nondiabetic patients + any of two components	Any of three out five components	Insulin resistance + any other component	Obesity + at least two components	At least three components	Any three components
Components of MetS							
Obesity	Waist/hip ratio >0.9 in males and >0.85 in females or BMI >30 kg/m^2	Waist circumference ≥94 cm in males and ≥80 cm in females	Waist circumference >102 cm in males and >80 cm in females	BMI >25 kg/m^2	BMI >30 kg/m^2 or specific gender and ethnicity waist circumference cutoffs	Waist circumference >40 inches in males and >35 inches in females	Raised waist circumference (population and country-specific definitions)
Elevated triglycerides	TG ≥150 mg/dL	TG ≥150 mg/dL or treatment of this lipid abnormality	TG ≥150 mg/dL or treatment of this lipid abnormality	TG ≥150 mg/dL	TG ≥150 mg/dL or treatment of this lipid abnormality	TG ≥150 mg/dL or treatment of this lipid abnormality	TG ≥150 mg/dL or treatment of this lipid abnormality
Decreased HDL	• HDL <35 mg/dL: Males • <39 mg/dL: Females	HDL <39 mg/dL: Males and females or treatment of this lipid abnormality	• HDL <40 mg/dL: Males • <50 mg/dL: Females or specific treatment for this lipid abnormality	• HDL <40mg/dL: Males • <50 mg/dL Females	• HDL <40mg/dL: Males • <50 mg/dL females: Females or specific treatment for this lipid abnormality	• HDL <40 mg/dL: Males • <50 mg/dL: Females or specific treatment for this lipid abnormality	• HDL <40 mg/dL: Males • <50 mg/dL: Females or specific treatment for this lipid abnormality

Continued

Continued

	WHO 1998	EGSIR 1999	ATP III 2001	AACE 2003	IDF 2005	AHA/NHLBI 2005	AHA/NHLBI+ IDF 2009
Hypertension	BP ≥140/90 mm Hg	BP ≥140/90 mm Hg or anti-hypertensive medication	SBP ≥130 or DBP ≥85 mm Hg or taking medication for hypertension	BP ≥130/85 mm Hg	SBP ≥130 or DBP ≥85 mm Hg or treatment of pre-viously diagnosed hypertension	BP ≥130/85 mm Hg or taking medication for hypertension	BP ≥130/85 mm Hg or taking medication for hypertension
Hyperglyce-mia	Impaired glucose tolerance, impaired fasting glucose, or lowered insulin sensitivity	Fasting plasma glucose >110 mg/dL	Fasting plasma glucose >110 mg/dL (modified in 2004) or taking medicine for high glucose	Impaired glucose tolerance or impaired fasting glucose (but not diabetes)	Fasting plasma glucose >100 mg/dL or previously diagnosed type 2 diabetes mellitus	Fasting plasma glucose >100 mg/dL or taking medicine for high glucose	Fasting plasma glucose >100 mg/dL or taking medicine for high glucose
Other	Urine albumin ≥20 µg/min or albumin: Creatinine ratio ≥30 mg/g	None	None	Other features of insulin resistance (family history of diabetes, polycystic ovary syndrome, sedentary lifestyle)	None	None	None

(AACE: American Association of Clinical Endocrinologists; AHA/NHLBI: American Heart Association/National Heart, lung and Blood institute; ATP: Adult Treatment Panel; BMI: body mass index; BP: blood pressure; DBP: diastolic blood pressure; EGSIA: European Group for the Study of Insulin Resistance; HDL: high-density lipoprotein; IDF: International Diabetes Federation; MetS: metabolic syndrome; SBP: systolic blood pressure; TG: triglycerides; WHO: World Health Organization)

It has been proposed that increase secretion of interleukin-6 (IL-6) and tumor necrosis factor-alpha (TNF-α) by adipose tissue in obesity-induced insulin resistance, could underlie the associations of insulin resistance with endothelial dysfunction and coagulopathy. Metabolic syndrome and its components are significantly associated with the susceptibility to SARS-CoV-2 infection and severity of COVID-19. Enhanced ACE2 expression, pre-existing endothelial dysfunction, and procoagulant state induced by adipocytokines dysregulation in metabolic syndrome may play a crucial role for the development of severe COVID-19.

PATHOPHYSIOLOGY

Obesity, particularly central obesity with accumulation of visceral fat leading to secondary development of insulin resistance is believed to be included in the risk factors of the metabolic syndrome primarily.[17] The accumulation of abdominal fat increases with the development of obesity.[18] A predictor of insulin resistance has been found to strongly associated with this increase in abdominal fat, specifically visceral adipose.[18,19] Glucose disposal has been found to be decreased with the increased amount of adipose tissue by Banerji et al. examining the relationship between glucose metabolism and fat distribution in diabetic men and women.[20] This study concluded the abdominal fat to be the best predictor of impaired glucose regulation inspite of gender or subcutaneous fat.[20] As per the beliefs, the increased body fat increases the rate of lipolysis leading to mobilization of the free fatty acids (FFAs) from the adipose tissue to the blood stream.[17] These FFAs enters in the liver and muscles[17] and oxidize leading to decreased glucose utilization in the muscles and increased hepatic glucose production.[21] This whole mechanism explains the contribution of the FFAs released from the adipose tissue to the development of hyperglycemia and subsequent impaired glucose tolerance.[17,21] In the response to the hyperglycemia, the insulin-producing beta cells of the pancreas initially release more insulin to maintain blood glucose levels[21,22] but over time, the sensitivity of insulin-sensitive tissue of the body decreases to the increased levels of circulating insulin resulting in development of insulin resistance.[20] The inability of the beta cells of the pancreas to produce enough insulin to maintain required blood glucose levels leads to rising glucose levels and subsequently to a prediabetes state and later overt T2DM.[21,22]

The central role of the adipose tissue in the development of risk factors for CVD and overt T2DM[19] is collectively suggested by increased production of small dense low-density lipoprotein (LDL) cholesterol, decreased production of HDL in the liver[17] and the increased hepatic production of triglycerides.[23] The association of even relatively small reductions in overall body weight has been reported with a significant beneficial effect on insulin-mediated glucose disposal.[20] Further, the decrease in the plasma glucose levels, glycated hemoglobin (HbA1c), and triglycerides and further delay in the progression of prediabetes to diabetes has been shown with a decrease in body weight of >5-7%.[24,25] Many of the key organs regulating glucose levels, i.e., the adipose tissue, the liver, the muscles, and the pancreas become sites for inflammation in obese individuals.[26]

The immune cells are believed to secrete proinflammatory cytokines resulting from a shift from anti-inflammation state to proinflammation state in the tissues of these organs interfering with the peripheral insulin signaling and inducing beta cells dysfunction causing later insulin deficiency.[26] The prothrombotic signaling pathways are activated in vascular cells by the chronic inflammation related to obesity resulting in dysregulation of endogenous anticoagulants and therefore increasing the risk of thrombosis and consequently CVD.[27-33]

MANAGEMENT OF METABOLIC SYNDROME

The adoption of a healthy lifestyle, weight loss, and the control of comorbidities (i.e., dyslipidemia, hyperglycemia, and arterial hypertension) are the main treatment targets of metabolic syndrome (**Fig. 1**).[34] The prevention of T2DM, cardiovascular events, and other metabolic syndrome-related outcomes (i.e., chronic liver disease and dementia) is the long-term goals.

Lifestyle Modification

The cornerstone of metabolic syndrome treatment is the adoption of a healthy which includes diet, physical activity, sleep, emotion control, peer support, and avoidance of tobacco, alcohol, and other drugs/medications altering satiety, or body weight as the key targets (**Fig. 1**). A systematic assessment and a patient-centered intervention plan are required by each component. There is need to evaluate each target for knowledge, beliefs, fears, barriers to achieve adherence to therapy, and motivation to change.[35] The major environmental and sociodemographic factors determining the health-related conduct are not altered by the intervention resulting in persistence of unhealthy behaviors.

Weight Loss

Weight loss is a prime objective. An improvement has been reported in several metabolic syndrome components by even a small weight loss (3% or more). This improvement could be most likely due to the high turnover rate of the intra-abdominal fat depots resulting in reduction in liver exposure to fatty acids and other proinflammatory mediators by a slight weight loss. Reversal of glucose intolerance, arterial hypertension, and several lipoprotein abnormalities are possible by a sustained weight loss >10%.

The prominent role of weight loss in the treatment of metabolic syndrome is best proved by bariatric surgery showing the capability of 30–40% weight loss in the reversal of majority of the metabolic syndrome abnormalities,[36] although this action is not exclusive to bariatric surgery.[37] Although few cases succeed to attain ideal body weight or maintain weight loss over time, weight loss is an unmet need for many metabolic syndrome cases despite of all the above facts.

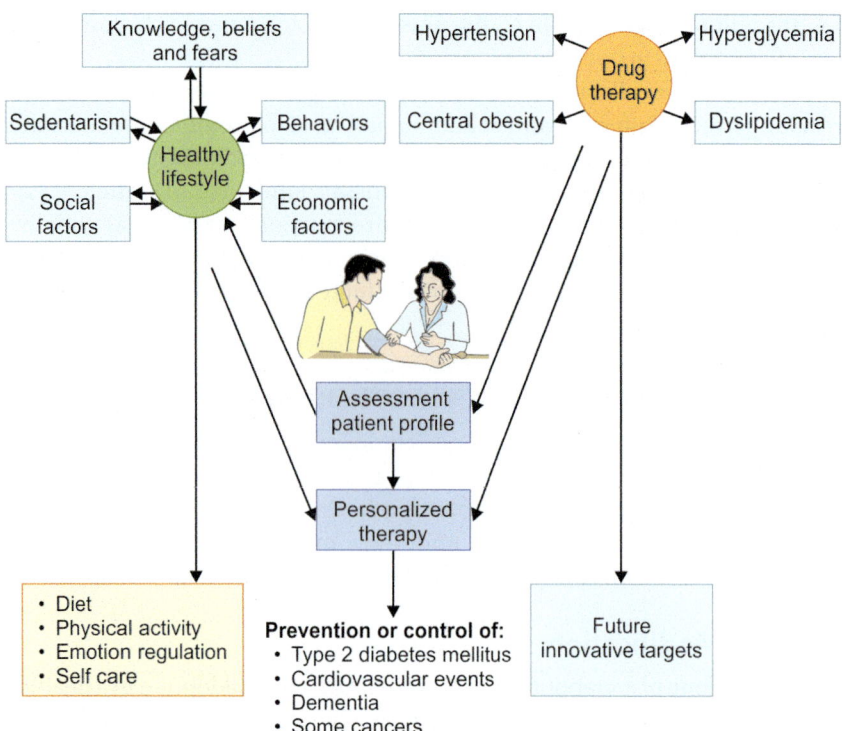

FIG.1: Treatment of metabolic syndrome. A personalized approach should be applied in the adoption of a healthy lifestyle and in the prescription of drug therapy. Adherence is a major challenge that could be overcome by identifying the patient profile, estimating the empowerment and addressing the main or most common barriers to include therapy in the daily routine.

Pharmacological Therapy for Obesity

Orlistat is a gastric and pancreatic lipase inhibitor and is approved by the Food and Drug Administration for the treatment of obesity in adolescents >12 years of age. This agent acts by decreasing the absorption of FFA and cholesterol. A significant improvement in the weight management in adolescents has been shown by Orlistat, 120 mg three times daily with meals along with diet, exercise, and behavior modification.

Sibutramine, a serotonin and adrenaline reuptake inhibitor, is approved for use in adolescents >16 years of age. It reduces food intake by decreasing appetite.

Noradrenergic drugs, i.e., phentermine, phenylpropanolamine, chlorphentermine and amphepramone (diethylpropion) also act by decreasing appetite and therefore reduced food intake without having any specific effects on macronutrient selection.

Once weekly semaglutide injection: The effect of semaglutide has been shown by a randomized, double-blind, placebo-controlled trial conducted at 129 sites in 16 countries including Asia, Europe, North America, and

South America. A mean weight loss of 14.9% from baseline was found in adults (with obesity or overweight with one or more weight-related condition) without diabetes with the use of semaglutide in addition to lifestyle intervention.

Human chorionic gonadotropin (HCG) plan—An accelerated weight loss along with suppressed appetite is caused by daily injections of HCG. This plan involves guided nutrition with no change in daily activities or exercise.

Lipotropic injections plan—Lipotropic injections contain fat-burning and vital agents, i.e., amino acids, minerals, and vitamins. This plan also involves guided nutrition but with an exercise regimen.

Octreotide acts by suppressing pancreatic insulin secretion. This agent is used in the treatment of obesity with the rationale to decrease insulinemia and insulin hypersecretion.

Topiramate, a novel broad-spectrum anticonvulsant drug, is used in children and adults. Although the exact mechanism of action is unknown, the weight loss in normal-weight and obese patients with the use of topiramate has been believed to be associated with decrease in food intake.

Control of Comorbidities

The control of comorbidities is the third treatment target. Availability of effective drug therapies for the treatment of hyperglycemia, arterial hypertension, and dyslipidemia suggests the accomplishment of this target to be the most likely approach to be implemented in primary care centers for the prevention of metabolic syndrome-related outcomes. The most frequently used drugs to treat these comorbidities include metformin, statins, ACE inhibitors, and angiotensin receptor blockers. New drugs derived from the identification of innovative treatment targets have been introduced in the market in the last few decades. These drugs include glucagon-like peptide 1 (GLP-1) agonists, sodium-glucose cotransporter-2 (SGLT-2) inhibitors, and dipeptidyl peptidase 4 (DPP-4) inhibitors.[38-40]

NEW APPROACHES

New potential treatment targets are under study. This is the case with farnesoid X receptor (FXR) agonists,[41] new peroxisome proliferator-activated receptor (PPAR)-gamma or PPAR-alpha modulators,[42,43] glucose-dependent insulinotropic polypeptide (GIP)/GLP-1 dual agonists,[44] dual SGLT-1/SGLT-2 inhibitors,[45] G protein-coupled receptor (GPCR/GPR) agonists,[46] apical sodium-dependent bile acid transporter (ASBT) inhibitors,[47] chemokine receptor 2 and 5 antagonists, fibroblast growth factor 19 agonists[48-50] and modulators of microbiota or their products among many others metabolic syndrome treatment is an area under intense investigation (**Table 3**). However, owing to long-term safety issues, the introduction of new agents is not as fast as needed.

TABLE 3: Treatment recommendation for the metabolic syndrome.

Criterion of the metabolic syndrome	Treatment targets	Management
Dyslipidemia: • Elevated triglycerides • Reduced HDL-C	**Lower-risk patients:** • <190 mg/dL **Moderate-risk patients:** • <160 mg/dL **Moderately high-risk patients:** • <160 mg/dL • Consider a more stringent therapeutic target <130 mg/dL **High-risk patients:** • <130 mg/dL • Consider a more stringent target <100 mg/dL for very high-risk patients	• Maximize lifestyle therapies • Intensify LDL-lowering therapy with 　○ Statins • If non-HDL remains elevated after maximum tolerated high intensity statin, might consider adding: 　○ Ezetimibe or PCSK9 inhibitor[a] 　○ Fibrate[b] • If triglycerides ≥500 mg/dL, treat the triglycerides first by initiating: 　○ Fibrate • If HDL is reduced maximize lifestyle therapies and consider initiating: 　○ Statins 　○ Fibrates, nicotinic acid, or CETP inhibitors added to statin therapy have not proven additional CV benefits
Elevated blood pressure	Reduce blood pressure to: • <140/90 • For patients with type 2 diabetes mellitus (T2DM) or high risk <130/80	1. Maximize lifestyle therapies 2. Initiate treatment with antihypertensive medication
Elevated fasting plasma glucose	Impaired fasting glucose: • Delay progression to T2DM T2DM: • Ensure good glycemic control: HbA1c <7.0%	1. Maximize lifestyle therapies 2. Consider antidiabetic medication according to ADA treatment guidelines

Continued

Continued

Criterion of the metabolic syndrome	Treatment targets	Management
Overweight/ Obesity: Elevated waist circumference	Reduce abdominal obesity by: • Reduce body weight by 7–10% within the first year • Achieve a BMI <25 kg/m²	1. Maximize lifestyle therapies 2. Considers anti-obesity medication

[a] Based on ACC 2016 Expert Consensus Decision Pathway on the Role of Non-Statin Therapies for LDL-Cholesterol Lowering in the Management of Atherosclerotic Cardiovascular Disease Risk.

[b] Possible particular benefits in patients with atherogenic dyslipidemia, although the effect on general or cardiovascular mortality could not be proven.

(ACC: American College of Cardiology; ADA: American Diabetes Association; AHA: American Heart Association; BMI: body mass Index; CETP: cholesteryl ester transfer protein; CV: cardiovascular; HbA1c: glycated hemoglobin; HDL: high-density lipoprotein; HDL-C: high-density lipoprotein cholesterol; LDL: low-density lipoprotein; LDL-C: low-density lipoprotein cholesterol; PCSK9: proprotein convertase subtilisin/kexin type 9; T2DM: type 2 diabetes mellitus)

ABCDE Approach to Metabolic Syndrome (Box 1)

Refer **Box 1**.

Box 1: ABCDE approach to metabolic syndrome.

A: Assessment
- Calculate Framingham Risk Score
- Make diagnosis of metabolic syndrome, using new criteria

A: Aspirin
- High risk—aspirin definitely beneficial
- High-intermediate risk (10–20%)—aspirin likely to be beneficial
- Low-intermediate risk (6–10%)—individualized decision-making, depending on sex, and risk of bleeding

B: BP control
- Aim for BP 125–135/80 mm Hg
- ACE inhibitors/ARBs first line, may reduce incident diabetes mellitus
- Dihydropyridine calcium channel blockers second line
- Beta-blockers and thiazides third line may have an adverse effect on impaired glucose tolerance but outweighed by benefits of reaching BP goal if first-line and second-line agents insufficient

C: Cholesterol
- First target: LDL
  ○ Statins to achieve LDL-C <100 mg/dL in high-risk, <130 mg/dL in intermediate-risk (≥6% 10-year risk) patients

Continued

Continued

- Second target: Non-HDL
  - Statin intensification, consider niacin and omega-3 fatty acids once statin maximized
  - Consider further reduction in LDL with statin therapy to mitigate risk of low HDL, consider niacin
- Third target: HDL
  - Consider fibrates, especially for those with combined hypertriglyceridemia/low HDL
- Fourth target: CRP
  - Statin therapy for those with hsCRP ≥ 2 mg/dL

D: Diabetes prevention/diet
- Intensive lifestyle modification is the most important therapy
- Weight loss, reduction in salt intake
- Mediterranean diet: Increase omega-3 fatty acids, fruits, vegetables, fiber, nuts
- Consider dietary supplementation with polyunsaturated fatty acids
- Metformin is second line in delaying the onset of diabetes mellitus
- Thiazolidinediones, alpha-glucosidase inhibitors, and incretin mimetics have shown benefit in smaller studies and are therefore third line

E: Exercise
- Daily vigorous activity
- Recommend use of pedometer with goal >10,000 steps/day

(ACE: angiotensin-converting enzyme; ARB: angiotensin receptor blocker; HDL: high-density lipoprotein; hsCRP: high-sensitivity C-reactive protein; LDL: low-density lipoprotein)

REFERENCES

1. Sarafidis PA, Nilsson PM. The metabolic syndrome: a glance at its history. J Hypertens. 2006;24:621-26.
2. Dawber TR, Meadors GF, Moore FE Jr. Epidemiological approaches to heart disease: the Framingham study. Am J Public Health Nations Health. 1951;41:279-81.
3. Wilson PW, D'Agostino RB, Levy D, Belanger AM, Silbershatz H, Kannel WB. Prediction of coronary heart disease using risk factor categories. Circulation. 1998;97(18):1837-47.
4. Eckel RH, Alberti KG, Grundy SM, Zimmet PZ. The metabolic syndrome. Lancet. 2010;375(9710):181-3.
5. Kaur J. A comprehensive review on metabolic syndrome. Cardiol Res Pract. 2014;2014:943162:1–21.
6. Stern MP, Haffner SM. Body fat distribution and hyperinsulinemia as risk factors for diabetes and cardiovascular disease. Arteriosclerosis. 1986;6:123-30.
7. Reaven GM. Banting lecture 1988. Role of insulin resistance in human disease. Diabetes. 1988;37(12):1595-607.
8. Benedict M, Zhang X. Non-alcoholic fatty liver disease: an expanded review. World J Hepatol. 2017;9:715-32.

9. Patil R, Sood GK. Non-alcoholic fatty liver disease and cardiovascular risk. World J Gastrointest Pathophysiol. 2017;8:51-8.
10. Uzunlulu M, Telci CO, Oguz A. Association between metabolic syndrome and cancer. Ann Nutr Metab. 2016;68:173-9.
11. Delitala AP, Capobianco G, Delitala G, Cherchi PL, Dessole S. Polycystic ovary syndrome, adipose tissue and metabolic syndrome. Arch Gynecol Obstet. 2017;296(3):405-19.
12. Koren D, Dumin M, Gozal D. Role of sleep quality in the metabolic syndrome. Diabetes Metab Syndr Obes. 2016;9:281-310.
13. Shabanzadeh DM, Sorensen LT, Jorgensen T. Determinants for gallstone formation - a new data cohort study and a systematic review with meta-analysis. Scand J Gastroenterol. 2016;51:1239-48.
14. Cameron AJ, Shaw JE, Zimmet PZ. The metabolic syndrome: prevalence in worldwide populations. Endocrinol Metab Clin North Am. 2004;33:351-75.
15. Alberti KG, Eckel RH, Grundy SM, Zimmet PZ, Cleeman JI, Donato KA, et al. Harmonizing the metabolic syndrome: a joint interim statement of the International Diabetes Federation Task Force on Epidemiology and Prevention; National Heart, Lung, and Blood Institute; American Heart Association; World Heart Federation; International Atherosclerosis Society; and International Association for the Study of Obesity. Circulation. 2009;120(16):1640-5.
16. Alberti KG, Zimmet P, Shaw J. The metabolic syndrome-a new worldwide definition. Lancet. 2005;366:1059-62.
17. Pi-Sunyer FX. The obesity epidemic: pathophysiology and consequences of obesity. Obes Res. 2002;10(Suppl 2):97S-104S.
18. Smith U, Kahn BB. Adipose tissue regulates insulin sensitivity: role of adipogenesis, de novo lipogenesis and novel lipids. J Intern Med. 2016;280:465-75.
19. Neeland IJ, Turer AT, Ayers CR, Powell-Wiley TM, Vega GL, Farzaneh-Far R, et al. Dysfunctional adiposity and the risk of prediabetes and type 2 diabetes in obese adults. JAMA. 2012;308(11):1150-9.
20. Banerji MA, Lebowitz J, Chaiken RL, Gordon D, Kral JG, Lebovitz HE. Relationship of visceral adipose tissue and glucose disposal is independent of sex in black NIDDM subjects. Am J Physiol. 1997;273:E425-32.
21. Kahn SE, Cooper ME, Del PS. Pathophysiology and treatment of type 2 diabetes: perspectives on the past, present, and future. Lancet. 2014;383:1068-83.
22. Nathan DM. Diabetes: advances in diagnosis and treatment. JAMA. 2015;314:1052-62.
23. Anstee QM, Targher G, Day CP. Progression of NAFLD to diabetes mellitus, cardiovascular disease or cirrhosis. Nat Rev Gastroenterol Hepatol. 2013;10:330-44.
24. Olefsky JM, Farquhar JW, Reaven GM. Reappraisal of the role of insulin in hypertriglyceridemia. Am J Med. 1974;57:551-60.
25. American Diabetes Association. Obesity management for the treatment of type 2 diabetes. Diabetes Care. 2017;40:S57-63.
26. Esser N, Legrand-Poels S, Piette J, Scheen AJ, Paquot N. Inflammation as a link between obesity, metabolic syndrome and type 2 diabetes. Diabetes Res Clin Pract. 2014;105(2):141-50.
27. Blokhin IO, Lentz SR. Mechanisms of thrombosis in obesity. Curr Opin Hematol. 2013;20:437-44.
28. Ridker PM, Buring JE, Cook NR, Rifai N. C-reactive protein, the metabolic syndrome, and risk of incident cardiovascular events: an 8- year follow-up of 14,719 initially healthy American women. Circulation. 2003;107(3):391-7.
29. Colotta F, Jansson B, Bonelli F. Modulation of inflammatory and immune responses by vitamin D. J Autoimmun. 2017;85:78-97.

30. Reis JP, Von MD, Miller ER III, Michos ED, Appel LJ. Vitamin D status and cardiometabolic risk factors in the United States adolescent population. Pediatrics. 2009;124(3):e371-9.
31. Stancakova A, Laakso M. Genetics of metabolic syndrome. Rev Endocr Metab Disord. 2014;15:243-52.
32. Kristiansson K, Perola M, Tikkanen E, Kettunen J, Surakka I, Havulinna AS, et al. Genome-wide screen for metabolic syndrome susceptibility Loci reveals strong lipid gene contribution but no evidence for common genetic basis for clustering of metabolic syndrome traits. Circ Cardiovasc Genet. 2012;5(2):242-9.
33. Stirnadel H, Lin X, Ling H, Song K, Barter P, Kesäniemi YA, et al. Genetic and phenotypic architecture of metabolic syndrome-associated components in dyslipidemic and normolipidemic subjects: the GEMS study. Atherosclerosis. 2008;197(2):868-76.
34. Grundy SM. Metabolic syndrome update. Trends Cardiovasc Med. 2016;26(4): 364-73.
35. Aspry KE, Van Horn L, Carson JAS, Wylie-Rosett J, Kushner RF, Lichtenstein AH, et al. Medical Nutrition Education, Training, and Competencies to Advance Guideline-Based Diet Counseling by Physicians: A Science Advisory From the American Heart Association. Circulation. 2018;137(23):e821-41.
36. de Toro-Martín J, Arsenault BJ, Després JP, Vohl MC. Precision Nutrition: A Review of Personalized Nutritional Approaches for the Prevention and Management of Metabolic Syndrome. Nutrients. 2017;9(8):913.
37. Madsbad S, Dirksen C, Holst JJ. Mechanisms of changes in glucose metabolism and bodyweight after bariatric surgery. Lancet Diabetes Endocrinol. 2014;2(2):152-64.
38. Halperin F, Ding SA, Simonson DC, Panosian J, Goebel-Fabbri A, Wewalka M, et al. Roux-en-Y gastric bypass surgery or lifestyle with intensive medical management in patients with type 2 diabetes: feasibility and 1-year results of a randomized clinical trial. JAMA Surg. 2014;149(7):716-26.
39. Bethel MA, Patel RA, Merrill P, Lokhnygina Y, Buse JB, Mentz RJ, et al. Cardiovascular outcomes with glucagon-like peptide-1 receptor agonists in patients with type 2 diabetes: a meta-analysis. Lancet Diabetes Endocrinol. 2018;6(2):105-13.
40. Hussein H, Zaccardi F, Khunti K, Seidu S, Davies MJ, Gray LJ. Cardiovascular efficacy and safety of sodium-glucose co-transporter-2 inhibitors and glucagon-like peptide-1 receptor agonists: a systematic review and network meta-analysis. Diabet Med. 2019;36(4):444-52.
41. Bozadjieva N, Heppner KM, Seeley RJ. Targeting FXR and FGF19 to Treat Metabolic Diseases-Lessons Learned From Bariatric Surgery. Diabetes. 2018;67(9):1720-8.
42. Chikara G, Sharma PK, Dwivedi P, Charan J, Ambwani S, Singh S. A Narrative Review of Potential Future Antidiabetic Drugs: Should We Expect More? Indian J Clin Biochem. 2018;33(2):121-31.
43. Li Z, Zhou Z, Deng F, Li Y, Zhang D, Zhang L. Design, synthesis, and biological evaluation of novel pan agonists of FFA1, PPARγ and PPARδ. Eur J Med Chem. 2018;159:267-76.
44. Frias JP, Bastyr EJ, Vignati L, Tschöp MH, Schmitt C, Owen K, et al. The Sustained Effects of a Dual GIP/ GLP-1 Receptor Agonist, NNC0090-2746, in Patients with Type 2 Diabetes. Cell Metab. 2017;26(2):343-52.e2.
45. Rendell MS. Sotagliflozin: a combined SGLT1/SGLT2 inhibitor to treat diabetes. Expert Rev Endocrinol Metab. 2018;13(6):333-9.
46. Neelamkavil SF, Stamford AW, Kowalski T, Biswas D, Boyle C, Chackalamannil S, et al. Discovery of MK-8282 as a Potent G-Protein-Coupled Receptor 119 Agonist for the Treatment of Type 2 Diabetes. ACS Med Chem Lett. 2018;9(5):457-61.

47. Hu YB, Liu XY, Zhan W. Farnesoid X receptor agonist INT-767 attenuates liver steatosis and inflammation in rat model of nonalcoholic steatohepatitis. Drug Des Devel Ther. 2018;12:2213-21.
48. Tiessen RG, Kennedy CA, Keller BT, Levin N, Acevedo L, Gedulin B, et al. Safety, tolerability and pharmacodynamics of apical sodium-dependent bile acid transporter inhibition with volixibat in healthy adults and patients with type 2 diabetes mellitus: a randomised placebo-controlled trial. BMC Gastroenterol. 2018;18(1):3.
49. Engin AB, Engin ED, Engin A. Two important controversial risk factors in SARS-CoV-2 infection: obesity and smoking. Environ Toxicol Pharmacol. 2020;78:103411.
50. Yudkin JS. Abnormalities of coagulation and fibrinolysis in insulin resistance. Evidence for a common antecedent? Diabetes Care. 1999;22(Suppl 3):C25-30.

20. Nonalcoholic Fatty Liver Disease: What is in the Name?

Suhas Erande

INTRODUCTION

In 1980s, an entity named as nonalcoholic fatty liver disease (NAFLD) or nonalcoholic steatohepatitis (NASH), resembled histopathologically with alcoholic liver disease (ALD).[1,2] Even then, the biochemical and clinical features of NAFLD and ALD were noted as distinct from each other. Association of NAFLD with type 2 diabetes mellitus (T2DM) and obesity was described in 1970.[3] When Ludwig first used the term NASH, this association was noted, however, this was largely ignored over years allowing NAFLD to be the established nomenclature. But researchers were struggling to pinpoint evolution of inflammation in NASH until Day and James proposed their two hits model,[4] suggesting oxidative stress as driver of inflammation. Insulin resistance came into picture when Marchesini showed NAFLD association with it even in lean individuals.[5] This paved way to link NAFLD as a part of metabolic syndrome subsequently.[6] Last 2 decades have clearly shown that NAFLD is a progressive, metabolic disease the prevalence parallel to T2DM and obesity and liver manifestations as a part of multisystem entity. In this background lies the recent nomenclature metabolic-associated fatty liver disease (MAFLD).[7,8] The change is more than semantic-catalyzing process to better conceptualize the disease for health promotion, patient orientation, case identification, ongoing clinical trials and healthcare delivery. The definition needs hepatic steatosis to be accompanied by obesity/overweight, T2DM, or metabolic dysregulation. At least two components should be present in metabolic dysregulation (1) waist circumference >90/80 cm in men/women, (2) prediabetes, (3) raised high-sensitive C-reactive protein (hsCRP), (4) elevated blood pressure (BP) or on treatment, (5) decreased high-density lipoprotein cholesterol (HDL-C), (6) increased triglyceride (TG), (7) homeostatic model assessment for insulin resistance (HOMA-IR) score >2.5. MAFLD and not NAFLD also de-emphasizes alcohol from the picture.

Nonalcoholic fatty liver disease is historically defined as excess accumulation of triglyceride droplets in hepatocytes >5% on histopathology or >5% proton density fat fraction on magnetic resonance imaging (MRI), in people who consume little or no alcohol (it is to be noted that other liver diseases or other etiologies of steatosis need to be ruled out). Some experts

TABLE 1: Summarization of a battery of tests.	
Hepatic steatosis	Fatty Liver Index, Hepatic Steatosis Index, NAFLD Liver Fat Score, and NAFLD Ridge score
Necroinflammation	Inflammation PAI-1, apoptosis CK18, adipocytokines-adiponectin, leptin, resistin, ghrelin, and lipid oxidation OxNASH score
Fibrosis	Scores—NAFLD fibrosis score, FIB-4, APRI, fibrometer, BARD score, and BAAT score
Evolving areas	Genomics, proteomics, lipidomics, metabolomics, and gut microbiome

(APRI: aspartate transaminase (AST)-to-platelet ratio index; ALT: alanine transaminase; BAAT: BMI, ALT, age and triglycerides; BARD: body mass index (BMI), AST/ALT ratio and diabetes; CK: cytokeratin; FIB-4: fibrosis-4; NAFLD: nonalcoholic fatty liver disease; oxNASH: oxidized nonalcoholic steatohepatitis; PAI: plasminogen activator inhibitor)

also say that these features should be accompanied by lack of hepatocellular injury (ballooning of hepatocytes and lobular inflammation) to be defined as steatosis. Liver biopsy is the gold standard for diagnosis and staging of whole spectrum of NAFL-NASH-fibrosis-cirrhosis and hepatocellular carcinoma (HCC). A number of noninvasive tests (biochemical and imaging) are used obviously to avoid biopsy. A battery of tests are summarized in the following table, most of these being research tools (**Table 1**).[9,10]

All scores are available on smartphone or Google.

No markers of fibrosis approved in United States of America (USA). Alpha test or enhanced liver fibrosis test approved in Europe.

Nonalcoholic Fatty Liver Disease Fibrosis Score (NFS) is computed using platelet count, albumin, aspartate transaminase (AST)/alanine transaminase (ALT) and three clinical parameters-age, body mass index (BMI), and glucose intolerance. It performs well to assess likelihood of advanced fibrosis or cirrhosis [AUROC 0.85, sensitivity 90%, specificity 60%, negative predictive value (NPV) 88%, and positive predictive value (PPV) 82%]. Lesser specific but implementable are fibrosis-4 (FIB-4) (platelet count, ALT, AST, and age-based computation) or AST-to-Platelet Ratio Index (APRI) (platelets and ALT). A new best fitting multivariable logistic regression model based on liver stiffness FibroScan and AST-called as fibroscan AST (FAST) can better identify at risk NASH and progression to cirrhosis.[11] FIB-4 value <1.3 implies low risk and >1.3 suggests need of transient elastography or magnetic resonance (MR) studies. MR elastography reading > 3.3 kpa and FIB-4 value >1.6 has PPV (NASH and fibrosis) > 90%.

A simple risk score of conversion of NAFLD→ NASH is based on hypertension, T2DM, obstructive sleep apnea (OSA), ALT > 27, and AST > 27 (each scoring 1) and black race scoring 2. Total 0–2 carries less risk and total >6 or 7, higher risk of conversion.

Nonalcoholic fatty liver (NAFL) is slowly progressive disease but in ~20% people it can progress to NASH faster (conversion rate ~14%).

NASH→fibrosis→cirrhosis→HCC is even slower, however, T2DM obese people convert/deteriorate faster.

An evolving area of studies looks at nonobese or lean people with NAFLD, having some different features than obese NAFLD and emphasizing need to approach NAFLD independent of BMI.[12] NAFLD prevalence in T1DM is also on the rise given the increasing lifespan of these patients.[13]

EPIDEMIOLOGY OF NAFLD—GLOBAL ASIAN INDIAN[14]

Nonalcoholic fatty liver disease is the umbrella term for liver diseases characterized primarily by excess fat accumulation in hepatocytes because of perturbations of homeostatic mechanisms regulating synthesis versus utilization of fat in liver. NAFLD has become the leading cause of liver disease across the Western World-pooled global prevalence 25.24% with high geographical variations, e.g., 30% in Middle East and South America by USG and 13% in Africa, 24-25% in North America and Europe. In developing Asian countries, smaller studies reveal NAFLD prevalence as 10% to >50%, depending on rural/urban locations or by methods (USG or biomarkers). A study from Hongkong using MR spectroscopy revealed incidence of NAFLD over 3-5 years as 13.5%. Rising global prevalence of obesity, T2DM, sedentary lifestyles, and excess calorie consumption (calorie dense fatty foods, sugar sweetened beverages, and high corn fructose syrup) underlie rise in NAFLD. Even childhood/adolescent obesity/overweight culminates in NAFLD. Effects of such foods on gut microbiota—both by pregnant mothers or by children-may result in NAFLD which could be independent of BMI.

NAFLD AND T2DM AN INTRICATE BIDIRECTIONAL ASSOCIATION

SPRINT study[15] from Indian T2DM patients revealed NAFLD prevalence to be 56.5% against general population prevalence of 9-32%. Remission of T2DM over 2 years was less common in those with NAFLD at baseline (USG based), compared to those without (8.7 vs. 13.1%).[16] Hepatic steatosis and fibrosis are associated with significant left ventricular (LV) dysfunction in T2DM patients due to impaired myocardial glucose uptake.[17] Professor V. Mohan in his CURES study subgroup of 541 patients, noted overall prevalence of NAFLD 32%-but-it was 54.5% in T2DM patients. He showed increasing prevalence of NAFLD with increasing degree of glucose intolerance.[18] Drivers of NAFLD (obesity, dyslipidemia, sedentary habits, excess calorie intake, systemic inflammation and insulin resistance, and metabolic syndrome) also are drivers of T2DM and cardiovascular disease (CVD). Angiopoietin like protein 8 (ANGPTL 8) is increased in NAFLD and is associated with hepatic lipid content independent of obesity, insulin resistance (IR), and liver injury. It could prove as biomarker to assess severity of NAFLD in T2DM. Over years, the old two hit theory (excess fat accumulation in liver, i.e., steatosis + one more trigger like drugs or lipid peroxidation) has understandably evolved into multiple hits theory (impaired mitochondrial

ATP activity, depletion of mitochondrial glutathione, hypoxia associated with impaired blood flow or obesity related OSA, dysregulated adipokine production, effects of high fructose diet, and rapid weight loss). Role of gut microbiota and genetic markers (PNPLA3) is being researched in.

Nonalcoholic Fatty Liver Disease and Cardiovascular Disease

Insulin resistance, dyslipidemia, obesity, excess visceral fat, and systemic low grade chronic inflammation (metabolic syndrome) are common soil for both NAFLD and CVD. Nuclear factor (NF) kappa beta and c-Jun NH2-terminal kinase (JNK) pathway activation in NAFLD drives IR, dyslipidemia, procoagulant states, proinflammatory [interleukin 1 alpha (IL-1α), beta-IL-18, IL-33, and tumor necrosis factor-alpha (TNF-α)] condition and, hence, CVD. Numerous studies have shown liver fibrosis scores incrementally linked with increased CVD risk. The Framingham Risk Score is validated to calculate CVD risk in NAFLD.

WHOM TO SCREEN FOR NAFLD? HOW TO FOLOW?

Since, NAFLD does not have Food and Drug Administration (FDA) approved drug treatment as yet, is it necessary to give importance to it? (NAFLD worsening to NASH, fibrosis, cirrhosis or HCC and end-stage liver disease, accompanying MetSyn T2DM CVD). Different associations recommend against universal screening, but, active surveillance is advised in obese T2DM people (EASL, NICE, and Asia-Pacific AASLD). USG, liver enzymes, and transient elastography modalities are advised for the same.[19] American Association for the Study of Liver Diseases (AASLD) feels that mass screening is not cost effective and the benefits in long-term are unclear.

Though gold standard, liver biopsy is advised only if advanced fibrosis is suspected-(the Asian guidelines differing from American and European). Scores based on biomarkers/USG/elastography can be followed and if worsening, biopsy is recommended.

LIFESTYLE MODIFICATION IN NAFLD TREATMENT

Dietary restrictions/modifications, physical exercise aimed at weight loss are recommended by all guidelines to treat NAFLD. Low cal (~1200–1500/day), very-low-calorie diet (VLCD) (450 or 800 cal/day), low carb (<20–45%), low fat (20–27%), DASH diet or Mediterranean Diet, intermittent fasting have favorable effects on weight loss, liver enzyme reduction, USG improvement, hepatic TG reduction on magnetic resonance spectroscopy (MRS) and even biopsy proved NAFLD/NASH improvement.[20]

DRUG TREATMENT FOR NAFLD

A variety of drugs are under investigations to treat NAFLD. Those which improve fibrosis and histopathology are more important than those (viz. statins) which improve only liver enzymes. Amongst antidiabetic drugs, pioglitazone and saroglitazar can be used (the latter DCGI approved label)- so also liraglutide injection. Sodium-glucose cotransporter-2 (SGLT-2) inhibitors hold some promise in small studies. Vitamin E 800 mg/day can be used for nondiabetic/noncirrhotic NAFLD. Farnesoid receptor agonist (obeticholic acid, cilofexor, tropifexor, and EDP-305) inhibitors of de novo lipogenesis (Armachol, Firsocostat, and PF-05221304) are also being studied.[21] Bariatric surgery can remarkably improve NAFLD, wherever appropriate.

Note: Readers may refer to illustrious publications by Professor Anoop Misra and Late Dr Deepak Amrapurkar for in depth NAFLD research in Indian population.

REFERENCES

1. Ludwig J, Viggiano T R, McGill DB, Oh BJ. Nonalcoholic steatohepatitis; Mayo clinic experiences with a hitherto unnamed disease. Mayo Clin Proc. 1980;55(7):434-8.
2. Fleming KA Morton JA, Barbatis C, Burns J, Canning S, McGee JO. Mallory bodies in alcoholic and nonalcoholic liver disease contain a common antigenic determinant. Gut. 1981;22(5):341-4.
3. Beringer A, Thaler H. Relationship between diabetes mellitus & fatty liver. Dtsch Med Wochenschr. 1970;95(15):836-8.
4. Day CP, James OF. Steatohepatitis: a tale of "two hits"? Gastroenterology. 1998;114:842-5.
5. Marchesini G, Brizi M, Morselli-Labate AM, Bianchi G, Bugianesi E, McCullough AJ, et al. Association of nonalcoholic fatty liver disease with insulin resistance Am J Med. 1999;107(5):450-5.
6. Marchesini G, Brizi M, Bianchi G, Tomassetti S, Bugianesi E, Lenzi M, et al. Nonalcoholic fatty liver disease: a feature of metabolic syndrome. Diabetes. 2001;50(8):1844-50.
7. Eslam M, Newsome PN, Sarin SK, Anstee QM, Targher G, Romero-Gomez M, et al. A new definition of metabolically associated fatty liver disease: An International expert consensus statement. J Hepatol. 2020;73(1):202-9.
8. Eslam M, Sanyal AJ, George J; International Consensus Panel. MAFLD: A consensus driven proposed nomenclature for metabolic associated fatty liver disease. Gastroenterology. 2020;158(7):1999-2014.e1
9. Tincopa MA. Diagnostic and interventional circulating biomarkers in nonalcoholic steatohepatitis. Endocrinol Diabetes Metab. 2020;3(4):e00177.
10. Angulo P, Hui JM, Marchesini G, Bugianesi E, George J, Farrell GC, et al. The NAFLD fibrosis score: a noninvasive system that identifies liver fibrosis in patients with NAFLD. Hepatology. 2007;45(4):846-54.
11. Newsome PN, Sasso M, Deeks JJ, Paredes A, Boursier J, Chan WK, et al. Fibroscan-AST (FAST) score for non-invasive identification of patients with NASH with significant activity and fibrosis: A prospective derivation and global validation study. Lancet Gastroenterol Hepatol. 2020;5(4):362-73.
12. Ren TY, Fan JG. What are clinical settings and outcomes of lean NAFLD? Nature Rev Gastroenterol Hepatol. 2021;18(5):289-90.
13. de Vries M, Westerink J, Kaasjager KHAH, de Valk HW. Prevalence of NAFLD in patients with T1DM: a systematic review and meta-analysis. J Clin Endocrinol Metab. 2020;105(12):3842-53.
14. Mitra S, De A, Chowdhury A. Epidemiology of non-alcoholic and alcoholic fatty liver. Transl Gastroenterol Hepatol. 2020;5:16.

15. Kalra S, Vithalani M, Gulati G, Kulkarni CM, Kadam Y, Pallivathukkal J,, et al. Study of Prevalence of nonalcoholic fatty liver disease (NAFLD) in type 2 diabetes patients in India (SPRINT). J Assoc Physicians India. 2013;61(7):448-53.
16. Hajime Yamazaki et al. Inverse association of fatty liver at baseline Ultrasonography and remission of Type 2 Diabetes over 2-years follow-up period. Clin Gastroenterol Hepatol. 2021;19(3):556-64.e5.
17. Lee M, Kim KJ, Chung TH, Bae J, Lee YH, Lee BW, et al. Nonalcoholic fatty liver disease, diastolic dysfunction, and impaired myocardial glucose uptake in patients with type 2 diabetes. Diabetes Obes Metab. 2021;23(4):1041-51.
18. Mohan V, Farooq S, Deepa M, Ravikumar R, Pitchumoni CS. Prevalence of non-alcoholic fatty liver disease in urban south Indians in relation to different grades of glucose intolerance & metabolic syndrome. Diabetes Res Clin Pract. 2009;84(1):84-91.
19. Leoni S, Tovoli F, Napoli L, Serio I, Ferri S, Bolondi L. Current guidelines for management of NAFLD: A systematic review and comparative analysis. World J Gastroenterol. 2018;24(30):3361-73.
20. Viveiros K. The Role of Life Style Modifications in Comprehensive Non-Alcoholic Fatty Liver Disease treatment. Clin Liver Dis. 2021;17(1):11-4.
21. White PJ, Abdelmalek MF. Insights into metabolic mechanisms and their application in the treatment of NASH. Clin Liver Dis (Hoboken).2021;17(1):29-32.

21. Vagal Nerve Stimulation and Baroreceptor Activation Therapy: An Emerging Modality for Refractory Heart Failure

Kamal Sharma

INTRODUCTION

Despite many recent advances like novel drugs and medicines like sodium-glucose cotransporter 2 (SGLT-2)-inhibitors, angiotensin receptor neprilysin inhibitor (ARNI) and device therapies like cardiac resynchronization therapy (CRT)/automatic implantable cardioverter-defibrillator (AICD), there is still a huge burden of refractory heart failure (HF) with high unmet needs both in terms of quality of life and life expectancy. Despite the modern advances, median survival in symptomatic HF is around meager 5 years only. Amongst HF patients with narrow electrocardiogram (ECG) (QRS) complex, medicines were the only avenue as devices like CRT show no benefit in quality of life or longevity.

Vagus nerve (10th cranial nerve) is the source of electrical supply from brain to heart through it's network of cardiac plexus. The impact of yoga, meditation, and exercise are all mediated and regulated through these neural networks also known as "autonomic regulation" of heart. The vagus nerve is part of the autonomic nervous system that plays vital role in functions including heart rate and respiratory control apart from gastric secretion, speech, and intestinal motility. Increased sympathetic and decreased parasympathetic activity contribute to HF symptoms and disease progression. Baroreceptor activation therapy (BAT) results in centrally-mediated reduction of sympathetic outflow and increased parasympathetic activity. Vagus nerve stimulation (VNS) refers to technique that stimulates the Vagus nerve, with electrical stimulation. VNS and/or BAT is a novel approach of regulating the autonomic innervation and supply of the heart by an implanted pacemaker generator under the chest wall just like a pacemaker. The implantation technique needs additional tunneling of the lead to vagus nerve in the neck for intermittent activation of the vagus nerve via the electrode wrapped around it in the carotid sheath in the neck for cyclic stimulation to it. Implantable devices for VNS have long been approved therapy for refractory epilepsy and for treatment-resistant depression. In HF, implantable VNS has been shown to be beneficial in both preclinical and clinical studies. Adverse effects of implantable VNS therapy systems are generally associated with the implantation procedure or continuous on-off stimulation.[1]

RESEARCH AND DATA

The ANTHEM study was first ever innovative therapy that evaluated VNS in patients who were refractory HF cases despite optimal medical therapy with narrow ECG complex and hence, not eligible for CRT device. ANTHEM-HF evaluated a novel autonomic regulation therapy (ART) via either left or right VNS in patients with HF and reduced ejection fraction (HFrEF). About 60 patients in New York Heart Association (NYHA) II-III with left ventricular ejection fraction (LVEF) ≤ 40%, left ventricular end-diastolic diameter ≥ 50 mm to < 80 mm on optimal pharmacologic therapy were randomized at 10 sites on the left ($n = 31$) or right ($n = 29$) vagus nerve. After 6 months of ART, the adjusted left-right differences in LVEF, left ventricular end-systolic volume (LVESV), and left ventricular end-systolic diameter (LVESD) were 0.2%, 3.7 mL, and 1.3 mm, respectively. In the combined population, absolute LVEF improved by 4.5%, LVESV improved by –4.1 mL, and LVESD improved by –1.7 mm. Heart rate variability improved by 17 ms (95% CI 6.5–28) with minimal left-right difference. A 6-minute walk (6 MWD) distance improved an average of 56 m with NYHA functional class improving in 77% of patients from baseline.[2] Author who was also the principal investigator for the ANTHEM study did the "world's first ever" VNS device implant in such a refractory case of HF.

INOVATE-HF was a multinational, randomized trial involving 85 centers including patients with chronic HF, NYHA functional class III symptoms and ejection fraction ≤40%. Patients were assigned to device implantation to provide VNS (active) or continued medical therapy (control) in a 3:2 ratios. The primary efficacy endpoint was composite of death from any cause or first event for worsening HF were 30.3% versus 25.8%. Quality of life, NYHA functional class, and 6 MWD improved by VNS ($p < 0.05$) but LVESV index was not different ($p = 0.49$).[3]

In a more recently published ANTHEM-HF long-term data of continuous cyclic VNS, the echocardiographic parameters and HF symptoms were assessed throughout a follow-up period of at least 42 months. At 42 months, there was significant improvement from baseline in LVEF, NYHA class, 6 MWD, and Minnesota Living with Heart Failure questionnaire (MLHFQ) score. However, these improvements at 42 months were not significantly different from mean values at 6 and 12 months. The study established, ART as durable, safe, and was associated with beneficial effects on LVEF and 6 MWD and well-tolerated in patients with HFrEF.[4]

In another study aimed to evaluate cost-utility of BAT using the Barostim NEO™ device (CVRx Inc., Minneapolis, MN, USA) compared with optimized medical management in patients with advanced chronic HF (NYHA class III) who were not eligible for treatment with CRT from a statutory health insurance perspective in Germany over a lifetime horizon, patients were enrolled at 45 centers were randomly assigned to receive ongoing guideline-directed medical therapy (GDMT) alone (control group) or ongoing GDMT plus BAT (treatment group) for 6 months. Of 70 patients in control and 76 to BAT arm, patients assigned to BAT had improvements in the 6 MWD, quality-of-life score, and NYHA functional class ranking. BAT significantly reduced N-terminal probrain natriuretic peptide ($p = 0.02$) and was associated with a trend toward fewer days hospitalized for HF ($p = 0.08$) making BAT safe and improves functional status, quality of life, exercise capacity, N-terminal probrain natriuretic peptide, and possibly the burden of HF hospitalizations in patients with GDMT-treated NYHA functional class III HF [Barostim Neo System in the Treatment of Heart Failure; NCT01471860; Barostim HOPE4HF (Hope for Heart Failure) Study; NCT01720160].[5]

Baroreceptor activation therapy also led to an incremental cost of €33,185 and incremental benefits of 1.78 life-years and 1.19 quality-adjusted life-years (QALYs). This resulted in an incremental cost-effectiveness ratio of €27,951/QALY (95% CI €21,357-82,970). BAT had a 59% probability of being cost-effective at a willingness-to-pay threshold of €35,000/QALY thus establishing BAT can be cost-effective in European settings in those not eligible for CRT among patients with advanced HF.[6]

SUMMARY

Last decade has seen various newer modalities of therapy emerge both in novel medicines like ARNI and SGLT-2-inhibitors and device therapies like CRT and AICD. VNS/BAT offers a new hope to those with refractory symptoms despite optimal treatment and are not suitable or eligible for CRT. BAROSTIM-NEO device is now United States Food and Drug Administration (US FDA) approved therapy for refractory HF despite optimal medical treatment and not eligible for CRT.

REFERENCES

1. Akdemir B, Benditt DG. Vagus nerve stimulation: An evolving adjunctive treatment for cardiac disease. Anatol J Cardiol. 2016;16(10):804-10.
2. Premchand RK, Sharma K, Mittal S, Monteiro R, Dixit S, Libbus I, et al. Autonomic regulation therapy via left or right cervical vagus nerve stimulation in patients with chronic heart failure: results of the ANTHEM-HF trial. J Card Fail. 2014;20(11):808-16.
3. Gold MR, Van Veldhuisen DJ, Hauptman PJ, Borggrefe M, Kubo SH, Lieberman RA, et al. Vagus Nerve Stimulation for the Treatment of Heart Failure: The INOVATE-HF Trial. J Am Coll Cardiol. 2016;68(2):149-58.
4. Sharma K, Premchand RK, Mittal S, Monteiro R, Libbus I, DiCarlo LA, et al. Long-term Follow-Up of Patients with Heart Failure and Reduced Ejection Fraction Receiving Autonomic Regulation Therapy in the ANTHEM-HF Pilot Study. Int J Cardiol. 2021;323:175-8.
5. Abraham WT, Zile MR, Weaver FA, Butter C, Ducharme A, Halbach M, et al. Baroreflex Activation Therapy for the Treatment of Heart Failure With a Reduced Ejection Fraction. JACC Heart Fail. 2015;3(6):487-96.
6. Borisenko O, Müller-Ehmsen J, Lindenfeld J, Rafflenbeul E, Hamm C. An early analysis of cost-utility of baroreflex activation therapy in advanced chronic heart failure in Germany. BMC Cardiovasc Disord. 2018;18(1):163.

22. A Century of Basal Glucose Regulation: From Longer to Flatter to more Predictable Insulins

Ganpathi Bantwal

INTRODUCTION

The discovery of insulin became one of the greatest innovations in medical history which gave hope to all the people suffering from diabetes. It was a series of experiments by Frederick Banting and his assistant Charles Best who were able to unlock the mystery for the world. After 40 years the discovery of insulin, quoting the words of Prof Elliot Josline "40 years with insulin and 4,000 years without. Today, there must be 3 million people with diabetes whose life span has increased on an average at least by 10 years each. This makes a total of 30 million years of productive human life in one country alone" landmarking how miraculous this molecule has been in transforming the lives of people with diabetes.

In healthy individuals, normal insulin response is biphasic in nature. The first phase is a sharp release of insulin which begins within 1-2 minutes after glucose administration and lasts approximately 10 minutes. This is followed by a more prolonged second phase which starts at approximately 10 minutes and lasts 1-2 hours. The goal of exogenous insulin therapy is to mimic normal endogenous insulin secretion which adapts to fasting and prandial conditions, and the main role of basal insulin secretion is to limit hepatic glucose production and lipolysis in the fasting state, particularly overnight, without impairing glucose availability for brain function.

When insulin therapy was first introduced for clinical use, it was available only as a short-acting formulation requiring multiple daily injections. This meant that, from the outset, there was a drive to develop new formulations of insulin and explore different routes of administration to make insulin treatment easier for people to manage and tolerate. The first breakthrough happened when Hans Christian Hagedorn, in 1936, discovered that the addition of strongly basic proteins like protamine could prolong the effects of injected insulin. This led to the development of longer acting insulin formulations like protamine zinc insulin. Subsequently, the Lente family of insulins (semiLente, Lente, and ultraLente) were created by complexing neutral insulin suspensions with small amounts of zinc ions in the absence of any added foreign proteins or synthetic compounds.

Over the years, several strategies have been employed to prolong the action of insulin. (1) Modification of the insulin molecule to achieve a low solubility at physiological pH was achieved with insulin glargine (IGlar); (2) The other strategy used was the addition of a fatty-acid chain of variable length to the insulin molecule which can bind to albumin, forming a circulating depot from which the insulin analog is slowly released, e.g., are the insulins detemir and degludec. An interesting new research is the human immunoglobulin (IgG) Fc fusion technology which comprises of attaching to an IgG Fc fragment which helps with a longer pharmacokinetic profile of the drug.

BASAL INSULINS THROUGH THE AGES

In 1946, neutral protamine Hagedorn (NPH) insulin, an intermediate-acting insulin developed by Hans Christian Hagedorn, became available. This was a stable "protamine zinc insulin" modification that combined insulin and protamine in "isophene" proportions (i.e., no excess of insulin or protamine) at neutral pH in the presence of a small amount of zinc and phenol or phenol derivatives. When injected, the protamine/insulin crystals dissolve slowly, delaying the dissociation of insulin hexamers, and thus slowing the absorption of insulin monomers into the circulation. However, despite the longer duration, basal insulin coverage was insufficient which therefore meant that it needed to be administered twice daily. Moreover, the time-action profile of NPH insulin can differ between individuals based on their physiological factors. Because NPH insulin is a precipitate with protamine and zinc, it needs to be resuspended by rolling it gently 12–15 times prior to injection. If this resuspension process is not followed, it can add significantly to the day-to-day variability. The discernible peak plasma concentrations after subcutaneous (SC) injection, led to an increased risk of hypoglycemia (in particular, nocturnal hypoglycemia). Therefore, in an attempt to avoid the shortcomings of conventional basal insulin therapies, long-acting basal insulin analog were developed. IGlar was first approved in the United States in the year 2000. IGlar differs from human insulin in that the amino acid asparagine in position A21 was substituted with glycine and 2 arginine (glargine) residues were added at positions B31 and B32. This led to a relatively flat PK profile compared to NPH.

The next innovation came in the year 2005 when insulin detemir was developed by covalently attaching a fatty acid to the insulin molecule. The chemical structure of insulin detemir is derived from human insulin with the omission of the threonine at position B30 and attachment of a 14-carbon fatty acid (tetradecanoic acid also called myristic acid) at position B29 by acylation. Insulin is injected as hexamers. In the subcutis, it forms dihexamers and binds to albumin. As zinc eludes out with a $t_{1/2}$ of 2–3 hours, insulin detemir hexamers dissociate into dimers. This leads to a slow steady absorption from the depot. In the bloodstream, 98.8% of insulin detemir is bound to albumin. This leads to further protraction, and also acts as a buffer, further increasing the stability of insulin concentration with insulin detemir.

However, despite these advances, some challenges were still left unanswered. The first-generation analog were not truly peakless. They needed to be administered more than once daily. They were associated with higher variability which led to fluctuations and also a higher risk of nocturnal hypoglycemia. Besides, they needed to be administered at a fixed time during the day, thus leading to poor adherence to regimen affecting efficacy and safety of the insulins.

The continued search for a basal insulin with a longer than 24-hour duration of action and a flatter insulin profile led to the development of insulin degludec. In the insulin degludec molecule, the B30 threonine is omitted and the recombinant DesB30 human insulin is acylated at the LysB29 residue with a hexadecandioyl-γ-L-Glu sidechain. The diacyl side chain of insulin degludec, in the presence of zinc and phenolic preservative, promotes association into dihexamers under formulation conditions. After injection and dilution of the phenolic preservative in the SC space, the dihexamers self-associate forming multihexamer complexes. This higher-order structure significantly slows hexameric dissociation and subsequent monomer absorption. The binding of monomers to albumin in the circulation also slows the disposition of degludec to peripheral tissues and clearance from the body, leading to a protracted time-action profile.

Continuing with innovations, a threefold concentrated version of IGlar was developed to prolong the duration of action. The higher concentration of glargine delivered in the same volume further slows the dissolution of the glargine precipitate in the SC space, leading to a better basal insulin. The concentrated IGlar U300 profile has a lower peak and a longer duration of action compared to IGlar U100.

LOOKING AT THE EVIDENCE FROM STUDIES

In a pharmacokinetic study by Tim Heise et al., insulin degludec has shown much lesser day-to-day variability compared to both GlarU100 and GlarU300. During the development program, insulin degludec has undergone intensive evaluation and study through several phase 3 studies like BEGIN, SWITCH, DEVOTE, CONCLUDE, etc., which consistently showed benefits in terms of efficacy in glycemic control and good safety profile with lower rates of overall symptomatic hypoglycemia, severe hypoglycemia, and nocturnal hypoglycemia. The SWITCH 2 study in type 2 diabetes mellitus (T2DM) patients comparing insulin degludec with insulin glargine U100 over 32 weeks showed statistically significant 30% lower overall symptomatic hypoglycemia and 42% lower nocturnal hypoglycemia with insulin degludec in comparison to insulin glargine U100. Real-world evidence studies conducted in India, the TRUST (Tresiba Real-World Use Study) study, have reconfirmed the evidence seen in clinical trials with good glycated hemoglobin (HbA1c) reduction, fasting plasma glucose (FPG) reduction, and lower hypoglycemia rates with insulin degludec when used as part of routine clinical practice. Recent evidence from the SWITCH PRO study observed that insulin degludec compared with IGlar U100 provided more time in glycemic target range, and less nocturnal time below range, using flash glucose monitoring techniques, in basal insulin-experienced people with T2DM at increased risk of hypoglycemia.

Basal insulins have evolved and transformed their path in changing the lives of people with diabetes, bringing solutions with innovations in molecular structure for a longer acting, more stable and predictable profiles with lower glycemia variability, better time in range, and minimal hypoglycemia offering the best glycemic control through simple and easily adaptable regimens.

SUGGESTED READINGS

1. Marso S, McGuire D, Zinman B, et al. Efficacy and Safety of Degludec versus Glargine in Type 2 Diabetes. New England Journal of Medicine. 2017;377(8):723-32. doi:10.1056/nejmoa1615692.
2. Wangnoo SK, Chowdhury S, Rao PV. Treating to target in type 2 diabetes: the BEGIN trial programme. J Assoc Physicians India. 2014;62(1 Suppl):21-6. PMID: 25330628.
3. Wysham C, Bhargava A, Chaykin L, et al. Effect of Insulin Degludec vs Insulin Glargine U100 on Hypoglycemia in Patients With Type 2 Diabetes: The SWITCH 2 Randomized Clinical Trial. JAMA. 2017;318(1):45-56. doi:10.1001/jama.2017.7117.
4. Philis-Tsimikas A, Klonoff D, Khunti K, et al. Risk of hypoglycaemia with insulin degludec versus insulin glargine U300 in insulin-treated patients with type 2 diabetes: the randomised, head-to-head CONCLUDE trial. Diabetologia. 2020;63(4):698-710. doi:10.1007/s00125-019-05080-9.
5. Kesavadev J, Murthy L, Saboo B, et al. One-Year Safety and Effectiveness of Insulin Degludec in Patients with Diabetes Mellitus in Routine Clinical Practice in India—TRUST (Tresiba Real-World Use Study). Diabetes. 2018;67(Supplement 1):1019-P. doi:10.2337/db18-1019-p
6. Goldenberg RM, Aroda VR, Billings LK, et al. Effect of insulin degludec versus insulin glargine U100 on time in range: SWITCH PRO, a crossover study of basal insulin-treated adults with type 2 diabetes and risk factors for hypoglycaemia. Diabetes Obes Metab. 2021 doi: 10.1111/dom.14504. Epub ahead of print. PMID: 34322967.

23 Pyrexia of Unknown Origin

Asha N Shah

INTRODUCTION

The term pyrexia of unknown origin (PUO) or fever of unknown origin (FUO) is used to describe prolonged febrile illnesses without an established etiology in spite of intensive evaluation and diagnostic testing. Fever of unknown origin is more frequently an atypical presentation of a common disease and not an unusual disease. The differential diagnosis may include a list of >200 diseases but in most cases in adults there would be limited possible causes. Diagnostic advances continuously modify the spectrum of FUO-causing diseases; e.g., serologic tests have reduced the importance of human immunodeficiency virus (HIV) and numerous rheumatic diseases. Modern imaging techniques such as ultrasound (USG), computed tomography (CT) scan, and magnetic resonance imaging (MRI) enable early detection of abscesses and solid tumors that were once difficult to diagnose. Typical subgroups used in the differential for classical FUO are infection (20-40%), malignancy (20-30%), noninfectious inflammatory diseases (NIID) (10-30%), miscellaneous (10-20%), and undiagnosed (up to 30%). NIID commonly include connective tissue diseases, vasculitides, and granulomatous diseases. In developed countries, the NIIDs and undiagnosed groups comprise a higher proportion of FUO cases. Underdeveloped countries have higher rates of infection (43%) and neoplasm. Drug fever is implicated in 1-3% of FUO cases. Comprehensive history and examination is must along with looking for potentially diagnostic clues (PDCs) for evaluation of PUO.

DEFINITION

Old definition: Petersdorf and Beeson defined PUO in 1961 as an illness of >3 weeks duration with fever of ≥38.3°C (101°F) on two occasions and diagnosis remains uncertain despite 1 week of inpatient evaluation and three outdoor visits.

The definition of PUO was modified by excluding immunocompromised patients, because they require an entirely different diagnostic and therapeutic approach.

New definition:
- Fever > 38.3°C (101°F) on at least two occasions
- Duration of illness ≥ 3 weeks

- No known immunocompromised state
- Diagnosis remains uncertain even after a detailed history taking, general physical examination, and the obligatory investigations which are as follows: Hemoglobin, total and differential leukocyte count, platelet count, erythrocyte sedimentation rate (ESR), C-reactive protein level (CRP); renal function test (RFT) like electrolytes and creatinine, liver function test (LFT) (total protein, alkaline phosphatase, alanine aminotransferase, and aspartate aminotransferase), lactate dehydrogenase (LDH), creatine kinase, ferritin, antinuclear antibodies (ANA), and rheumatoid factor; protein electrophoresis; urine examination and urine culture, three blood cultures; chest X-ray, USG abdomen, and tuberculin skin test (TST).

DIFFERENTIAL DIAGNOSIS

The differential diagnosis for PUO is extensive, but it is important to remember that PUO is far more often caused by an atypical presentation of a rather common disease than by a very rare disease. There are large number of bacterial infections with some unusual bacterial infections, viral infections, parasitic infections, noninfectious autoimmune diseases, vasculitis, autoinflammatory diseases, granulomatous diseases, malignancy, solid tumors, or defective thermoregulatory causes. The list is quite long but all the causes need to be kept in mind. The definition and the causes in pediatric populations are different. Causes may also differ as per geographical variation, economic development, or availability of the diagnostic facilities. So, travel-related causes must be thought of.

Indian context: In a study from south India, 100 cases of PUO were evaluated in 10 years, 64 were males and 36 were females with peak incidence in 30–40 years. Etiological basis was as follows, infection 60 cases (45 with tuberculosis), collagen vascular disease 24, neoplasms 10, and miscellaneous 6. While, PUO in eastern India showed that amongst 100 patients, infections, especially tuberculosis was the most dominant cause (53%), followed by neoplasms (17%), and collagen vascular disorders (11%), miscellaneous causes in 5% cases, and in 14% the cause was not found.

Factitious fever is due to administration of pyrogenic substances (bacterial suspensions) which is observed in young women with connection to health care, often nurses. While in fraudulent fever thermometer manipulation using external heat or substitute thermometer is the cause.

APPROACH TO PATIENT (FLOWCHART 1)

The first and very most important step in the diagnostic workup is to search for PDCs by complete and repeated history taking, detailed physical examination, and the obligatory investigations. PDCs are defined as all localizing symptoms, signs, and any abnormalities which potentially points toward a diagnosis.

Factitious fever or fraudulent fever should be ruled out.

Pyrexia of Unknown Origin

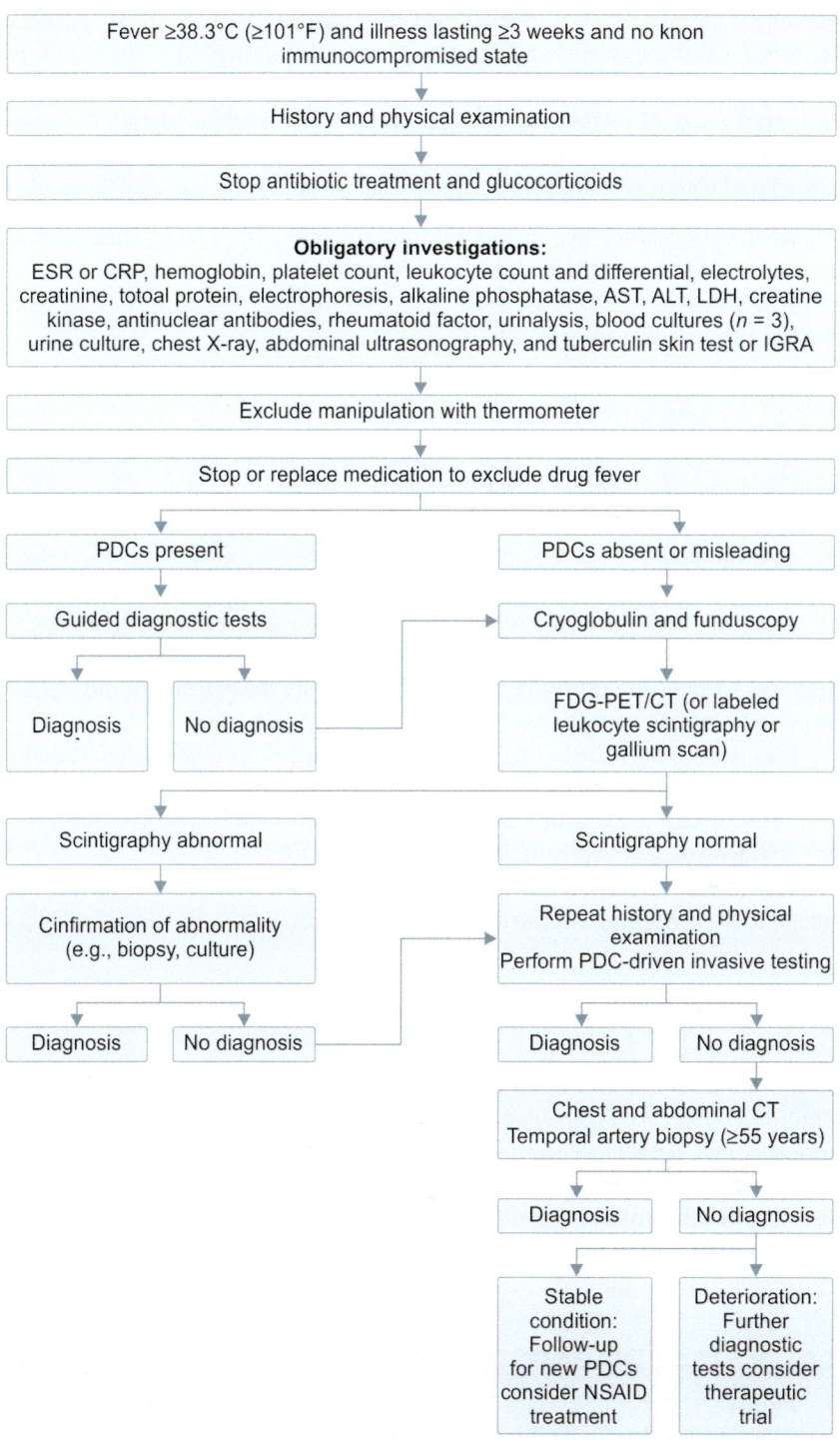

(CRP: C-reactive protein level; CT: computed tomography; ESR: erythrocyte sedimentation rate; FDG: fluorodeoxyglucose; NSAIDs: nonsteroidal anti-inflammatory drugs; PDC: potentially diagnostic clues; PET: positron emission tomography)

FLOWCHART 1: Pyrexia of unknown origin (PUO) approach.

History: The history should include information about the fever pattern (continuous or recurrent) and duration, previous medical history of surgery or implant, history of drug use which also includes over the counter drugs or herbal drugs or recreational drugs, family history, sexual history, country of origin, recent and remote travel, unusual environmental exposures associated with travel or hobbies, and animal contacts.

Physical examination: Special attention to the eyes, oral ulcers, sinus or calf tenderness, tender tooth, lymph nodes, temporal arteries, liver, spleen, sites of previous surgery, entire skin surface, and mucous membranes, nails, and detailed systemic examination.

FIRST STAGE DIAGNOSTIC TESTS

- Obligatory investigations as mentioned in definition and as per PDCs
- Cerebrospinal fluid (CSF) for FUO with headache
- Cryoglobulin and fundus
- Scintigraphy
- Fluorodeoxyglucose-positron emission tomography (FDG-PET)

The diagnostic yield of sinus radiography, echocardiography, endoscopic or radiologic evaluation of the gastrointestinal tract, and bronchoscopy is very low without the presence of PDCs. That is why these tests should not be used as screening procedures.

It is necessary to rule out factitious or fraudulent fever, especially in patients without signs of inflammation in laboratory investigations. All nonprescription drugs and nutritional supplements should be discontinued to exclude drug fever early in the evaluation.

In patients who have no PDCs or misleading PDCs, fundoscopy may be useful in the early stage of the diagnostic workup.

Scintigraphy:
- It is noninvasive, delineation of foci on basis of functional changes in tissues is observed and it uses ^{67}Ga citrate and ^{111}In or ^{99m}Tc labeled leukocyte and allows whole body imaging.

Fluorodeoxyglucose-positron emission tomography: It is established imaging procedure in FUO. FDG accumulates in tissues with a high rate of glycolysis which occurs in malignant cells and in activated leukocytes. It has high resolution and greater sensitivity in chronic low-grade infection. It can be used in integration with CT (FDG-PET/CT) but the problem is that it is expensive and has limited availability.

LATER STAGE DIAGNOSTIC TESTS

- Biopsy
- Chest and abdominal CT
- Temporal artery biopsy
- Bone marrow aspiration
- Review of lab tests and imaging

TREATMENT

The focus in patients with PUO is on continued observation and repeated examination with avoidance of empirical therapy as it is nonspecific, underlying disease may remit spontaneously or the PUO may not respond totally or there would be delay in specific diagnosis or drug side effects can be misleading. However, empirical therapy is indicated if there is instability in vital signs or neutropenia.

If Mantoux test is strongly positive and granulomatous disease or miliary tuberculosis is suspected (and sarcoid seems unlikely), or if the patient is immunocompromised or elderly, then a therapeutic trial for tuberculosis can be undertaken with treatment continued for up to 6 weeks and observe. Though nowadays, with the advent of GeneXpert, the chances of diagnosis of tuberculosis are very high if tissue sample is available. A failure of the fever to respond over this period suggests other alternative diagnosis. Empiric drug trial for suspected culture endocarditis can be considered in patients with new or changing murmur or peripheral signs of endocarditis or suspected infection with difficult to culture bacteria. Colchicine is used for preventing attacks of familial Mediterranean fever.

Rheumatic fever and Still's disease may respond to aspirin and nonsteroidal anti-inflammatory drugs (NSAIDs) dramatically and so is the effect of glucocorticoids on temporal arteritis, polymyalgia rheumatica, and granulomatous hepatitis. Recombinant interleukin 1 receptor antagonist anakinra is extremely effective for autoinflammatory syndromes and for patients whose PUO is not diagnosed after later stage diagnostic test and it is without side effects of steroids.

OUTCOME

Patients with undiagnosed FUO (5–15% of cases) generally have a benign long-term course when fever is not accompanied by substantial weight loss, other signs of a serious underlying disease, or malignancy.

CONCLUSION

Initiating empirical therapy, doesn't mark the end of the diagnostic work-up, rather it commits the physician to continued thoughtful re-examination and evaluation. Compassion, patience, serenity, careful observation, and flexible attitude are indispensable attributes for the physician in dealing successfully with PUO. The challenges are extensive list of diseases causing PUO, geographical and travel-related variation, misleading PDCs and the fact that only rarely biochemical tests lead to definitive diagnosis in absence of PDCs and diagnostic pointers are numerous and diverse and missed on initial examination.

SUGGESTED READINGS

1. Jameson JL, Fauci AS, Kasper DL, Hauser SL, Longo DL, Loscalzo J. Harrison's textbook of medicine, 20th Edition. [online] Available from: https://accessmedicine.mhmedical.com/book.aspx?bookID=2129 (Last accessed August, 2020).
2. Hersch EC, Oh RC. Prolonged Febrile Illness and Fever of Unknown Origin in Adults. Am Fam Physician. 2014;90(2):91-6.
3. Cunha BA, Lortholary O, Cunha CB. Fever of Unknown Origin: A Clinical Approach. AJM Online Rev. 2015;128(10):E1-15.
4. The Association of Physicians of India. [online] Available from: https://www.apiindia.org/pdf/pg_med_2004/chapter_52.pdfct (Last accessed August, 2020).
5. Salla SR, Raghupatruni P, Yerra R, Betha TP. Study of spectrum of pyrexia of unknown origin patients in a tertiary care hospital in coastal Andhra Pradesh. 2017;4(74):4372-81.
6. Kejariwal D, Sarkar N, Chakraborti SK, Agarwal V, Roy S. Pyrexia of unknown origin: a prospective study of 100 cases. J Postgrad Med. 2001;47(2):104-7.

24. Evolving Epidemiology of COVID, Clinical Presentation, and Triage

Niteen D Karnik, Aditi S Patankar, Gauri Pathak-Oak

EVOLVING EPIDEMIOLOGY

Novel coronavirus disease 2019 (COVID-19) is caused by ribonucleic acid (RNA) virus belonging to coronaviridae family. Epicenter of the outbreak was seafood market in Wuhan city in China in December, 2019. World Health Organization (WHO) declared this outbreak as a "Public Health Emergency of International Concern" (PHEIC) on January 30, 2020 and subsequently declared it a pandemic on March 11, 2020. By March 21, the virus had spread to 183 countries with 2 lakh confirmed cases worldwide with Italy being the worst affected. The first case of COVID-19 in India was detected in Kerala on January 30, 2020. Using the United States of America (USA) mathematical model, Center for Disease Dynamics Economics and Policy (CDDEP) projected about 30 crore cases in India. However, a nationwide lockdown helped to reduce case positivity and death rate. The USA, Brazil, and India were the hardest hit by the pandemic. By late September, Europe especially United Kingdom saw the start of second wave of COVID-19 with peak in mid-October. The second wave in US and Europe saw record daily new cases and fatalities by mid-November (**Fig. 1**). India is witnessing a second wave beginning February end (**Fig. 2**).

As of March 23, 2021, globally cases stand at 125 million with 2 million deaths with a case fatality ratio (CFR) of 1.6. In India, there are 11 million cases as of March 23, 2021 with 1.6 lakh deaths with a CFR of 1.4. State of Maharashtra is maximally affected.

Transmission is through respiratory droplets released during coughing, sneezing, talking, and aerosol generating procedures such as suctioning, nebulization, intubation, noninvasive ventilation (NIV), and high-flow nasal oxygen (HFNO). Incubation period ranges from 5 to 14 days postexposure. Asymptomatic patients can transmit disease in this period. Period of infectivity varies from 10 to 14 days. Protective neutralizing antibodies occur by day 14 in convalescent plasma. Positive reverse transcription polymerase chain reaction (RT-PCR) in swab during recovery may be due to shedding of dead virus. The major risk factors for severe illness are age >60 years (increasing with age), underlying comorbidities such as diabetes, hypertension, ischemic heart disease (IHD), chronic lung disease, cerebrovascular disease, chronic kidney disease, cancer, obesity, and immunocompromised state.

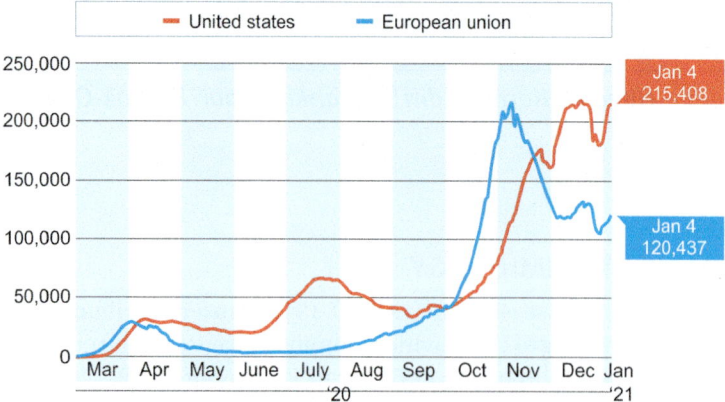

FIG. 1: Evolving epidemiology of coronavirus disease (COVID), clinical presentation, and triage: Trend of cases during the second wave in Europe and the United States with peak in October.

Source: Johns hopkins unoversity

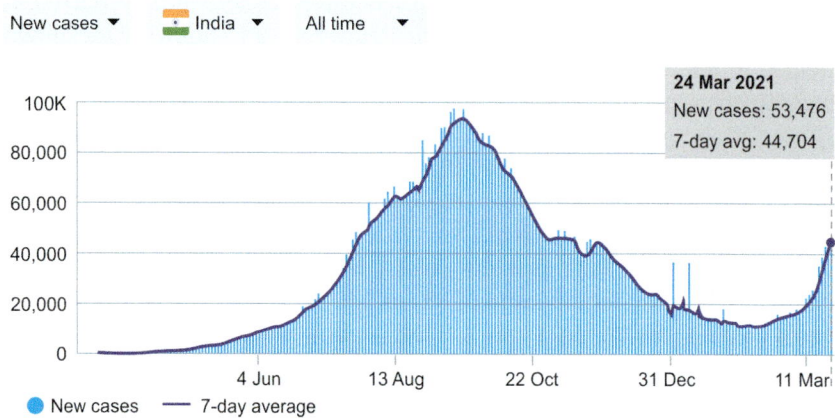

FIG. 2: Evolving epidemiology of coronavirus disease (COVID), clinical presentation, and triage: Trend of cases in India with peak of first wave in September and start of the second wave by February end.

EVOLVING CLINICAL PRESENTATIONS

The clinical spectrum of COVID-19 varies from being asymptomatic or paucisymptomatic to severe manifestations like respiratory distress requiring mechanical ventilation, multiorgan dysfunction, and septic shock. It is estimated that 80% of infections are mild or asymptomatic, 15% are severe and requiring oxygen, and 5% are critical and requiring ventilation.

April to June 2020

We became familiar with standard clinical presentations of COVID-19. Fever is present in 99% of symptomatic cases. Patients have fatigue, anorexia, dry cough, sore throat, nasal congestion, malaise, myalgia, headache, new loss of taste and/or smell, diarrhea, and vomiting. Elderly and immunosuppressed patients present with atypical symptoms such as fatigue, reduced alertness, diarrhea, loss of appetite, and delirium. Fever is typically absent. COVID lungs are major morbidity and mortality determinants. Pneumonia appears to be the most frequent serious manifestation. Patients present with cough, fever, dyspnea and hypoxia (SpO_2 90–94% on room air). Two phenotypes of lungs were observed. Type L is characterized by low elastance, low ventilation to perfusion ratio, low lung weight and low recruitability. The near normal compliance explains why some patients present without dyspnea; a novel concept called as "happy hypoxia". Type H is characterized by high elastance, high lung weight, and high recruitability which is typical of acute respiratory distress syndrome (ARDS) lung. ARDS, which is characterized by new-onset respiratory failure or acute worsening in a case of pneumonia, was found in 20% of cases. Acute kidney injury (AKI) is seen in 5–40% of patients with COVID-19 possibly due to hemodynamic compromise causing prerenal AKI or direct tubular injury by the virus due to overexpression of angiotensin-converting enzyme (ACE) receptors in tubular membrane. In a study on "impact of COVID-19 on maintenance hemodialysis in chronic kidney disease patients" ($n = 37$), 27% presented with severe symptoms while 56.7% were asymptomatic or had mild disease.[1] 30% of patients presented with extended dialysis break due to logistic and social issue. Overall, 23 (62.1%) had a successful outcome and 14 (37.8%) died. Patients with pre-existing end-stage renal disease (ESRD) are at increased risk of severe COVID-19 infections with 14–16 times higher mortality.

In the early part of COVID-19 pandemic, concept of "cytokine storm" was recognized.[2] The onset of cytokine storm is heralded by unremitting fever, worsening of hypoxia, hypotension, deterioration in renal, and liver function tests with worsening of hyperglycemia/appearance of diabetic ketoacidosis. Blood investigations may reveal cytopenias (bicytopenia or pancytopenia), elevated inflammatory markers like ferritin, erythrocyte sedimentation rate (ESR) and C-reactive protein (CRP), and D-dimer. The cytokines incriminated include interleukin (IL)-2, IL-6, interferon-γ, tumor necrosis factor (TNF)-α as well as certain chemokines. Secondary bacterial infections such as pyogenic liver abscess, bacterial sepsis, and mucormycosis due to transient paralysis of immune system became recognized.[3] Treatment with tocilizumab an IL-6 inhibitor used in cytokine storm of COVID-19 was associated with increased incidence of bacterial and fungal sepsis. Septic shock was a contributory factor in the mortality of COVID-19.

July to September 2020

Clinical features were expanded to include thrombotic complications such as acute myocardial infarction (AWMI/AMI), acute cerebrovascular events, cortical venous sinus thrombosis, deep vein thrombosis, and pulmonary thromboembolism (PTE) due to hypercoagulable state. When patients of AWMI were screened for COVID-19, an association of 8–12% was noted. Pulmonary embolism was reported to occur in 2.6–8.9% of COVID-19 patients. Coagulopathy in COVID-19 has mild thrombocytopenia and high levels of D-dimer. D-dimer levels correlate with disease severity and risk of thrombosis. Patients with established cardiovascular disease have high vulnerability to develop serious COVID-19. Viral myocarditis and arrythmias have been reported. Concomitant use of azithromycin and hydroxychloroquine was found to cause corrected QT (QTc) prolongation and sudden cardiac arrest. Neurological features are myriad and include anosmia, ageusia, headache, altered sensorium, dizziness, encephalitis, stroke, epilepsy as well as Guillain–Barré syndrome. Delirium was recognized as presenting feature of COVID-19 in elderly population. Skin manifestations such as erythematous rashes and COVID toes were reported.[4] Conjunctivitis, iridocyclitis, papilledema, and subconjunctival hemorrhage were ocular manifestations. Severe acute respiratory syndrome coronavirus 2 (SARS-CoV-2) induced damage of pancreatic β-cells resulted in "acute new-onset diabetes" in patients with COVID-19. Hyperinflammation causing stress-induced hyperglycemia led to uncontrolled sugars and diabetic ketoacidosis. Gastrointestinal symptoms such as diarrhea, epigastric pain, nausea, and vomiting became increasingly recognized as initial manifestations.

Symptoms of COVID-19 differ in children with most being asymptomatic. Fever and cough are frequent. <3.5% of children who were hospitalized needed intensive unit care (ICU). Mortality rate was only 0.09% in pediatric population.

October to December 2020

There was a gradual decline in patient load. This period saw incidental COVID RT-PCR positives on a background of comorbidities. Special outpatient units were started to handle the load of post-COVID patients. These patients had severe persistent fatigue, myalgia, arthralgia, and new-onset depression. This new entity was outlined as "post-COVID fatigue syndrome".[5] This superimposed on a residual hypoxic state due to post-COVID fibrosis reduced the effort tolerance and made few patients dependent on home oxygen therapy. Patients presenting with thromboembolic complications such as AWMI, PTE, and strokes few weeks after discharge despite adequate anticoagulation were a major concern.[6]

January 2021 Onward

India is currently facing a second wave. With new mutant strains being detected, infectivity has increased. However, due to early detection and treatment with antivirals, steroids, anticoagulants, and increased ventilators, mortality has decreased. Vaccination has been started in full gear. Patients are presenting with abdominal pain and loose motions without fever, cough, cold, or breathlessness. Clinicians are reporting COVID pneumonia in younger patients with discordance between clinical symptoms (almost absent) and computed tomography (CT) chest (high CT severity index). Myocarditis is a frequent complication seen in these patients. Interestingly, the conundrum of COVID-19-like but COVID RT-PCR negative cases with immunoglobulin M (IgM) COVID antibody positivity (possibly because of mutant strains) are being reported.

TRIAGE

Triage is important in COVID-19 given the limited resources. Classification of COVID-19 is based on clinical criteria, clinical scoring system, laboratory assessment, and radiological assessment like high-resolution CT (HRCT) based scores.
- *Clinical classification:* Task force of Maharashtra state endorsed a clinical staging system:
  - Stage I mild (early infection)—Group A, B, and C
    - Group A includes patients who are asymptomatic but RT-PCR positive for COVID-19.
    - Group B includes patients who are mildly symptomatic (fever, myalgia, diarrhea, anosmia, loss of taste, and dry cough) without any comorbidities.
    - Group C includes patients who are mildly symptomatic but with comorbidities such as diabetes, hypertension, IHD, chronic kidney disease, chronic obstructive pulmonary disease (COPD), obesity, immunocompromised state, immunosuppressive drugs, and age >60 years.
  - Stage IIa moderate (pulmonary involvement without hypoxia)—Group D: Group D includes patients who have pneumonia without respiratory failure.
  - Stage IIb moderate (pulmonary involvement with hypoxia)—Group E: Group E includes patients who have pneumonia with respiratory failure.
  - Stage III severe (pulmonary involvement with hypoxia with sepsis/septic shock/multiorgan dysfunction)—Group F.

Patients belonging to Group A, B, and C can be admitted in Covid Care Centers (CCC), those in Group D are directed to Dedicated Covid Health Center (DCHC) whereas those in Group E and F need to be admitted in Dedicated Covid Hospital (DCH) with ICU facilities. In all groups, red flag signs like neutrophil lymphocyte ratio >3.5, PaO_2/FiO_2 (P:F) ratio <300, 3–4-minute exercise-induced deoxygenation, resting tachycardia, and raised serum CRP/serum ferritin/D-dimer/lactate dehydrogenase (LDH)/triglycerides are watched for.
- *National Early Warning Score 2 (NEWS2):* NEWS2 is a standardized clinical scoring system developed to improve detection of deterioration in acutely ill patients. It is based on aggregate scoring of six physiological parameters (**Table 1**). In addition, two points are added for patients requiring supplementary oxygen treatment. A NEWS2 score of 5 or 6 is

TABLE 1: Evolving epidemiology of coronavirus disease (COVID), clinical presentation, and triage: National Early Warning Score 2 (NEWS2).

Physiological parameter	3	2	1	0	1	2	3
Respiration rate (per minute)	≤8		9–11	12–20		21–24	≥25
SpO_2 Scale 1 (%)	≤91	92–93	94–95	≥96			
SpO_2 Scale 2 (%)	≤83	84–85	86–87	88–92 ≥93 on air	93–94 on oxygen	95–96 on oxygen	≥97 on oxygen
Air or oxygen?		Oxygen		Air			
Systolic blood pressure (mm Hg)	≤90	91–100	101–110	111–219			≥220
Pulse (per minute)	≤40		41–50	51–90	91–110	111–130	≥131
Consciousness				Alert			CVPU
Temperature (°C)	≤35.0		35.1–36	36.1–38.0	38.1–39.0	≥39.1	

TABLE 2: Evolving epidemiology of coronavirus disease (COVID), clinical presentation, and triage: COVID-19 Reporting and Data System (CO-RADS) Score.

	CO-RADS	
	Level of suspicion COVID-19 infection	
		CT Findings
CO-RADS 1	No	Normal or noninfectious abnormalities
CO-RADS 2	Low	Abnormalities consistent with infections other than COVID-19
CO-RADS 3	Indeterminate	Unclear whether COVID-19 is present
CO-RADS 4	High	Abnormalities suspicious for COVID-19
CO-RADS 5	Very High	Typical COVID-19
CO-RADS 6	PCR +	

considered a key threshold that may indicate clinical deterioration with a sensitivity and specificity of 80% and 84.3%, respectively.
- Radiology based scoring systems:
  - COVID-19 Reporting and Data System (CO-RADS) score: CO-RADS assesses the suspicion for pulmonary involvement of COVID-19 on a scale from 1 (very low) to 5 (very high) (**Table 2**).

- Computed tomography severity index: It is calculated for each of the five lobes considering the extent of anatomical involvement, as follows: 0, no involvement; 1, <5% involvement; 2, 5–25% involvement; 3, 26–50% involvement; 4, 51–75% involvement; and 5, >75% involvement. The resulting global CT score is the sum of each individual lobar score (0–25). *A CT score ≥18 has shown to be highly predictive of patient's mortality in short-term follow-up.*

REFERENCES

1. Trivedi M, Shingada A, Shah M, Khanna U, Karnik ND, Ramachandran R. Impact of COVID-19 on maintenance haemodialysis patients: The Indian scenario. Nephrology. 2020;25(12):929-32.
2. Fajgenbaum DC, June CH. Cytokine Storm. In: Longo DL (ed). N Engl J Med. 2020;383(23):2255-73.
3. Gokhale Y, Patankar A, Holla U, Shilke M, Kalekar L, Karnik ND, et al. Dermatomyositis during COVID-19 Pandemic (A Case Series): Is there a Cause Effect Relationship? J Assoc Physicians India. 2020;68(11):20-4.
4. Nalbandian A, Sehgal K, Gupta A, Madhavan MV, McGroder C, Stevens JS, et al. Post-acute COVID-19 syndrome. Nat Med. 2021;27(4):601-15.
5. Soman R, Sunavala A. Post COVID-19 Mucormycosis - from the Frying Pan into the Fire. J Assoc Physicians India. 2021;69(1):13-4.
6. Sripadma PV, Jain RS, Vyas A, Sharma B, Srivastava T, Murarka S, et al. Isolated Acute Cerebrovascular Involvement in COVID-19 without Fever and Respiratory Symptoms: An Indian Perspective. J Assoc Physicians India. 2021;69.

25 COVID-19 and Diabetes Mellitus

Sudhir Bhandari

INTRODUCTION

Severe acute respiratory syndrome coronavirus 2 (SARS-CoV-2), the novel coronavirus that causes coronavirus disease 2019 (COVID-19), was first reported in Wuhan, China, in December 2019 and has spread worldwide. Type 2 diabetes mellitus (T2DM) is majorly known as disease of aging and, hence, if it is risk factor for COVID-19 is not clear. Good number of studies are ongoing in this filed to clear this ambiguous situation of inter-relation of diabetes and COVID-19.

PREVALENCE OF DIABETES IN CORONAVIRUS DISEASE 2019

A large number of studies across the globe have provided evidence suggesting high prevalence of diabetes in patients with COVID-19. **Table 1** summarizes prevalence data from several countries around the world.

TABLE 1: Data from several countries summarizes prevalence of diabetes in patients with COVID-19.

Author	Country	Sample size (*n*)	Diabetes prevalence (%)
Chinese Center for Disease Control and Prevention[1]	China	20,982	5.3
Center for Disease Control[2]	USA	7,162	10.9
Grasselli et al.[3]	Italy	1,043	17.3
Docherty et al.[4]	UK	20,133	20.7
Prieto–Alhambra et al.[5]	Spain	121,263	9.8
Bello–Chavolla et al.[6]	Mexico	51,633	18.3
Almazeedi et al.[7]	Kuwait	1,096	14.1
Bhandari et al.[8]	India	522	39.7

RELATIONSHIP BETWEEN CORONAVIRUS DISEASE 2019 AND DIABETES

With the growing data reporting poor clinical outcomes in patients with COVID-19 having diabetes and metabolic dysfunction, latest reports point in the opposite direction wherein COVID-19 infection also impacts diabetes outcomes, e.g., exacerbation of acute metabolic complications of diabetes such as diabetic ketoacidosis and hyperglycemia. There may be several mechanisms responsible for this bidirectional relationship between COVID-19 and diabetes; however, these remains to be fully elucidated. One possible mechanism might include the ubiquitous expression of angiotensin converting enzyme 2 (ACE2) receptor, a crucial receptor for attachment of the SARS-CoV-2, in several metabolic organs including the pancreas, and in β-cells in particular (**Box 1**). The potential of SARS-CoV-2 tropism for β-cells could lead to acute impairment of insulin secretion or damage of β-cells ultimately causing development of new-onset diabetes, or triggering hyperglycemia, and ketoacidosis. The SARS-CoV-2 infection also has potential to cause sustain hyperglycemia at hospital admission.[9] These outcomes along with new-onset diabetes, hyperglycemia at admission, and acute metabolic deterioration, in turn, can further worsen COVID-19 outcomes. The combined action of β-cell dysfunction, inflammatory cytokine storm, and counter-regulatory hormonal responses can trigger further acute metabolic complications (diabetic ketoacidosis or hyperglycemic hyperosmolar syndrome).

Bidirectional Relationship between Diabetes and Coronavirus Disease 2019 (Flowchart 1)

See **Flowchart 1**.

POTENTIAL MECHANISMS

Potential pathogenic mechanisms in patients with T2DM and COVID-19: There are multiple suggestive potential mechanisms in patients with T2DM and COVID-19. There is an increase observed in levels of inflammatory mediators like endotoxins [lipopolysaccharide (LPS)] and toxic metabolites in presence of infection with SARS-CoV-2. Over and above this, SARS-CoV-2 also increases reactive oxygen species (ROS) production and its activity.

Box 1: Mechanisms through which diabetes increases the SARS-CoV-2 morbidity and mortality.

- Increased cellular binding affinity and efficient viral entry
- Decreased viral clearance
- Reduced T-cell function
- Increased susceptibility to hyperinflammation and cytokine storm

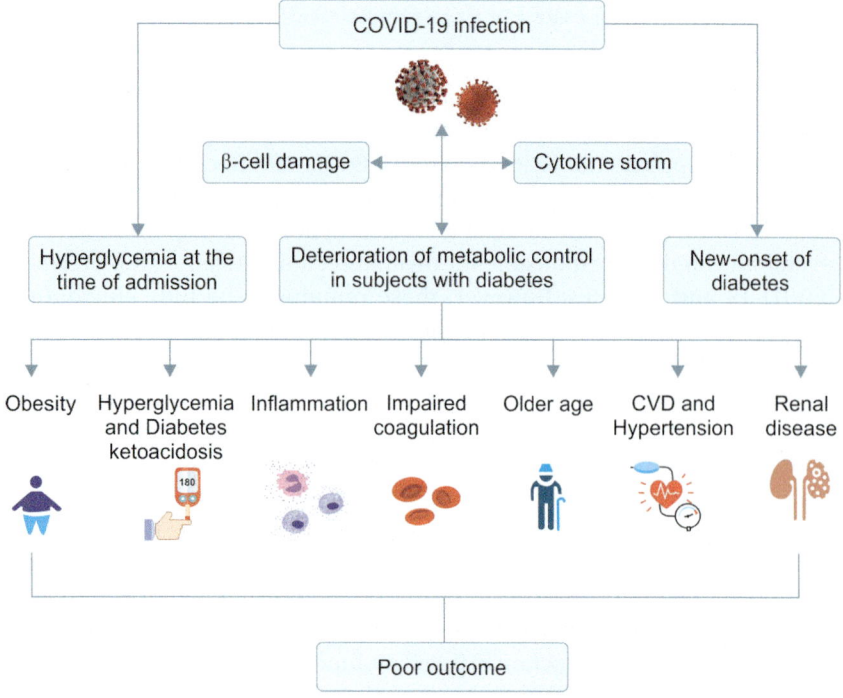

(COVID-19: coronavirus disease 2019; CVD: cardiovascular disease)

FLOWCHART 1: Bidirectional relationship between diabetes and COVID-19.
Source: Adapted from Apicella M, et al. Lancet Diabetes Endocrinol. 2020;8(9):782-92.

All this increase in inflammatory markers leads to a severe damage to lungs by lung fibrosis leading to acute respiratory distress syndrome (ARDS). Further, these inflammatory markers and viral activation of renin–angiotensin–aldosterone system (RAAS) causes insulin resistance, hyperglycemia, and vascular endothelial damage all of this further contributes to cardiovascular (CV) events, thromboembolism, and coagulation. This infection also leads to increase in clotting components, resulting in increased blood viscosity, vascular endothelial damage, further associated with CV events.

Infection with Severe Acute Respiratory Syndrome Coronavirus 2 (Flowchart 2)

Some patients with severe COVID-19 experience a cytokine storm, which is a dangerous and potentially life-threatening event. A retrospective study of 317 patients with laboratory-confirmed COVID-19 showed the presence of active inflammatory responses (IL-6 and lactate dehydrogenase) within 24 hours of hospital admission, which were correlated with disease severity. Several mechanisms have been proposed by which virally-induced inflammation increases insulin resistance. For example, in COVID-induced pneumonia, such as SARS and Middle East respiratory syndrome (MERS), inflammatory cells infiltrate the lungs, leading to acute lung injury, ARDS and/or death. This large burden of inflammatory cells can affect the functions of skeletal muscle

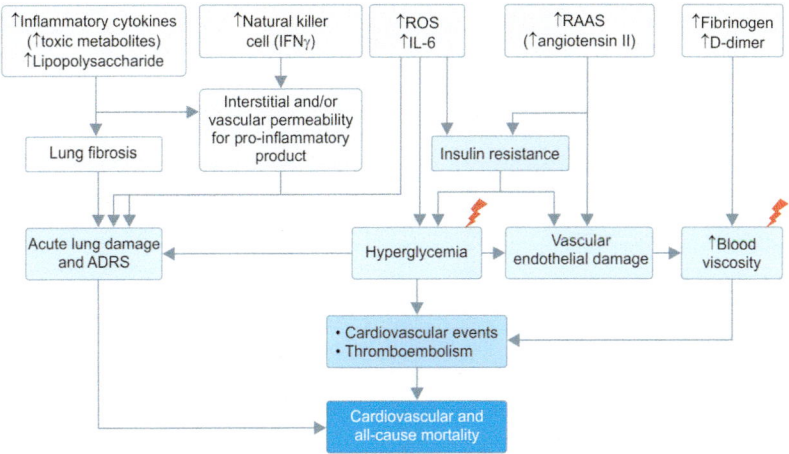

(IFN: interferon; IL: interleukin; RAAS: renin–angiotensin–aldosterone system; ROS: reactive oxygen species; SARS-CoV-2: severe acute respiratory syndrome coronavirus 2)

FLOWCHART 2: Infection with SARS-CoV-2.

and the liver, the major insulin-responsive organs that are responsible for the bulk of insulin-mediated glucose uptake.

IMMUNOMODULATION

It is recognized that mechanisms linking COVID-19 and both type 1 diabetes mellitus (T1DM) and T2DM overlap with pathways that regulate immune function. For example, age is the strongest risk factor for developing T2DM and the effect of ageing on immune function might be equally important for COVID-19 susceptibility and severity. Hyperglycemia can affect immune function; conversely, a dysregulated immunological status is linked to macrovascular complications of diabetes mellitus (DM). Thus, T2DM is associated with immunological dysregulation, which is potentially equivalent to accelerated ageing, and could therefore potentially explain the poor prognosis in patients with DM and COVID-19.

RENIN–ANGIOTENSIN–ALDOSTERONE SYSTEM

As a part of the RAAS, ACE2 has already received much attention as it can also serve as an entry receptor for SARS-CoV as well as SARS-CoV-2. ACE2 was initially reported to be predominantly expressed in the respiratory system. However, a more sophisticated study using immunohistochemical analyses found that ACE2 is expressed mainly in the intestines, kidneys, myocardium, vasculature, and pancreas, but expression is limited in the respiratory system. Evidence therefore suggests that ACE2 is expressed in many human cells and tissues, including pancreatic islets. Furthermore, infection with SARS-CoV can cause hyperglycemia in people without pre-existing DM. This finding and the localization of ACE2 expression in the endocrine pancreas together suggest that coronaviruses might specifically damages islets, potentially leading to hyperglycemia (**Flowchart 3**).

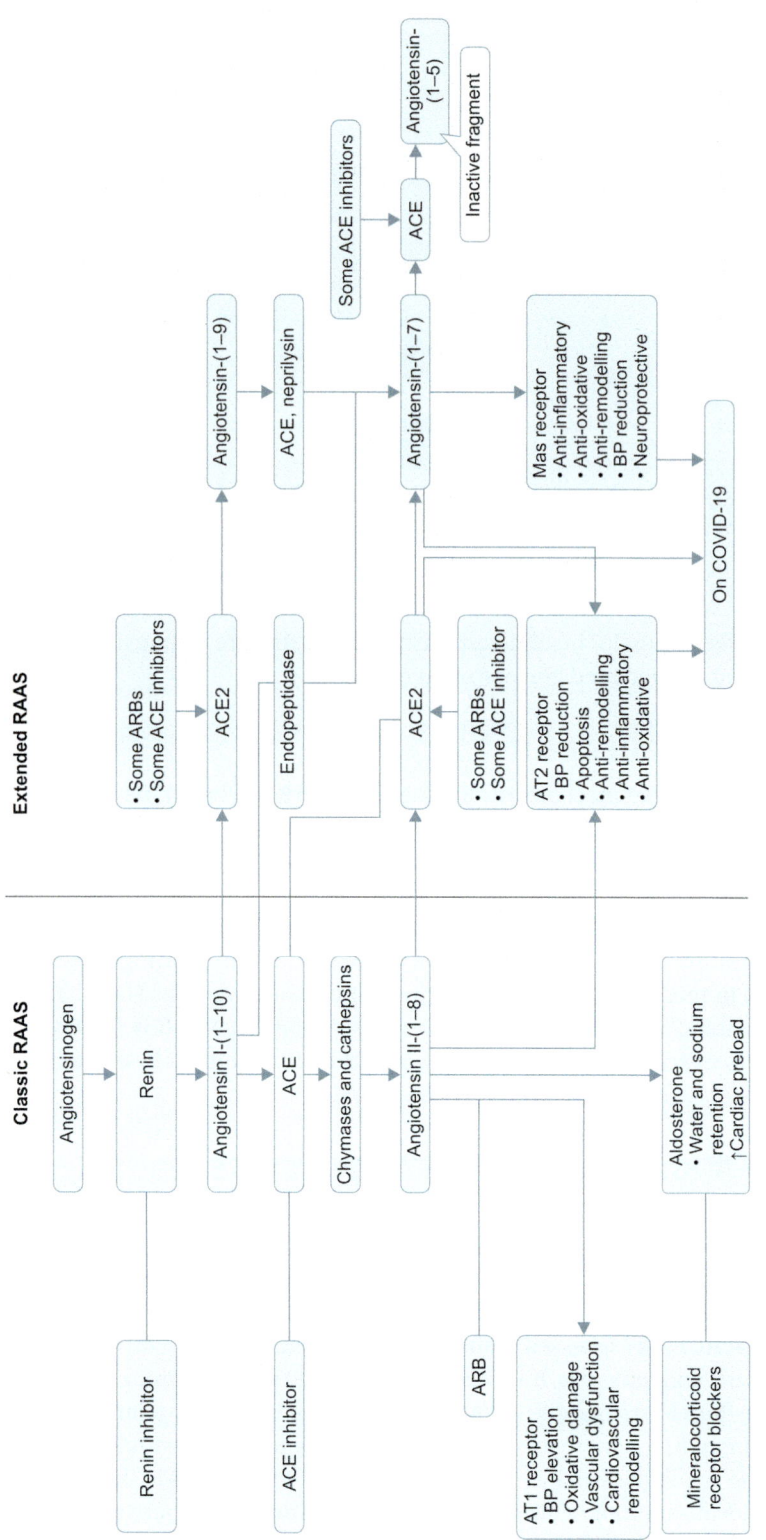

FLOWCHART 3: Renin–angiotensin–aldosterone system (RAAS).

(ACE: angiotensin-converting enzyme; ARB: angiotensin II receptor blockers)

INCREASED CORONAVIRUS DISEASE 2019 SEVERITY

There was increased diabetes prevalence observed in patient case scenarios admitted to intensive care units (ICUs) being critically ill because of COVID-19. The high prevalence rate suggests a clear link between severe COVID-19 and diabetes mellitus. The potential pathogenic mechanisms for this increased prevalence were already described, includes glucotoxicity, endothelial damage, oxidative stress, and cytokine storm lead to thromboembolic complications which further leads to damage to various vital organs. Furthermore the drugs used to treat COVID-19 might also deteriorate and worsen the hyperglycemic episode.

A multicenter retrospective study from China found that high fasting glucose levels (≥126 mg/dL) at admission was an independent predictor of increased mortality in patients with COVID-19 who did not have diabetes mellitus. Therefore, it is important to focus on glucose levels and to treat worsening hyperglycemia in patients with progression to severe states of COVID-19.

GLUCOSE-LOWERING DRUGS

Glucose-lowering medications commonly used to treat DM might have effects on COVID-19 pathogenesis and these effects could have implications for the management of patients with DM and COVID-19 (**Fig. 1**).

USE OF ANTIDIABETIC MEDICATIONS IN PATIENTS WITH TYPE 2 DIABETES MELLITUS AND CORONAVIRUS DISEASE 2019

Insulin is mainly recommended and used in critically ill patients with diabetes mellitus and also infected with SARS-CoV-2. Use of continuous insulin infusion for optimal glucose control can significantly reduce endotoxins and can improve COVID-19 severity. Metformin can only be used in uninfected or with mild COVID-19. It is not recommended to be used in critically ill patients. Similar recommendations are there for sulfonylureas and thiazolidinediones (TZDs). Dipeptidyl peptidase-4 (DPP-4) inhibitors with their established safety profile can be recommended for wide severity of COVID-19. Glucagon-like peptide-1 (GLP-1) analogs also comes with good safety profile and are recommended in patients with T2DM at the risk of comorbid situations of cardiovascular disease (CVD) and kidney disease. Mechanism of action of sodium-glucose cotransporter-2 (SGLT-2) inhibitors are such which potentiates risk factors for acute kidney injury (AKI) and ketoacidosis. As such, SGLT-2 inhibitors are not recommended in critically ill patients and are recommended to be withdrawn presurgery.

THROMBOEMBOLIC RISK IN PATIENTS WITH DIABETES MELLITUS

Several publications have reported an increased thromboembolic risk among patients with DM outside the specific situation of SARS-CoV-2 infection. For

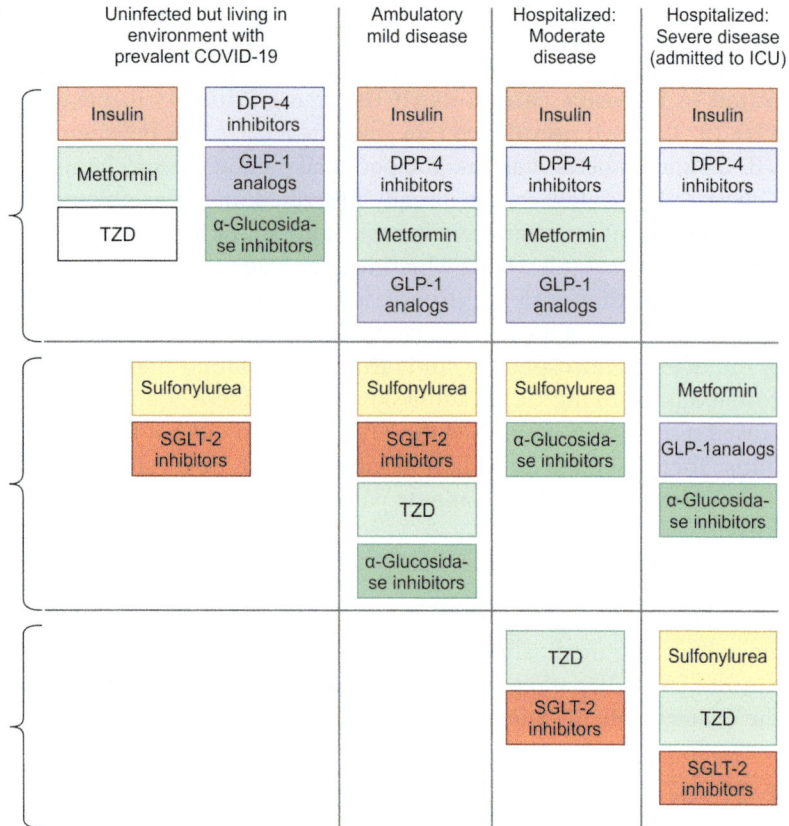

(DPP-4: dipeptidyl peptidase-4; GLP-1: glucagon-like peptide-1; SGLT-2: sodium-glucose cotransporter-2; TZD: thiazolidinediones)

FIG. 1: Glucose-lowering drugs.

example, a population-based study found that patients with T2DM exhibited an increased risk of venous thromboembolism compared with controls (HR1.44; 95% CI 1.27–1.63). Furthermore, the risks of pulmonary embolism were greater in the patients with T2DM than in the controls (HR 1.52; 95% CI 1.22–1.90).

To prevent such complications, patients with DM who are at risk of SARS-CoV-2 infection should try not to be sedentary for long periods, as regular physical activity is associated with decreased incidence of thromboembolism. Instead, these individuals should try to engage in physical activity to improve blood circulation. Antiplatelet or anticoagulant (low molecular weight heparin) is recommended to be used in addition in these patients to prevent the complications related to thromboembolic risk (mechanism discussed earlier).

CONCLUSION

In this pandemic situation, patients with DM should acknowledge the fact that COVID-19 may further lead to increase in blood glucose levels and more strict adherence to guidelines and treatment is recommended. A general guidance and recommendation for both physician and healthcare providers: Patients with DM should sincerely follow the prescribed medications and regularly monitor their blood glucose levels than earlier. At any point of time a consistently higher blood glucose levels posing risk of severity of disease, an immediate consultation with the physician is recommended. Healthcare providers on the other hand should give utmost priority to control the blood glucose levels by emphasizing more on diet and lifestyle modification. Patients experiencing dry cough, fever, sudden increase in blood glucose are suggested to immediately take opinion from their physician. A general precaution should be strictly followed by both patients and healthcare providers, such as using masks, physical distancing, regular washing of hands, and regular sanitization. These could be further ways to minimize the risk of SARS-CoV-2 transmission and at the same time provide continued and safe medical care to the general public.

REFERENCES

1. Epidemiology Working Group for Ncip Epidemic Response. The epidemiological characteristics of an outbreak of 2019 novel coronavirus diseases (COVID-19) in China. Chin J Epidemiol 2020;41(2):145e51.
2. Preliminary estimates of the prevalence of selected underlying health conditions among patients with coronavirus disease 2019—United States, February 12-march 28, 2020.CDC COVID-19 response team. https://www.cdc.gov/mmwr/volumes/69/wr/mm6913e2.htm.
3. Grasselli G, Zangrillo A, Zanella A, et al. Baseline characteristics and outcomes of 1591 patients infected with SARS-CoV-2 admitted to ICUs of the lombardy region. Italy. Jama 2020;6:6.
4. Docherty AB, Harrison EM, Green CA, Hardwick H, Pius R, Norman L, et al. Features of 20133 UK patients in hospital with COVID-19 using the ISARIC WHO Clinical Characterisation Protocol: prospective observational cohort study. BMJ 2020;369:m1985. https://doi.org/10.1136/bmj.m1985.
5. Preito-Alhambra D, Ballo E, Coma E, Mora N, Aragon M, Prats-Uribe A, et al. Hospitalization and 30-day fatality in 121,263 COVID-19 outpatient cases. medRxiv preprint, https://doi.org/10.1101/2020.05.04.20090050; 2020.
6. Bello-Chavolla OY, Bahena-Lopez JP, Antonio-Villa NE, Vargas-Vazquez A, Gonzalez-Diaz A, Mequez-Salinas A, et al. Predicting mortality due to SARS CoV-2: a mechanistic score relating obesity and diabetes to COVID-19 out comes in Mexico. J Clin Endocrinol Metab 2020;105(8):1e10.
7. Almazeedi S, Al-Youha S, Jamal MH, et al. Characteristics, risk factors and outcomes among the first consecutive 1,096 patients diagnosed with COVID 19 in Kuwait. Lancet EClinicalMedicine 2020. https://doi.org/10.1016/j.eclinm.2020.100448 [Epub ahead of print].
8. Bhandari S, Singh A, Sharma R. Characteristics, treatment outcomes and role of hydroxychloroquine among 522 COVID-19 hospitalized patients in Jaipur city: an epidemio-clinical study. J Assoc Phys India 2020;68(6):13e9.
9. Clark AL, RG Mirmira. SARS-CoV-2 infection of islet β cells: Evidence and implications. Cell Rep Med. 2021;2(8):100380. doi: 10.1016/j.xcrm.2021.100380.

26. Digital Outreach: Reaching the Unreached

S Arulrhaj, Aarathy Kannan, Chandra Sekar, Faizur Rahman, Manikandan

DIGITAL OUTREACH

WHAT IS DIGITAL HEALTH?
World Health Organization (WHO) defines as below:
- The use in the health sector of digital data-transmitted, stored, and retrieved electronically—in support of healthcare, both at the local site and at a distance (WHO 2003).
- Digital health is the convergence of the digital and genomic revolutions with health, healthcare, living, and society.
- Digital health is empowering people to better track, manage, and improve their own and their family's health, live better, more productive lives, and improve society.

TERMINOLOGIES
- e-Health
- m-Health
- i-Health
- TeleHealth
- Digital Health

TYPES OF DIGITAL HEALTH
Types of e-health: e-health has diverse applications including:
- *Electronic health records:* Patient data stored on computers enabling the communication of patient data between different healthcare professionals [general practitioners (GPs), specialists, etc.].
- *E-prescribing*: Prescription options, printed prescriptions, and sometimes electronic transmission of prescriptions from doctors to pharmacists.
- *Telemedicine*: Physical and psychological treatments provided over networks including telemonitoring of patients' functions.
- *Consumer health informatics*: Use of electronic medical resources by healthy individuals or patients.

- *Health knowledge management*: For example, providing an overview of latest medical journals, best practice guidelines, or epidemiological tracking (e.g., physician resources such as Medscape and MDLinx).
- *m-health*: Includes the use of mobile devices in collecting aggregate and patient-level health data; providing healthcare information to practitioners, researchers and patients, real-time monitoring of patient vitals, and direct provision of care via mobile telemedicine.
- *Medical research using grids*: Powerful computing and data management capabilities for handling large amounts of heterogeneous data.
- *Health care information systems*: Software solutions for appointment scheduling, patient data management, work schedule management, and other administrative tasks surrounding health.

WHY DIGITAL OUTREACH?
- Connecting care givers and patients-nullifies distance
- Round the clock monitoring
- Reduces travel and waiting
- Reduces cost
- Shortfall of health workforce (HWF) compensated
- Quality healthcare
- Uniform health system

Connecting Doctors with Patients

Challenges Facing Indian Healthcare
- *Missing five A's:* Availability, accessibility, affordability, acceptability and accountability.
- *Capacity:* Physical infrastructure, human resources, and financing medical care (**Table 1**).
- Low public sector spending 25–30% as compared to private sector.
- Very low per capita healthcare spent (US$ 50 as compared to US$ 250 in China and US$ 850 in Brazil).
- *Low healthcare insurance penetration*: 7–8% only.

TABLE 1: Health infrastructure in India in comparative with WHO.		
	WHO	India
Doctor	1/1,000 population	1/1,600 population
Doctor patient ratio	1:1,600	• 1:1,700 urban area • 1:25,000 rural area
Beds	1.9/1,000 population	0.9/1,000 population
Patient bed ratio	0.9 bed/1,000	0.3 bed/1,000
Nurses	2.4 million	3.72 lakhs/10.43 lakhs
Patient nurses ratio	1.25 nurses for every 1,000 people	0.17 nurses for every 1,000 people

HOW TO MATCH?

How Humans Adapted to Technology?
- Over 860 million individuals worldwide are suffering from chronic diseases.
- Chronic diseases are representing 63% of all annual deaths.
- Up to 80% of healthcare costs are related to chronic diseases.

Benefits to Patients
- Easy access to specialized healthcare services by rural, underserved, semiurban, and in remote areas.
- Early diagnosis and quick treatment.
- Reduced visits to specialty hospitals.
- Reduced travel expenses.
- Reduced burden of morbidity.

DOCTOR IN YOUR POCKET

Benefits to Healthcare Professionals
- Providing services to as many patients as possible
- Extend specialist resources to more locations
- *Convenience:* Doctor can be located anywhere
- Quick and timely follow up of patients getting discharged

DOCTORS MOBILITY RESTORED

Access to Continuing Medical Education (Fig. 1)

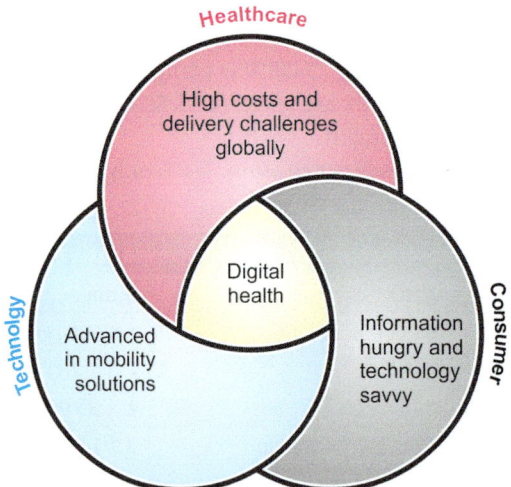

FIG. 1: Digital Health—Advantages.

Typical Telemedicine System (Figs. 2 and 3)

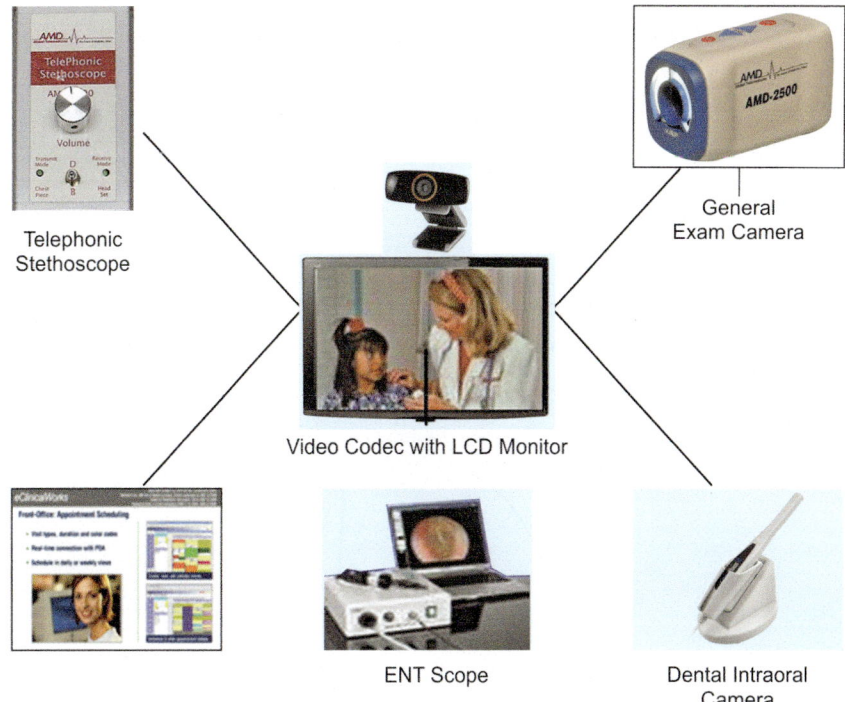

FIG. 2: Typical telemedicine system.

HOW m-HEALTH WORKS?
- *Wireless*—health, pulse, blood pressure (BP), O_2, blood stained liquor (BSL), temperature, weight, Treadmill Stress Test (TMT), pulmonary function test (PFT), walking, medication tracking
- *Devices*—body sensor, home sensor, and medical sensors
- Devices—Bluetooth/USB mobiles, i-pad and computertele health center health hub
- *What services*—emergencies, pregnancy status, rural health, and primary care.
- Hospitals/lab networking and Electronic Patient Record (EPR).

PHYSICIANS TOUCH CANNOT BE ELIMINATED
India initiatives in digital health outreach (**Table 2**).
- *Emergency Management and Research Institute (EMRI)*—innovative emergency response model
- *Health Management and Research Institute (HMRI)*—remote advice and mobile solutions

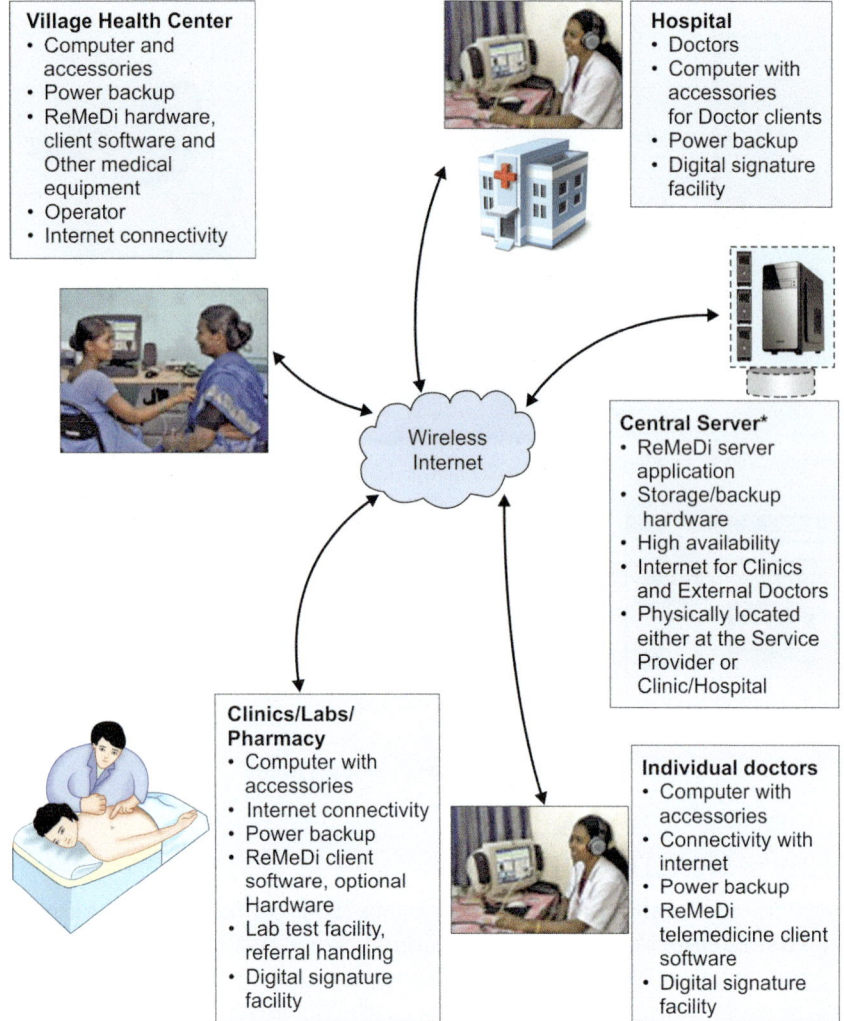

*Computer based data backup system which provides required information to the doctors about the patients which can be assessed from any location.

FIG. 3: Comprehensive rural e-healthcare network.

- *Aravind Eye*—low cost eye-care model leveraging telemedicine-diabetic retinopathy
- *Mobile based high-risk expectant mothers tracking system*—dropped by 93% and this is not enough
- The National Optical Fiber Network (NOFN) is a project to provide broadband connectivity to over 2 lakh (200,000) *Gram Panchayats* of India at a cost of ₹ 20,000 crore ($4 billion).
- Various categories of applications like e-health, e-education, and e-governance, etc., can also be provided by these operators.

TABLE 2: India initiatives in digital health outreach.	
eDhanwanthari—rural telemedicine facility (www.edhanwanthari.in):	mDhanwanthari—mobile telemedicine system:
• Connects rural/community hospitals with tertiary/speciality hospitals, along with videoconferencing • Interface of biomedical equipments with system • Creation, storage, and uploading of patient records • Supports telepathology, teleradiology, telecardiology, teleophthalmology, and tele-education • Deployed at eight PHC/CHCs and four specialty hospitals in Kerala • Accessible to 1.70 lakhs people in Tirur taluk of Kerala	• A unique system with its compact design that enables easy reach to rural location • Van integrated with medical equipments, i.e., X-ray, ultrasound, hematology analyzer, ECG with a suitable power back-up, and communication setup • Useful for early detection of diseases like TB, diabetes, and hypertension • Health awareness through video screening • Deployed at 22 locations of Cherthala taluk of Kerala • Accessible to 4.4 lakhs people of the taluk

- Pilots tried in seven states and National rollout in March 2014. Specialist care to villages (**Figs. 4** to **8**).

TELEMEDICINE—DEFINITION BY WORLD HEALTH ORGANIZATION AND MEDICAL COUNCIL OF INDIA

The delivery of health care services, where distance is a critical factor, by all health care professionals using information and communication technologies for the exchange of valid information for diagnosis, treatment, and prevention of disease and injuries, research and evaluation, and for the continuing education of health care providers, all in the interests of advancing the health of individuals and their communities.

TELEHEALTH

The delivery and facilitation of health and health-related services including medical care, provider and patient education, health information services, and selfcare via telecommunications and digital communication technologies.

Application Programming Interface Telemedicine Guidelines and Summary

- Application programming interface (API) supports the promotion and expanded role of telemedicine as a method of health care delivery that enhances patient-physician collaborations; improve health outcomes, increase access to care and members of a patient's health care team, and reduce medical costs—travel time when utilized as a component of a patient's all round as well as longitudinal care.

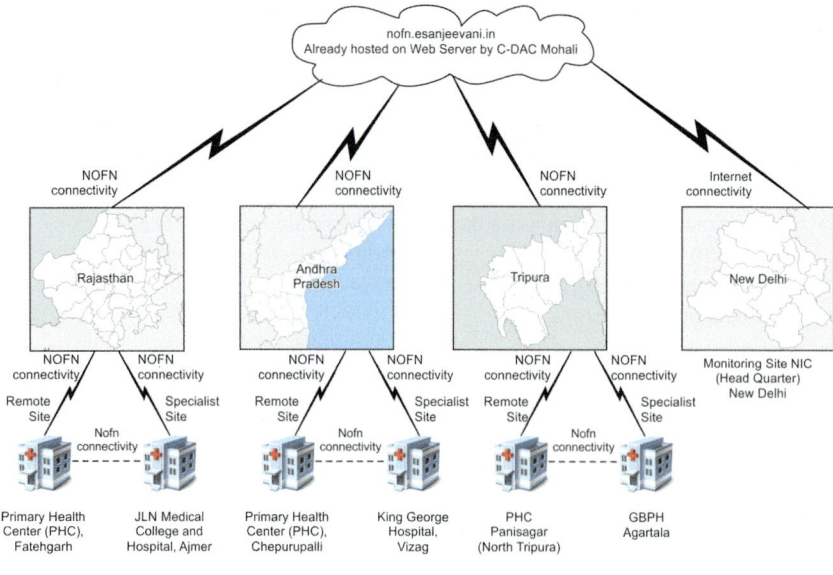
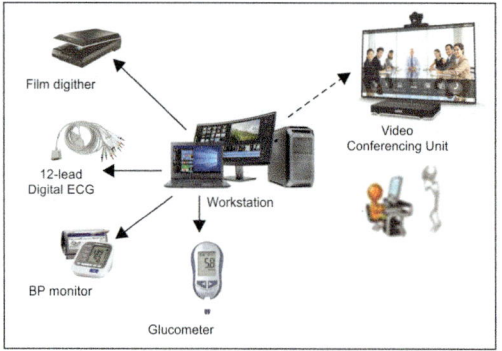

(NIC: National Informatics Centre; NOFN: National Optical Fibre Network)

FIG. 4: Specialist care to villages.

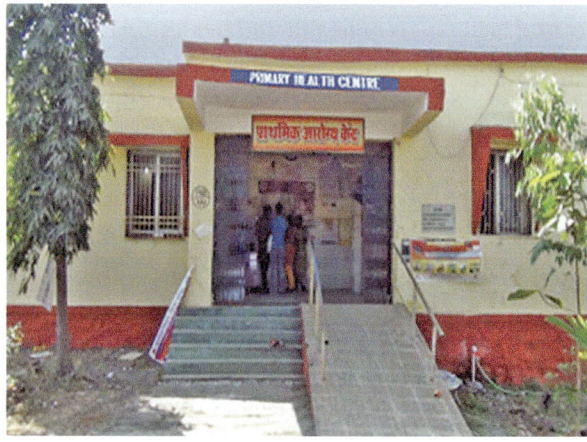

FIG. 5: m-Health Primary Health Center (PHC) Maharashtra.

Digital Outreach: Reaching the Unreached

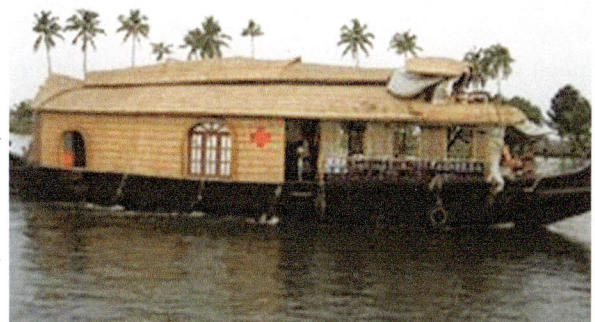

FIG. 6: Floating hospital, constructed by the state government under the National Rural Health Mission (NRHM).

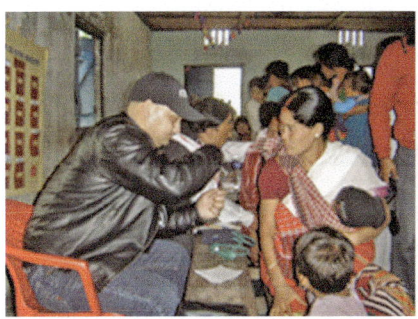 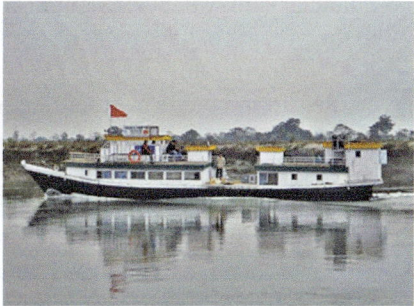

FIG. 7: Boat Clinic in ASSAM under National Rural Health Mission (NRHM).

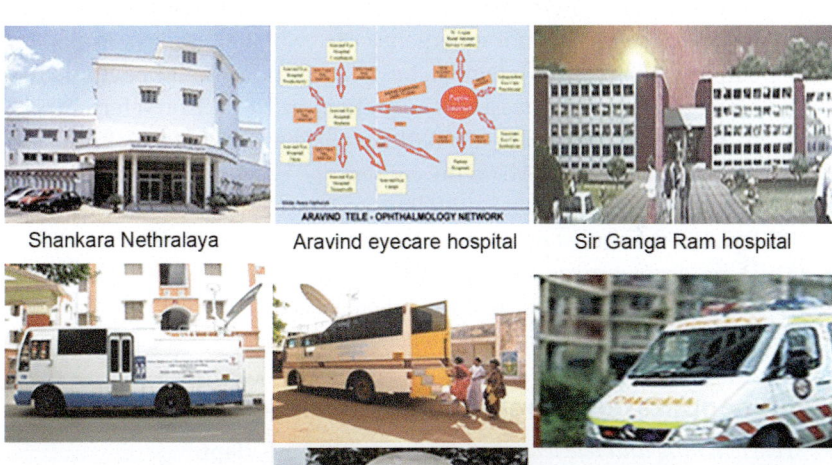

Shankara Nethralaya Aravind eyecare hospital Sir Ganga Ram hospital

Tele-Oncology Unit: Malabar Cancer Care Society Kannur, Kerala

FIG. 8: Mobile units teleophthalmology, mammography, and teleoncology.

- *Consent:* Patient consent is necessary for any telemedicine consultation. The consent can be implied or explicit depending on the following situations:
  - If the patient initiates the telemedicine consultation, then the consent is implied.
  - An explicit patient consent is needed, if: A health worker, registered medical practitioner (RMP), or a caregiver initiates a telemedicine consultation.

    An explicit consent can be recorded in any form. Patient can send an email, text, or audio/video message. Patient can state his/her intent on phone/video to the RMP (e.g., "Yes, I consent to avail consultation via telemedicine" or any such communication in simple words). The RMP must record this in his patient records.

    Ascertain age of patient, if required, with age proof; minor has to be accompanied with an adult parent or guardian.
- Data safety, data security and not sharing the personal information for financial gains or advertisements must be strictly prohibited by everyone in the process of telemedicine consultation.
- *For e-prescription*:
  - Registered medical practitioner can provide photo, scan, digital copy of a signed prescription, or e-prescription to the patient via email or any messaging platform.
  - Every RMP should display the registration number on the prescriptions and on the receipts, etc. given to patients.
- Emergency consult for immediate assistance or first aid, etc.
  - In case alternative care is not present, teleconsultation might be the only way to provide timely care. In such situations, RMPs may provide consultation to their best judgement. Telemedicine services should, however, be avoided for emergency care when alternative in-person care is available and telemedicine consultation should be limited to first aid, life-saving measure, counseling, and advice on referral.
  - In all cases of emergency, the patient must be advised for an in-person interaction with an RMP at the earliest.
- Therapy based telemedicine guidelines in 15 areas are identified by API.
- MEDICAL ethics must be strictly adhered to.
- Must be a structured teleconsultation—time of the day, duration, contents, recording, cost, etc. to avoid fake usage.
- Hippocrates touch cannot be replaced with telehealth.

Digital Application Programming Interface

- *Tele teaching and tele learning:* Listen, learn, and adapt.
- During COVID pandemic API was locked in.
- Member could not attend any meeting, conferences, clinic, etc.
- Science got stagnated. Patient not reachable.
- Then emerged digital API.
- Patient care through video conference/eSanjeevani app.
- All meetings both official and academic were on digital mode.

- Without boundaries physicians stated learning and exchanging knowledge.
- API-DIAS is one of the master continuing medical education (CME) of API. Became digital and reached to more than 100,000 physicians in India and South Asia region.
- APICON 2021 was conducted eAPICON2021 and all the faculties and members enjoyed the academic bonanza.

DIGITAL HEALTH REACHING THE UNREACHED

Healthcare

- Tele consultation
    - Voice call
    - Video call
    - Short message service (SMS)
    - Smart phone
    - First visit and follow up visits
    - Diagnosis made: E-prescription sent
    - Diet, physiotherapy, pills reminder
    - Visit reminder
    - Mental health counseling
    - Emergency consultant and guidelines are possible
    - During covid much needed
- Tele diagnosis
    - Tele X-ray, echocardiogram (ECG), computed tomography (CT) scan, echo biochemistry, etc.
    - Reality today
    - Coronary artery disease (CAD) over voice-vocal biomarkers
    - Heart failure (HF)—detection and monitoring
- Tele Monitoring
    - Based on sensor connectivity
    - Blood pressure, O_2, pulse rate, ECG BP, and blood sugar
    - Physical activity and diet, spirometry, and body composition
- Tele intervention/treatment
    - *ZOLL's LifeVest* is a wearable defibrillator worn by patients at risk of a heart attack. It monitors heart rhythms and in the event of a heart attack, releases conductive gel from its electrodes, and administers a life-saving electrical shock to restore normal heart rhythms.
    - Defibrillator-equipped drones could be first on scene in cardiac arrest.
    - A drone could get to a patient faster than emergency services and could increase survival rates.
    - Dispatching drones outfitted with defibrillators could cut response times and increase survival rates during cardiac arrest. Currently, only 10% of people survive a cardiac arrest that occurs outside a hospital (Ashley Burke/CBC).
    - Intracardiac catheter placement.

- Clinical outcome prediction-artificial intelligence.
- Electronic intensive care unit (eICU) a reality today.
- Therapy specific digital interventions
  - Cardiovascular diseases

Diagnostic	Therapeutics
• ECG—arrhythmias	• Detect dysrhythmia
• PA pressure—pre-LHF	• Defibrillator
• Lung fluid level—LHF	• HTN
• Pulse oximeter—hypoxia	• Hypotension
• BP—low or high BP	• Early cardiac failure
• Diet	
• Walking	
• Sleep	
• PFT	
• Drugs—remainder and adherence	

  - Diabetes

Monitor	Treatment
• Blood glucose	• Artificial pancreas
• BP	• Hypoglycemia
• Diet	• Cardiac arrhythmias
• Physical activities	
• Drugs—remainder and adherence	
• Walking	
• Drug administration	
• Sleep	

Medical Education

Tele learning/teaching.

Tele learning:
- e-Learning is used increasingly in health care to support the delivery of learning in outcome-based education. Broadly speaking, eLearning is considered to be the application and integration of educational technology to the learning process.
- Webinars, discussions, conference and eAPICON2021, and structured course—universities

E-medical education:
- Digital universities—permitted by UGC
- Statutory universities can add online university
- Webinars, conferences, and meeting are digital today
- Online classes for all students during COVID pandemic

Digital medical schools with skill labs are not far of:
- IMA eVarsity—2013
- University affiliated online courses
  - Certificate

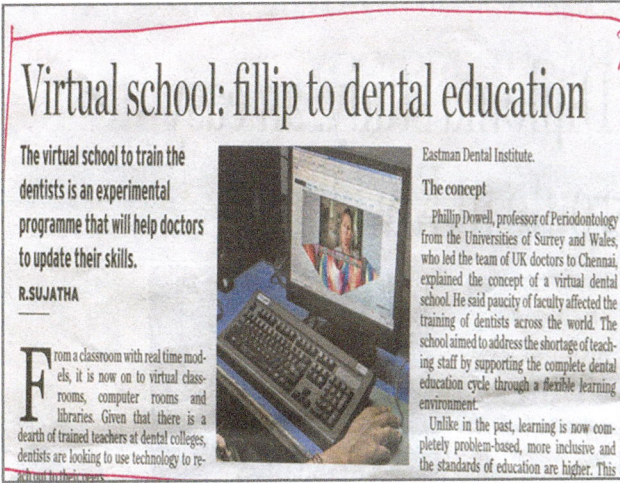

FIG. 9: Virtual school.

- ○ Fellowship
- ○ Diploma
- Virtual classroom teaching
  Commonwealth medical eVarsity launched on 13th October, 2015 (**Fig. 9**)

Future of Digital Outreach
- Pharmacogenomics
- Nutrigenomics
- Doctors inside
- Artificial intelligence
- Internet of things (IOT)
- Digital 3-dimension (3D) imaging

Digital outreach: Healthcare reaching the unreached
Medical knowledge reaching the unreached

SUGGESTED READINGS
1. WHO. Telehealth [Internet]. World Health Organization. [cited 2018 Dec 02]. Available from: https://apps.who.int/iris/bitstream/handle/10665/344249/9789240020924-eng.pdf
2. Teleophthalmology. Aravind Eye Care System [Internet]. Aravind.org. [cited 2019 Jan 20]. Available from: https://www.ncbi.nlm.nih.gov/pmc/articles/PMC6618173/
3. CENSUS OF INDIA. (2012). GOI. [online] Available from: http://censusindia.gov.in/2011-prov-results/paper2/data_files/india/Rural_Urban_2011.pdf [Last accessed August, 2021].
4. Ministry of External Affairs, Government of India. [online] Available from: http://www.mea.gov.in/ [Last accessed August, 2021].
5. Doctor patient ratio in India [Internet]. 164.100.47.190. 2018 [cited 2018 Dec 01]. Available from: https://www.ncbi.nlm.nih.gov/pmc/articles/PMC6259525/
6. Ministry of health and family welfare, Govt of India. National telemedicine portal. Telemedicine division. [online] Available from: http://nmcn.in/ [Last accessed August, 2021].

27. Asthma, Biologics, and Clinical Pharmacology

Shambo S Samajdar, Arijit Kayal, Shashank R Joshi

INTRODUCTION

Recent findings in last decade showed that asthma is not a single disease entity rather a collection of different conditions with overlapping symptomatology but diverse etiologies.[1] It is now important to identify the subphenotypes of asthma based on clinical, functional, or inflammatory parameters.[2-5] Diagnosis of asthma can be done by clinical history of cough, shortness of breath, and chest tightness, along with pulmonary function tests showing increased airway hyper-reactivity or reversible airflow limitation. In common practice, the asthma patients are characterized by the presence or absence of type 2 (T2) inflammations in the airways.

The inflammation of the airway mediated by eosinophils can occur in two different ways, allergic and nonallergic. The underlying pathogenesis of allergic asthma includes immunoglobulin E (IgE) switching of B-cells and mucous hypersecretion which is triggered by production of various interleukins (IL-4, IL-5, and IL-13), after allergens are presented to CD4+ T-cells with the help of dendritic cells. While in nonallergic eosinophilic asthma, antigen-independent activation of innate lymphoid cells (ILCs), mediated by IL-33, IL-25, and thymic stromal lymphopoietin (TSLP) via their specific receptors.

Type 2 inflammation is associated with expression of airway epithelial cell (*AEC*) gene signature which is contributory to atopy, eosinophilia, and high fractional exhaled nitric oxide (FeNO) observed in asthma. This is mainly mediated by eotaxin-3 (*CCL26*), a gene included in the *AEC* gene signature, and also an eosinophil chemokine.[6-8] *CCL26* gene expression in AECs is upregulated by IL-13 that results in eotaxin-3 hypersecretion and airway eosinophilia.[9] Maturation of eosinophilia is dependent on presence of IL-5 (**Fig. 1**).[10]

In childhood-onset allergic asthma and adult-onset nonallergic asthma, eosinophils are the predominant granulocytes involved that are upregulated on allergen exposure in two phase response. Degranulation of mast cells occurs in early phase followed by secondary infiltration of cells in the airways in late phase response.[11-14] Damage to the epithelial lining of airways, edema, increased production of mucus from goblet cells, and exaggerated response of bronchial muscles is mediated by proteins like major basic protein,

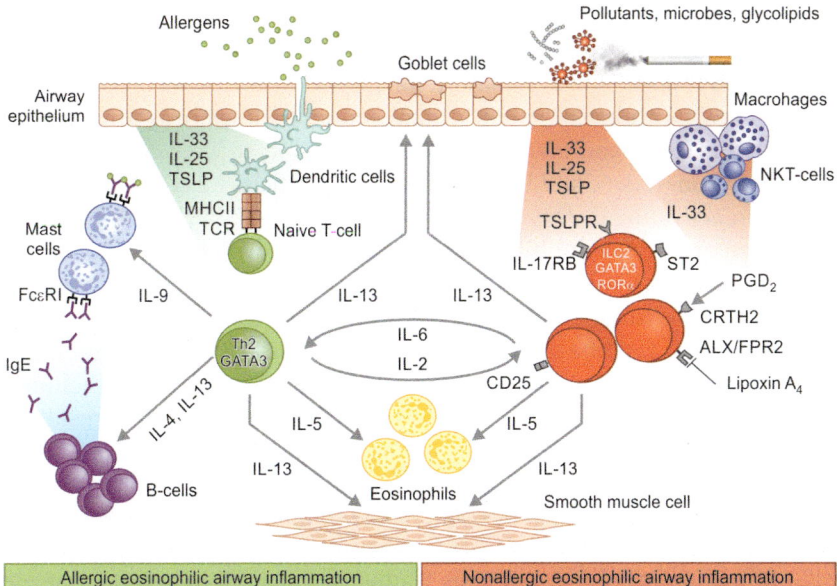

(FPR2: formyl peptide receptor 2; IL: interleukin; MHC: major histocompatibility complex; NKT: natural killer T; TSLP: thymic stromal lymphopoietin; CRTH2: chemoattractant receptor homologous molecule expressed on Th2 cells; ALX/FPR2: receptor for lipoxin A4; FcεRI: high-affinity receptor for IgE; GATA3: GATA-binding protein 3; PG: prostaglandin; ROR: retinoic acid receptor-related orphan receptor; NK: natural killer; MHC: major histocompatibility complex; TCR: T-cell receptor.)

FIG. 1: Showing the two different pathways that lead to inflammation in asthma. The left hand side shows allergic asthma where dendritic cells presents allergen to CD4+ T cells, thus inducing T- helper (Th)2 cells which again produce Interleukin IL-4, IL-5, IL-13 that causes IgE switching in B-cells, airway eosinophilia and mucous hypersecretion. The right hand side shows nonallergic eosinophilic asthma, air pollutants, microbes and glycolipids induce the release of epithelium-derived cytokines, including IL-33, IL-25 and thymic stromal lymphopoietin (TSLP) these leads to activation of innate lymphoid cells (ILCs) in an antigen-independent manner this happens via their respective receptors, i.e., IL-17 receptor B (IL-17RB), ST2 and TSLP receptor (TSLPR). Activated ILC2s leads to production of high amounts of IL-5 and IL-13 which leads to eosinophilia, mucus hypersecretion and airway hyperreactivity.

Source: de Groot JC, Ten Brinke A, Bel EH. Management of the patient with eosinophilic asthma: a new era begins. ERJ open research. 2015 May 1;1(1).

eosinophil cationic protein, neurotoxin, peroxidize, and other cytotoxic products released on degranulation of eosinophils.[14]

The association of genotype, phenotype, and endotype (i.e., underlying mechanism) is complex involving various factors of host and its interaction with the environment. An association between IL-33, human leukocyte antigen (HLA)-DQ, SMAD3, and IL2RB9 polymorphism and chromosome 17q21 having genes *ZPBP2*, *GSDMB*, and *ORMDL3* has been observed in asthmatic-population.[7,8] These genes were associated with dysregulation of both innate and adaptive immune responses along with epithelial barrier dysfunction seen in asthma.

Approximately, half of asthmatic adults have eosinophilic T2 airway inflammation.[15,16] However, its actual prevalence may be higher as suggested by presence of eosinophilic inflammation of airways in patients on corticosteroid withdrawal. Atopy is more common in severe asthma among children and childhood-onset asthmatic adults.[15,16]

Interleukin-4, IL-5, and IL-13 are formed by T helper 2 cells in presence of certain activating factors like epithelium-derived TSLP. This is followed by movement of eosinophils to the lung mucosa which is mediated via chemoattractants like C-C motif chemokine receptor 3 chemokines.[17]

In allergic eosinophilic asthma, B-cell switching and IgE synthesis is mediated by IL-4. While in nonallergic eosinophilic asthma, IL-5 and IL-13 are produced by ILCs in response to prostaglandin D2 and epithelium-derived alarmin, and IL-33, IL-25, and TSLP are released as a result of pollutants and microbes-induced epithelial damage.

Adult-onset asthma is more of eosinophilic phenotype as compared to childhood-onset asthma. While females are more commonly affected by adult asthma, eosinophilic asthma has no such gender predisposition.[18-21] Allergic symptoms are common in adults with asthma than in late-onset eosinophilic asthma.[18,21,22] Raised levels of total IgE, in absence of allergic symptoms may be attributed to hidden allergens like superantigens.[23,24] Increased sensitivity to aspirin has also been associated with late-onset eosinophilic asthma.[18,25] Late-onset eosinophilic asthma has a more severe disease course than noneosinophilic asthma.[26,27]

Level of eosinophils in sputum[28] and bronchial biopsies[29] has a positive correlation with severity as well as prognosis of asthma. High levels are associated with poor control, more severe exacerbations, and higher risk of being intubated.[30,31] Chronic rhinosinusitis and nasal polyposis are frequently associated with late-onset eosinophilic asthma.[32] Association between eosinophilia in peripheral blood, history of polyp, and asthma is well established, and could also linked to increased sensitivity to aspirin.[33-36]

The pathogenesis of noneosinophilic asthma is not well established. Neutrophilic predominance observed in these cases could be primarily attributed to macrophage activation and release of chemokines, or could be due to bacterial colonization observed in presence of other comorbid conditions.

DIAGNOSIS OF ASTHMA

History and physical examination are crucial in diagnosing asthma. Proper assessment of the type of asthma should be done by a specialist for a target-based approach to treatment.

Absence or <15 years of smoking history and absence of any occupational exposures, usually rules out chronic obstructive pulmonary disease (COPD), and other diagnosis should be considered. Eosinophilic asthma can taken into consideration, if there is history of nasal polyps or recurrent polypectomy surgeries.[37,38] Recurrent exacerbations on steroid withdrawal indicates steroid dependency which is also observed in eosinophilic asthma.[39,40]

Diagnosis of eosinophilic asthma can be done by sputum analysis.[5,41] However, appropriate sample collection is sometimes not feasible, so alternative tests like peripheral blood eosinophils, exhaled FeNO fraction, and serum IgE can be considered.[42-44] The results show that overall blood eosinophils, although FeNO, and IgE are only moderately accurate in predicting airway eosinophilia, FeNO when combined with blood eosinophils were better predictors of asthma than total IgE alone.[45] In a study, eosinophils $<0.09 \times 10^9$ L^{-1} was found to be highly predictive of no airway eosinophilia in majority of subjects. Also, similar percentage of subjects showed sputum eosinophils >3% with >0.41×10^9 L^{-1} eosinophil level.[45] Hence, blood eosinophilia is considered as the most useful surrogate marker to detect airway eosinophilia.[46,47]

BIOMARKERS IN SEVERE ASTHMA

Biomarkers can play a decisive role in selecting the biologics and predict their responsiveness. For instance, baseline blood eosinophilic count in severe eosinophilic asthma along with exacerbations can predict response to anti-IL-5 therapy. Response to omalizumab in severe allergic asthma can be predicted using total serum IgE level. Blood eosinophil counts is also a good biomarker to predict clinical efficacy of steroids in children. Sputum eosinophil count is a better outcome predictor of steroid therapy. FeNO (>19.5 ppb) and blood eosinophil count (>260 per µL) can be correlated with response to treatment in terms of reduction in incidence of asthma exacerbations (**Table 1**).

BIOLOGICS APPROVED GLOBALLY

Anti-immunoglobulin E Therapy (Omalizumab)

Omalizumab is a recombinant, DNA-derived humanized IgG1 k antibody that binds to the Fc region of IgE and blocks its binding to the high-affinity IgE receptor, FcεR1 (**Table 2**). Omalizumab reduces free IgE by 96%,[48-52] but total IgE levels increase after the first injection because of omalizumab: IgE complex formation. It is associated with less incidence of wheal and flare reactions and late allergic responses by down-regulating FcεRI receptors and basophils.[53]

Anti-interleukin-5 Therapy (Mepolizumab, Reslizumab, and Benralizumab)

Mepolizumab and reslizumab act by binding and destructing IL-5 cytokines that leads to decreased eosinophilia and airway inflammation, though exact mechanism is not well understood.[54,55] Benralizumab promotes eosinophilic destruction by binding to the alpha chain of IL-5 receptor in an irreversible manner and leads to near complete reduction in eosinophilia.[56,57] Response to treatment with these biologics can be better predicted from baseline status of eosinophilia in blood than sputum.[58]

TABLE 1: Biological markers commonly used in asthma.

	Association with treatment response	Invasiveness	Comments
FeNO	Corticosteroids, anti-interleukin-13, anti-interleukin-4 and anti-interleukin-13, and anti-IgE	Noninvasive	Easy, quick, not specific, cheap, and generally available; loses specificity in smokers[*]
Serum IgE	No association	Minimal	Although recommended, no clear association has been identified between IgE or allergy as a biomarker of treatment responses or clinical outcome[**]
Serum periostin	Anti-interleukin-13 and anti-IgE	Minimal	Effect shown with anti-interleukin-13, poor availability; confounded by growth in childhood, pregnancy, and dental disease
Blood eosinophil count	Oral corticosteroids and anti-interleukin-5	Minimal	Generally available, high clinical impact, predicts anti-interleukin-5 response[12] and response to inhaled corticosteroids in chronic obstructive pulmonary disease; associated with increased risk of lung attacks[***]
Sputum eosinophil count	Corticosteroids and anti-interleukin-5	Moderate	Available at specialist centers, tissue specific, time-consuming; good therapeutic marker for inhaled corticosteroids, oral corticosteroids, and biological drugs; established evidence of value as a monitoring tool

[*]Ahovuo-Saloranta A, Csonka P, Lehtimäki L. Basic characteristics and clinical value of FeNO in smoking asthmatics-a systematic review. Journal of breath research. 2019;13(3):034003. https://doi.org/10.1088/1752-7163/ab0ece.

[**]Korn S, Haasler I, Fliedner F, Becher G, Strohner P, Staatz A, Taube C, Buhl R. Monitoring free serum IgE in severe asthma patients treated with omalizumab. Respiratory medicine. 2012;106(11), 1494–1500. https://doi.org/10.1016/j.rmed.2012.07.010.

[***]Nakagome K, Nagata M. Involvement and possible role of eosinophils in asthma exacerbation. Frontiers in immunology. 2018;9:2220.

Anti-interleukin-4 and Anti-interleukin-13 Therapy (Dupilumab)

The dupilumab monoclonal antibody binds the IL-4 receptor a chain (IL-4Ra), blocking both IL-4 and IL-13 receptors and their signaling

TABLE 2: List of biologics approved for use in asthma along with their common adverse effects.

Drug	Indication	Dose	Frequency	Adverse effects
Omalizumab	Moderate-severe persistent asthma uncontrolled by ICS in ages 6 years positive for perennial aeroallergens	75–375 mg, SC, (dose is weight dependent)	2 or 4 weekly	• BBW: Anaphylaxis • 10%: Injection site reaction • 0.5%: Malignancies • 1–10%: Cardiovascular, dermatologic and neuromuscular effects
Mepolizumab	Add-on maintenance treatment for severe asthma in ages ≥12 years with eosinophilic phenotype	100 mg, SC	4 weekly	• 5%: headache, injection site reaction, back pain and fatigue • 3%: pruritus, eczema, muscle spasms and abdominal pain
Reslizumab	Add-on maintenance treatment for severe asthma in adults with eosinophilic phenotype	3mg/kg, IV infusion	4 weekly	• BBW: Anaphylaxis • 5%: Antibody development • 3%: Oropharyngeal pain
Benralizumab	Add-on maintenance treatment for severe asthma in ≥12 years with an eosinophilic phenotype	30 mg, SC	First three injections 4 weekly, then 8 weekly	Headache, pharyngitis and injection-site reactions
Dupilumab	Add-on maintenance treatment for moderate-to-severe asthma in >12 years with eosinophilic phenotype or with corticosteroid dependent asthma	400/600 mg SC loading dose followed by 300 mg SC alternate week	2 weekly	10%: Injection site reactions and conjunctivitis

(BBW: black box warning; ICS: inhaled corticosteroid; SC: subcutaneous)

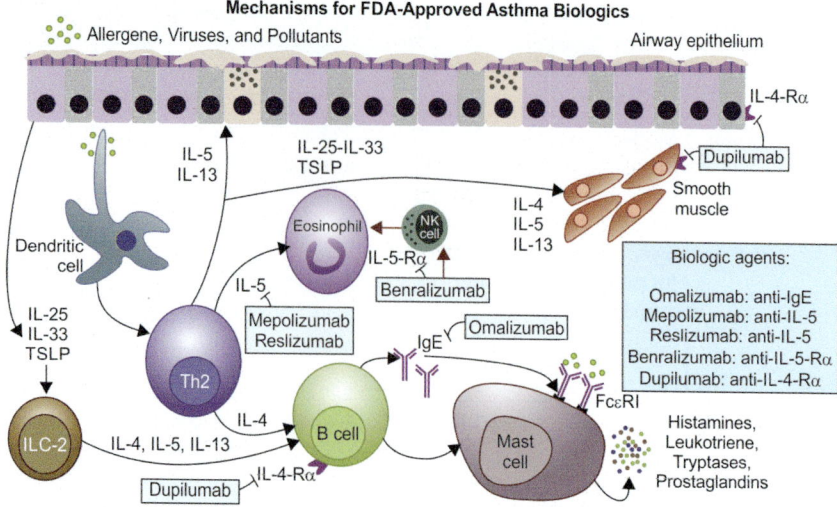

FIG. 2: Mechanism how biologics act on each of the pathway of airway inflammation thus preventing development of asthma.

(FDA: Food and Drug Administration; IL: interleukin; TSLP: thymic stromal lymphopoietin)

pathway.[1,38] Positive response to treatment with either IL-4 or IL-13 cytokines when used alone is unlikely due to biological redundancy of involved mechanism (**Fig. 2**) (**Table 3**).[59-61]

REDUCTION IN EXACERBATION WITH CURRENTLY USED BIOLOGICS

Treatment with omalizumab in symptomatic asthmatic patients who were being treated with medium- to high-dose ICS therapy could lead to reduction in the dose of ICS. This was observed in phase III trials conducted on patients aged 12–75 years. Moreover, exacerbations also reduced by 48% and 41% compared to placebo treated group.[53,62] Mepolizumab treatment was also associated with decreased incidence of exacerbations in a 3-arm phase II trial on patients receiving 75, 250, and 750 mg intravenous (IV) doses (reduction by 48%, 39%, and 52%, respectively, relative to placebo). The patients (12–74 years) were already on high-dose ICS use with atleast one of the following features: eosinophil in sputum ≥ 3%, FeNO ≥ 50 ppb, eosinophils in blood ≥ 300 cells/mL, or worsening of asthma after ≤ 25% decrease in maintenance steroids.[6]

Similarly, reslizumab reduced the incidence of exacerbations by 50–59% in two different phase III studies involving patients (12–75 years) on medium to high doses of ICS with an eosinophilic count ≥ 400 cells/mL blood and ≥1 asthma exacerbation in the previous year. Dupilumab treated groups have also experienced reduction in incidence of asthma exacerbations over 12-week treatment and 8-week follow up period, relative to placebo.

TABLE 3: Dosing and indication of commonly used biologics in asthma.

Drug	Indication	Dosing
Omalizumab	Add-on maintenance treatment for moderate-to-severe persistent asthma in those aged 6 years or older with a positive skin test or in vitro reactivity to a perennial aeroallergen and symptoms that are inadequately controlled with inhaled corticosteroids	75–375 mg SC every 2 or 4 weeks[a]
Mepolizumab	Add-on maintenance treatment of patients with severe asthma aged 6 years and older, and with an eosinophilic phenotype. Treatment of adult patients with eosinophilic granulomatosis with polyangiitis	100 mg SC every 4 weeks (patients aged 12 years and older); 40 mg SC every 4 weeks (patients aged 6 to 11 years)[b]
Reslizumab	Add-on maintenance treatment of patients with severe asthma, aged 18 years and older with an eosinophilic phenotype	3 mg/kg IV every 4 weeks
Benralizumab	Add-on maintenance treatment of patients with severe asthma aged 12 years and older with an eosinophilic phenotype	30 mg SC every 4 weeks 3 doses, then every 8 weeks
Dupilumab	Add-on maintenance treatment in patients with moderate-to-severe asthma aged 12 years and older with an eosinophilic phenotype or with oral corticosteroid dependent asthma	400 or 600 mg (two injections) SC followed by 200 or 300[c] mg every other week

Note: [a]Dose and frequency are determined by serum total IgE level (IU/mL) pretreatment and body weight (kg).
[b]Treatment for eosinophilic granulomatosis with polyangiitis is 300 mg as three separate 100 mg injections administered subcutaneously once every 4 weeks.
[c]300 mg (600-mg initial) dose is indicated for those with oral corticosteroid dependent asthma or with atopic dermatitis.

(SC: subcutaneous)

IMPROVEMENTS IN LUNG FUNCTION AND SYMPTOM SCORES

In the above mentioned studies, FEV1 improved from 68 to 72.5% in omalizumab-treated group and to 69% in the placebo group.[62-64] Also, there was an improvement of 98 mL and 100 mL from baseline in the subcutaneous (SC) and IV mepolizumab-treated groups, respectively when compared to placebo group.[65]

Reslizumab in its two major phase III trials, reslizumab treatment improved prebronchodilator forced expiratory volume (FEV1) from baseline in comparison with placebo by +126 mL for study 1 and for study 2 +90 mL, and +100 mL for the pooled data.[66]

Benralizumab in the CALIMA trial, the eosinophil-high group demonstrated prebronchodilator FEV1 improvements of +125 and +116 mL with the q4w and q8w dosing regimens, respectfully, relative to placebo showing improvement. Benralizumab in long-term extension trial featuring participants of CALIMA and SIROCCO, the BORA trial showed that improvements in prebronchodilator FEV1 were roughly maintained after 1 year.[67]

Dupilumab in the phase 2A study, dupilumab improved prebronchodilator FEV1 by +270 mL and reduced ACQ-5 by 0.73 points, both relative to placebo.[64] The Sino-Nasal Outcome Test (SNOT-22) showed an −8.5-point change relative to placebo with better outcome than that of placebo.

WHEN TO START A BIOLOGIC AND WHICH ONE TO CHOOSE

The clinician's decision to initiate and choose a biologic is usually governed by current disease status and response to current treatment plan. The Global Initiative for Asthma (GINA) 2019 guidelines recommend biologics as step 4 therapy and lay down basic guiding principles.[68]

Treatment with dupilumab, mepolizumab, or benralizumab can be taken into consideration, if oral steroids is being used for maintenance phase.

Inclusion criteria for biologic studies:
- Predicted prebronchodilator FEV1 40–80%
- ≥1 exacerbation/year in patients being treated with moderate-to-high dose ICS.

Before initiating a biologics, few points needs to be taken care of.

Patient must be complaint with step 4 therapy in GINA with complete lung function test results and with >3 days course of oral steroid in previous year. Any comorbidities gastroesophageal reflux, obesity must be identified and treated. Asthma-mimicking conditions like vocal cord dysfunction, COPD, and bronchiectasis must be excluded.

Only omalizumab and mepolizumab are currently approved for use in children < 12 years. While safety of omalizumab in children is almost established and mepolizumab has shown encouraging results in children aged 6–11 years of age.[69,70]

Any biologic can be considered for adolescents and adults with blood eosinophilia. Reslizumab is approved by Food and Drug Administration (FDA) only for >18 years of age. Dupilumab, mepolizumab, and reslizumab have demonstrated very optimizing results in reducing exacerbations, while benralizumab and dupilumab have shown promising results in reducing daily oral steroid dosage (**Table 4**). In patients who are not on maintenance steroids and are without blood eosinophilia, omalizumab has shown the ability to reduce ICS dose.

Dupilumab is useful in patients with exacerbations due to aspirin sensitivity and can also improve symptoms in patients with chronic rhinosinusitis with nasal polyps (CRSwNP; SINUS-24 trial phase III trial).[71,72]

TABLE 4: Dosing interval and routes of dosing for Biologics.

Biologic	Route	Dose
Benralizumab	Subcutaneous	Loading dose, then every 2 months
Mepolizumab	Subcutaneous	Monthly
Dupilumab	Subcutaneous	Every 15 days
Reslizumab	Intravenous	Monthly

CONCLUSION

Food and Drug Administration has currently approved five biologic therapies based on the clinical trial data from different sources for difficult-to-control asthma. It has been observed that the based on the aim of treatment, biologic can be chosen upon.

In a patient with blood eosinophilia, if reduction in clinically significant exacerbations is aimed, then dupilumab, mepolizumab, or reslizumab are better choices. If improvement in lung function is targeted, then dupilumab therapy should be preferred as it has shown consistent results across most of the trials. Benralizumab has also shown encouraging results, along with promising long-term effects. If reduction of daily oral steroids is needed, benralizumab and dupilumab should be preferred.

However, in the three steroid-sparing trials, analysis of data could be difficult as a significant difference was observed among the placebo groups in terms of dose reduction of steroids.

With these novel biologics drugs, one hopes that the greatest unmet needs in asthma will be eliminated and a new era of asthma treatment will begin.

REFERENCES

1. Wenzel SE. Asthma: defining of the persistent adult phenotypes. Lancet. 2006;368:804-13.
2. Hekking PP, Bel EH. Developing and emerging clinical asthma phenotypes. J Allergy Clin Immunol Pract. 2014;2:671-80.
3. Leynaert B, Sunyer J, Garcia-Esteban R, Svanes C, Jarvis D, Cerveri I, et al. Gender differences in prevalence, diagnosis and incidence of allergic and non-allergic asthma: a population-based cohort. Thorax. 2012;67(7):625-31.
4. Moore WC, Bleecker ER, Curran-Everett D, Erzurum SC, Ameredes BT, Bacharier L, et al. Characterization of the severe asthma phenotype by the National Heart, Lung, and Blood Institute's Severe Asthma Research Program. J Allergy Clin Immunol. 2007;119(2):405-13.
5. Simpson JL, Scott R, Boyle MJ, Gibson PG. Inflammatory subtypes in asthma: assessment and identification using induced sputum. Respirology. 2006;11(1):54-61.
6. Woodruff PG, Boushey HA, Dolganov GM, Barker CS, Yang YH, Donnelly S, et al. Genome-wide profiling identifies epithelial cell genes associated with asthma and with treatment response to corticosteroids. Proc Natl Acad Sci USA. 2007;104(40):15858-63.

7. Woodruff PG, Modrek B, Choy DF, Jia G, Abbas AR, Ellwanger A, et al. T-helper type 2-driven inflammation defines major subphenotypes of asthma. Am J Respir Crit Care Med. 2009;180(5):388-95.
8. Modena BD, Tedrow JR, Milosevic J, Bleecker ER, Meyers DA, Wu W, et al. Gene expression in relation to exhaled nitric oxide identifies novel asthma phenotypes with unique biomolecular pathways. Am J Respir Crit Care Med. 2014;190(12): 1363-72.
9. Larose MC, Chakir J, Archambault AS, Joubert P, Provost V, Laviolette M, et al. Correlation between CCL26 production by human bronchial epithelial cells and airway eosinophils: involvement in patients with severe eosinophilic asthma. J Allergy Clin Immunol. 2015;136(4):904-13.
10. Rothenberg ME, Hogan SP. The eosinophil. Annu Rev Immunol. 2006;24:147-74.
11. Bousquet J, Chanez P, Lacoste JY, Barnéon G, Ghavanian N, Enander I, et al. Eosinophilic inflammation in asthma. N Engl J Med. 1990;323(15):1033-9.
12. Pin I, Freitag AP, O'Byrne PM, Girgis-Gabardo A, Watson RM, Dolovich J, et al. Changes in the cellular profile of induced sputum after allergen-induced asthmatic responses. Am Rev Respir Dis. 1992;145:1265-9.
13. Durham SR, Craddock CF, Cookson WO, Benson MK. Increases in airway responsiveness to histamine precede allergen-induced late asthmatic responses. J Allergy Clin Immunol. 1988;82(5):764-70.
14. Aalbers R, Kauffman HF, Vrugt B, Koëter GH, de Monchy JG. Allergen-induced recruitment of inflammatory cells in lavage 3 and 24 h after challenge in allergic asthmatic lungs. Chest. 1993;103(4):1178-84.
15. Chung KF, Wenzel SE, Brozek JL, Bush A, Castro M, Sterk PJ, et al. International ERS/ATS guidelines on definition, evaluation and treatment of severe asthma. Eur Respir J. 2014;43(2):343-73.
16. Wenzel S. Severe asthma in adults. Am J Respir Crit Care Med. 2005;172(2):149-60.
17. Xue L, Salimi M, Panse I, Mjösberg JM, McKenzie AN, Spits H, et al. Prostaglandin D2 activates group 2 innate lymphoid cells through chemoattractant receptor-homologous molecule expressed on TH2 cells. J Allergy Clin Immunol. 2014;133(4):1184-94.
18. Miranda C, Busacker A, Balzar S, Trudeau J, Wenzel SE. Distinguishing severe asthma phenotypes: role of age at onset and eosinophilic inflammation. J Allergy Clin Immunol. 2004;113(1):101-8.
19. Haldar P, Pavord ID, Shaw DE, Berry MA, Thomas M, Brightling CE, et al. Cluster analysis and clinical asthma phenotypes. Am J Respir Crit Care Med. 2008;178(3):218-24.
20. Nair P, Pizzichini MM, Kjarsgaard M, Inman MD, Efthimiadis A, Pizzichini E, et al. Mepolizumab for prednisone-dependent asthma with sputum eosinophilia. N Engl J Med. 2009;360(10):985-93.
21. van Veen IH, Ten Brinke A, Gauw SA, Sterk PJ, Rabe KF, Bel EH. Consistency of sputum eosinophilia in difficult-to-treat asthma: a 5-year follow-up study. J Allergy Clin Immunol. 2009;124(3):615-7.
22. De Carvalho-Pinto RM, Cukier A, Angelini L, Antonangelo L, Mauad T, Dolhnikoff M, et al. Clinical characteristics and possible phenotypes of an adult severe asthma population. Respir Med. 2012;106(1):47-56.
23. Barnes PJ. Intrinsic asthma: not so different from allergic asthma but driven by superantigens? Clin Exp Allergy. 2009;39:1145-51.
24. Yoo HS, Shin YS, Liu JN, Kim MA, Park HS. Clinical significance of immunoglobulin E responses to staphylococcal superantigens in patients with aspirin-exacerbated respiratory disease. Int Arch Allergy Immunol. 2013;162:340-5.
25. Szczeklik A, Stevenson DD. Aspirin-induced asthma: advances in pathogenesis, diagnosis, and management. J Allergy Clin Immunol. 2003;111:913-21.

26. Amelink M, de Groot JC, de Nijs SB, Lutter R, Zwinderman AH, Sterk PJ, et al. Severe adult-onset asthma: a distinct phenotype. J Allergy Clin Immunol. 2013;132: 336-41.
27. Wenzel SE, Schwartz LB, Langmack EL, Halliday JL, Trudeau JB, Gibbs RL, et al. Evidence that severe asthma can be divided pathologically into two inflammatory subtypes with distinct physiologic and clinical characteristics. Am J Respir Crit Care Med. 1999;160:1001-8.
28. Romagnoli M, Vachier I, Tarodo de la Fuente P, Meziane H, Chavis C, Bousquet J, et al. Eosinophilic inflammation in sputum of poorly controlled asthmatics. Eur Respir J. 2002;20(6):1370-7.
29. Volbeda F, Broekema M, Lodewijk ME, Hylkema MN, Reddel HK, Timens W, et al. Clinical control of asthma associates with measures of airway inflammation. Thorax. 2013;68(1):19-24.
30. Meijer RJ, Postma DS, Kauffman HF, Arends LR, Koëter GH, Kerstjens HA. Accuracy of eosinophils and eosinophil cationic protein to predict steroid improvement in asthma. Clin Exp Allergy. 2002;32(7):1096-103.
31. Wenzel S. Severe/fatal asthma. Chest. 2003;123:405S-10S.
32. Jarvis D, Newson R, Lotvall J, Hastan D, Tomassen P, Keil T, et al. Asthma in adults and its association with chronic rhinosinusitis: the GA2 LEN survey in Europe. Allergy. 2012;67:91-8.
33. Samter M, Beers RF Jr. Concerning the nature of intolerance to aspirin. J Allergy. 1967;40:281-93.
34. Demoly P, Crampette L, Mondain M, Campbell AM, Lequeux N, Enander I, et al. Assessment of inflammation in noninfectious chronic maxillary sinusitis. J Allergy Clin Immunol. 1994;94:95-108.
35. Hamilos DL, Leung DY, Wood R, Cunningham L, Bean DK, Yasruel Z, et al. Evidence for distinct cytokine expression in allergic versus nonallergic chronic sinusitis. J Allergy Clin Immunol. 1995;96(4):537-44.
36. Harlin SL, Ansel DG, Lane SR, et al. A clinical and pathologic study of chronic sinusitis: the role of the eosinophil. J Allergy Clin Immunol. 1988;81:867-75.
37. Moneret-Vautrin DA, Jankowski R, Bene MC, Kanny G, Hsieh V, Faure G, et al. NARES: a model of inflammation caused by activated eosinophils? Rhinology. 1992;30:161-8.
38. Wu W, Bleecker E, Moore W, Busse WW, Castro M, Chung KF, et al. Unsupervised phenotyping of Severe Asthma Research Program participants using expanded lung data. J Allergy Clin Immunol. 2014;133:1280-8.
39. Pavord ID, Korn S, Howarth P, Bleecker ER, Buhl R, Keene ON, et al. Mepolizumab for severe eosinophilic asthma (DREAM): a multicentre, double-blind, placebo-controlled trial. Lancet. 2012;380(9842):651-9.
40. Bel EH, Wenzel SE, Thompson PJ, Prazma CM, Keene ON, Yancey SW et al. Oral glucocorticoid-sparing effect of mepolizumab in eosinophilic asthma. N Engl J Med. 2014;371:1189-97.
41. Sweeney J, Brightling CE, Menzies-Gow A, Niven R, Patterson CC, Heaney LG. Clinical management and outcome of refractory asthma in the UK from the British Thoracic Society Difficult Asthma Registry. Thorax. 2012;67(8):754-6.
42. Ten Brinke A, de Lange C, Zwinderman AH, Rabe KF, Sterk PJ, Bel EH. Sputum induction in severe asthma by a standardized protocol: predictors of excessive bronchoconstriction. Am J Respir Crit Care Med. 2001;164:749-53.
43. Pin I, Gibson PG, Kolendowicz R, Girgis-Gabardo A, Denburg JA, Hargreave FE, et al. Use of induced sputum cell counts to investigate airway inflammation in asthma. Thorax. 1992;47(1):259.

44. Korevaar DA, Westerhof GA, Wang J, Cohen JF, Spijker R, Sterk PJ, et al. Diagnostic accuracy of minimally invasive markers for detection of airway eosinophilia in asthma: a systematic review and meta-analysis. Lancet Respir Med. 2015;3: 290-300.
45. Westerhof GA, Korevaar DA, Amelink M, de Nijs SB, de Groot JC, Wang J, et al. Biomarkers to identify sputum eosinophilia in different adult asthma phenotypes. Eur Respir J. 2015;46(3):688-96.
46. Katz LE, Gleich GJ, Hartley BF, Yancey SW, Ortega HG. Blood eosinophil count is a useful biomarker to identify patients with severe eosinophilic asthma. Ann Am Thorac Soc. 2014;11(4):531-6.
47. Zhang XY, Simpson JL, Powell H, Yang IA, Upham JW, Reynolds PN, et al. Full blood count parameters for the detection of asthma inflammatory phenotypes. Clin Exp Allergy. 2014;44(9):1137-45.
48. Hochhaus G, Brookman L, Fox H, Johnson C, Matthews J, Ren S, et al. Pharmacodynamics of omalizumab: implications for optimised dosing strategies and clinical efficacy in the treatment of allergic asthma. Curr Med Res Opin. 2003;19(6):491-8.
49. Casale TB, Bernstein IL, Busse WW, LaForce CF, Tinkelman DG, Stoltz RR, et al. Use of an anti-IgE humanized monoclonal antibody in ragweed-induced allergic rhinitis. J Allergy Clin Immunol. 1997;100(1):110-21.
50. Galli SJ, TsaiM. IgE and mast cells in allergic disease. Nat Med. 2012;18(5):693-704.
51. Modena BD, Dazy K, White AA. Emerging concepts: mast cell involvement in allergic diseases. Transl Res. 2016;174:98-121.
52. Pelaia G, Gallelli L, Renda T, Romeo P, Busceti MT, Grembiale RD, et al. Update on optimal use of omalizumab in management of asthma. J Asthma Allergy. 2011;4:49-59.
53. Busse W, Corren J, Lanier BQ, McAlary M, Fowler-Taylor A, Cioppa GD, et al. Omalizumab, anti-IgE recombinant humanized monoclonal antibody, for the treatment of severe allergic asthma. J Allergy Clin Immunol. 2001;108(2):184-90.
54. Lampinen M, Carlson M, Håkansson LD, Venge P. Cytokine-regulated accumulation of eosinophils in inflammatory disease. Allergy. 2004;59(8):793-805.
55. Tan LD, Bratt JM, Godor D, Louie S, Kenyon NJ. Benralizumab: a unique IL-5 inhibitor for severe asthma. J Asthma Allergy. 2016;9:71-81.
56. Kolbeck R, Kozhich A, Koike M, Peng L, Andersson CK, Damschroder MM, et al. MEDI-563, a humanized anti-IL-5 receptor alpha mAb with enhanced antibody-dependent cell-mediated cytotoxicity function. J Allergy Clin Immunol. 2010;125(6):1344-53.
57. Kotsimbos AT, Hamid Q. IL-5 and IL-5 receptor in asthma. Mem Inst Oswaldo Cruz. 1997;92(Suppl 2):75-91.
58. Rothenberg ME. Eosinophilia. N Engl J Med. 1998;338(22):1592-600.
59. Kau AL, Korenblat PE. Anti-interleukin 4 and 13 for asthma treatment in the era of endotypes. Curr Opin Allergy Clin Immunol. 2014;14(6):570-5.
60. Akdis CA. Therapies for allergic inflammation: refining strategies to induce tolerance. Nat Med. 2012;18(5):736-49.
61. Bagnasco D, Ferrando M, Varricchi G, Passalacqua G, Canonica GW. A critical evaluation of anti-IL-13 and anti-IL-4 strategies in severe asthma. Int Arch Allergy Immunol. 2016;170(2):122-31.
62. Solèr M, Matz J, Townley R, Buhl R, O'Brien J, Fox H, et al. The anti-IgE antibody omalizumab reduces exacerbations and steroid requirement in allergic asthmatics. Eur Respir J. 2001;18(2):254-61.

63. Castro M, Wenzel SE, Bleecker ER, Pizzichini E, Kuna P, Busse WW, et al. Benralizumab, an anti-interleukin 5 receptor alpha monoclonal antibody, versus placebo for uncontrolled eosinophilic asthma: a phase 2b randomised dose-ranging study. Lancet Respir Med. 2014;2(11):879-90.
64. Wenzel S, Ford L, Pearlman D, Spector S, Sher L, Skobieranda F, et al. Dupilumab in persistent asthma with elevated eosinophil levels. N Engl J Med. 2013;368(26):2455-66.
65. Ortega HG, Liu MC, Pavord ID, Brusselle GG, FitzGerald JM, Chetta A, et al. Mepolizumab treatment in patients with severe eosinophilic asthma. N Engl J Med. 2014;371(13):1198-207.
66. Castro M, Zangrilli J, Wechsler ME, Bateman ED, Brusselle GG, Bardin P, et al. Reslizumab for inadequately controlled asthma with elevated blood eosinophil counts: results from two multicentre, parallel, double-blind, randomised, placebo-controlled, phase 3 trials. Lancet Respir Med. 2015;3(5):355-66.
67. Busse WW, Bleecker ER, FitzGerald JM, Ferguson GT, Barker P, Sproule S, et al. Long-term safety and efficacy of benralizumab in patients with severe, uncontrolled asthma: 1-year results from the BORA phase 3 extension trial. Lancet Respir Med. 2019;7(1):46-59.
68. Global Asthma Network. The Global Asthma Report 2014. (2014). [online] Available from http://globalasthmareport.org/2014/Global_Asthma_Report_2014.pdf (Last accessed September, 2020).
69. Gupta A, Pouliquen I, Austin D, Price RG, Kempsford R, Steinfeld J, et al. Subcutaneous mepolizumab in children aged 6 to 11 years with severe eosinophilic asthma. Pediatr Pulmonol. 2019;54(12):1957-67.
70. Gupta A, Ikeda M, Geng B, Azmi J, Price RG, Bradford ES, et al. Long-term safety and pharmacodynamics of mepolizumab in children with severe asthma with an eosinophilic phenotype. J Allergy Clin Immunol. 2019;144(5):1336-42.
71. Han JK, Bachert C, Desrosiers M, Laidlaw TM, Hopkins C, Fokkens WJ, et al. Efficacy and safety of dupilumab in patients with chronic rhinosinusitis with nasal polyps: results from the randomized phase 3 sinus-24 study. J Allergy Clin Immunol. 2019;143(2):AB422.
72. Dodge RR, Burrows B. The prevalence and incidence of asthma and asthma-like symptoms in a general population sample. Am Rev Respir Dis. 1980;122:567-75.

28

An Approach to Diabetic Autonomic Neuropathy

Shambo S Samajdar, Santanu K Tripathi, Shashank R Joshi

INTRODUCTION

Autonomic neuropathy is a complication of diabetes which we often forget to screen. As consequences of diabetes, both peripheral and autonomic nerves are damaged and lead to poor quality of life, increased expenditure, and mortality. It is very important to detect early the presence of autonomic neuropathy to prevent further progression and complications. Autonomic neuropathy is associated with multisystem involvement including cardiovascular, respiratory, genitourinary, gastrointestinal, ocular, sudomotor, and neurovascular systems. In presence of cardiac dysautonomia, 5 years mortality rate is increased by 5–6 times,[1] which seek urgent attention from the treating physician's perspective to offer treatment and necessary care to the patient after prompt diagnosis. Coexistence of autonomic neuropathy is associated with increased chance of life-threatening arrhythmia. Concomitant medications, hypokalemia, hypoglycemia, ischemic heart disease, and hypotension may aggravate the incidence of arrhythmia and following sudden cardiac death. Prevalence of cardiac autonomic neuropathy in type 1 diabetes mellitus (T1DM) ranging from 7.7% in newly diagnosed cases[2] to 90% in patients who are awaiting for pancreatic transplant.[3] In type 2 diabetes mellitus (T2DM), patients multiple studies had shown variable prevalence from 20 to 73%.[4,5] This variability was due to age, sex, duration of diabetes, and glycemic burden. Maximum patients with cardiac dysautonomia are asymptomatic, after prolong period with diabetes they have developed symptoms. If we not go for tests to evaluate autonomic nervous system function, we would fail to detect cases with subclinical autonomic dysfunction which is very commonly associated with diabetics.

BALANCE BETWEEN SYMPATHETIC AND PARASYMPATHETIC NERVOUS SYSTEM

Balance is the principle in every sectors of life. Sympathetic and parasympathetic nervous system should perform in a balancing way to perform well. In a brief, we know that sympathetic nervous system's function is "flight or fight response" whereas parasympathetic nervous system has "rest and digest response". When a deer is eating grasses in a forest, its parasympathetic nervous system is sitting in the pivotal chair but hearing the sound and anticipating the attack from a leopard while it starts running sympathetic nervous system is mainly driving its body physiology. Activation of sympathetic nervous system increases heart rate (HR) and sweating, dilates pupil, inhibits gastrointestinal movement, closes sphincters, and diverts blood from skin and gastrointestinal tract to skeletal muscles. Whereas parasympathetic nervous system functions predominate during "rest and digest" promotes digestion, increase gastrointestinal peristalsis, slows HR, constricts pupil, empties bladder, and relaxes sphincters. Regarding male sexual function erection is the function of parasympathetic nervous system and ejaculation is sympathetic nervous system activity. Autonomic neurointegrity is essential for existence and sustenance of human life.

DIABETIC AUTONOMIC NEUROPATHY SCREENING—INDICATIONS

1. According to the American Neurological Society guidelines, dysautonomia screening should be carried out immediately after the diagnosis of T2DM.
2. Screening is required 5 years after the diagnosis of T1DM or in presence of symptoms suggestive of dysautonomia.
3. Diabetics presented with poor glycemic control, micro- and macrovascular complications, and cardiovascular risk factors should be investigated for dysautonomia.
4. Yearly repetition of testing should be done even if cardiac autonomic neuropathy testing results are normal.
5. Before prescribing exercise, it is better to screen autonomic neuropathy.
6. Patients with diabetes requiring general anesthesia, need to be evaluated for dysautonomia.

DETECTION OF DIABETIC AUTONOMIC NEUROPATHY

Proper history taking and a few simple clinical tests can guide us to detect diabetic autonomic neuropathy (DAN). Vagus nerve, the longest parasympathetic nerve in human, which is responsible for two-thirds parasympathetic activity in our system, is suffered early by diabetes. Initially, parasympathetic activity is suffered and when sympathetic disturbances appear, we can address the case as advanced dysautonomia. Symptoms and signs of dysautonomia are depicted in **Box 1**.

CLINICAL TESTS FOR DYSAUTONOMIA

1. Resting HR >100 beats/min is abnormal and needs to be cautious.
2. Patient should abstain from drinking coffee overnight before test day. Dysautonomia testing should not be performed after overnight hypoglycemic episodes.
3. *Expiration:inspiration R-R ratio*[6↑↑↑↑]: When the patient lies supine and breathes 6 times per min, a difference in HR <10 beats/minute is abnormal. An expiration:inspiration R-R ratio <1.17 is abnormal

> **Box 1: Signs and symptoms of diabetic autonomic neuropathy.**
>
> - *Metabolic*:
>   - Hypoglycemia unawareness
>   - Hypoglycemia-associated autonomic failure
> - *Cardiovascular system (CAN)*:
>   - Loss of BP circad rhythm (nondipping)
>   - Resting tachycardia
>   - Exercise intolerance
>   - Intraoperative cardiovascular lability
>   - "Silent ischemia" and "painless" MI
>   - Diabetic cardiomyopathy
>   - Arrhythmias and sudden cardiac arrest
>   - Orthostatic hypotension
> - *Respiratory system*:
>   - Central dysregulation of breathing
>   - Reduced bronchial reactivity
> - *Pupillomotor*:
>   - Pupil dysfunction (decreased diameter of dark adapted pupil)
>   - Argyll–Robertson pupil
> - *Gastrointestinal system*:
>   - Dysfunction of the esophagus
>   - Gastroparesis
>   - Change in gut motility (constipation and diarrhea)
>   - Anorectal dysfunction (fecal incontinence)
> - *Genitourinary system*:
>   - Neurogenic bladder
>   - Erectile dysfunction
>   - Retrograde ejaculation
>   - Loss of vaginal lubrication
> - *Sudomotor*:
>   - Hyperhidrosis of upper limbs
>   - Gustatory sweating
>   - Anhidrosis of lower limbs and dry skin
>   - Heat intolerance
>   - Changes in skin blood flow (warm skin, varicose veins, and peripheral edema)

(BP: blood pressure; CAN: cardiac autonomic neuropathy; MI: myocardial infarction)

(age dependent index)* [E/I ratio lowest normal value*: 1.17 (age 20-24 years), 1.15 (25-29 years), 1.13 (30-34 years), 1.12 (35-39 years), 1.10 (40-44 years), 1.08 (45-49 years), 1.07 (50-54 years), 1.06 (55-59 years), 1.04 (60-64 years), 1.03 (65-69 years), and 1.02 (70-75 years)].

4. *Heart rate response to Valsalva maneuver*:[6] Patient would be asked to exhale forcibly into the mouthpiece of a manometer, exerting a pressure

REFERENCES

1. Spallone V, Ziegler D, Freeman R, Bernardi L, Frontoni S, Pop-Busui R, et al. Cardiovascular autonomic neuropathy in diabetes: clinical impact, assessment, diagnosis, and management. Diabetes Metab Res Rev. 2011;27(7):639-53.
2. Ziegler D, Gries FA, Spuler M, Lessmann F. The epidemiology of diabetic neuropathy. Diabetic Cardiovascular Autonomic Neuropathy Multicenter Study Group. J Diabetes Complications. 1992;6(1):49-57.
3. Kennedy WR, Navarro X, Sutherland DE. Neuropathy profile of diabetic patients in a pancreas transplantation program. Neurology. 1995;45(4):773-80.
4. Dimitropoulos G, Tahrani AA, Stevens MJ. Cardiac autonomic neuropathy in patients with diabetes mellitus. World J Diabetes. 2014;5:17-39.
5. American Diabetes Association. Report and recommendations of the San Antonio Conference on diabetic neuropathy (Consensus Statement). Diabetes. 1988;37(7):1000-4.
6. Vinik AI, Erbas T. Recognizing and treating diabetic autonomic neuropathy. Cleve Clin J Med. 2001;68:928-30.
7. Jameson JL, Fauci AS, Kasper DL, Hauser SL, Longo DL, Loscalzo J. Harrison's principles of internal medicine, 20th edition. New York: McGraw-Hill Education; 2020.
8. Ewing DJ, Martyn CN, Young RJ, Clarke BF. The value of cardiovascular autonomic function tests: 10 years experience in diabetes. Diabetes Care. 1985;8:491-8.
9. Gaede P, Lund-Andersen H, Parving HH, Pedersen O. Effect of a multifactorial intervention on mortality in type 2 diabetes. N Engl J Med. 2008;358:580-91.
10. Zieglar D, Gries FA. Alpha-lipoic acid in the treatment of diabetic peripheral and cardiac autonomic neuropathy. Diabetes. 1997;46:S62-6.
11. Athyros VG, Didangelos TP, Karamitsos DT, Papageorgiou AA, Boudoulas H, Kontopoulos AG. Long-term effect of converting enzyme inhibition on circadian sympathetic and parasympathetic modulation in patients with diabetic autonomic neuropathy. Acta Cardiol. 1998;53(4):201-9.
12. Tesfaye S. Neuropathy in diabetes. Medicine. 2010;38:649-55.
13. Pasina L, Djade CD, Lucca U, Nobili A, Tettamanti M, Franchi C, et al. Association of anticholinergic burden with cognitive and functional status in a cohort of hospitalized elderly: comparison of the anticholinergic cognitive burden scale and anticholinergic risk scale: results from the REPOSI study. Drugs Aging. 2013;30(2):103-12.

29. Pharmacokinetic Considerations in Prescribing Chronic Kidney Disease Patients

Shambo S Samajdar, Shashank R Joshi

INTRODUCTION

The term "pharmacokinetics" is derived from the Greek words *pharmakon* (drug) and *kinetikos* (movement).[1] Pharmacokinetics describe the time-course of drug concentration into, within, and out of the body.[2] It is characterized by: (1) Drug movement from the site of administration to the systemic circulation (input), and (2) Drug dispersal and removal from the systemic circulation (disposition). It includes the kinetics of absorption (A), distribution (D), metabolism (M), and excretion (E). In simple terms, it describes the fate of the drug within the body.[3,4] The course of drug action is, therefore, directly linked with the concentration of the drug in the systemic circulation and depends upon the ADME processes.[5]

Absorption is the transfer of a drug from administered route to the systemic circulation. The rate and extent of absorption rests on the route of administration, the formulation type and chemical characteristics of the drug, and physiological factors that can impact the site of absorption.[5] The bioavailability of a drug is the association between the drug dose and the amount of drug that finally reaches the bloodstream evading the presystemic metabolism or transport. Volume of distribution (Vd) is the "apparent" volume into which a drug must be allotted to match its concentration in plasma. Metabolism also known as biotransformation is the enzymatic conversion of a drug to a new chemical species which may be less or more active than the parent drug; sometimes more easily eliminated from the circulation.[6] Though liver proportionately leads the sites of biotransformation, gastrointestinal tract, and kidneys are also critical ones for several drugs. Any disease affecting these organs can affect the biotransformation process. The removal of the drug from the body is referred to as excretion; elimination refers to complete excretion and includes both the metabolism of the drug, and excretion of the drug. Majority drugs or their metabolites are excreted by the kidneys. Several factors affect renal excretion (**Box 1**). Few are also eliminated by the liver in the bile and excreted in feces. Enterohepatic circulation can occur (drug excreted in bile is absorbed by the gut and re-excreted by the liver in bile).[7] Some volatile substances (mainly gaseous anesthetics) can be excreted via the lungs. Saliva frequently contains negligible quantities of drug and this may be regarded as a mechanism of excretion though the amount

> **Box 1: Factors affecting renal excretion.[8,9]**
>
> - *Renal disease*: Since, the amount of proteins are lost, the proportion of unbound or free drug increases and may result in toxicity
> - *Urinary pH*: When the pH of blood becomes either too acidic or basic, the kidneys adjust the pH by regulating the amount of water removed through micturition and controlling sodium balance via carbonic anhydrase
> - *Alteration in renal blood flow*: Any change in the perfusion rate affects the time required for elimination of drug
> - *Concentration of drug in plasma*: Concentration of unbound drug, protein-binding affinity, water solubility, and pH affect the degree to which drug can be renally excreted
> - *Molecular weight of drug*: Glomerular filtration occurs with small molecules (<300 molecular weight) of free (unbound) drug. Large size, ionized state, and protein binding of drugs deters glomerular filtration

is insignificant. The gastrointestinal tract also eliminates some of the drugs. The removal of drugs into milk is a negligible excretion pathway, however, it could be clinically significant for the nursing neonate.[7]

RELATIONSHIP BETWEEN DOSING REGIMEN AND THE EFFECT OF A DRUG

The net effects of pharmacokinetic processes after drug administration can be observed using the concentration-time profile of a drug (**Fig. 1**). The clinical effect of a drug correlates with the maximum plasma concentration (C_{max}) and/or the area under the concentration (AUC)-time curve. Usually, the risk of adverse events increases with exposure to higher drug concentrations, while suboptimal exposure leads to inefficacy of the treatment. Hence, it is imperative to understand the changes in pharmacokinetic parameters with comorbid conditions like hepatic or renal impairment so that the dosing regimen is modified to optimize concentration-time profile for the subject.[10]

Rates of Reaction

Absorption, distribution, metabolism, and excretion are processes that are characterized by the rates or velocity at which they occur either a zero-order or first order. These are clinically useful in achieving a therapeutic level of medicines and predicting toxicity levels and employing treatment.[11] Most of the drugs are eliminated via first-order kinetics, however, fluidity may exist between these two types of elimination for a specific substance.[11] Elimination of substances which follow zero-order elimination depends only on time and not on the amount of drug intake. This means that zero-order kinetics undergo constant elimination irrespective of the plasma concentration, resulting in a linear elimination phase as the system becomes saturated. On the contrary substances eliminated by the first-order kinetics depend on

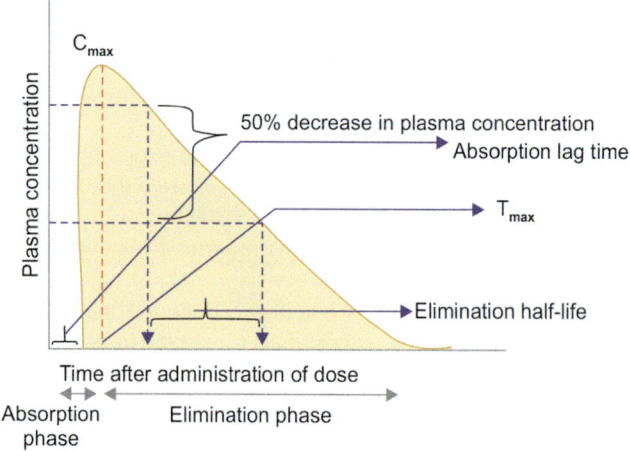

FIG. 1: Plasma-concentration profile after single dose administration.

the systemic drug concentration and not on time; thus, the rate increases with increase in plasma concentration.[11] Thus, first order kinetics result in exponential elimination and is never saturated.[11]

The equation for both zero and first-order kinetics is same.[11]

$$\Delta[drug]/\Delta[time] = -Kc[drug]^n$$

where,

Δ symbolizes the change, hence, the equation denotes the ratio of change in plasma concentration of the drug with time.

Kc denotes a constant/

"n" is 0 in case of zero-order and "1" for the first-order elimination reactions.

Accordingly, the graphical representation of zero-order kinetics would be a linear slope (**Fig. 2**), while it would be an exponential curve (**Fig. 3**) for the first order kinetics.[11]

The distribution half-life ($t_{1/2a}$) denotes the amount of time required for the plasma concentration to decrease by half during the distribution phase. Elimination half-life ($t_{1/2e}$) is generally the time required for one-half of a given amount of drug to be reduced to half its initial concentration in the body during its elimination phase (**Fig. 1**).[12] It is required for defining excretion rates and steady-state concentrations. Though majority drugs follow first-order kinetics, some do follow zero-order elimination (**Fig. 4**).[13]

The integral AUC-A indicates the total drug exposure over time. In the first-order kinetics, the curve follows a logarithmic decay.[13]

$$\ln[D1]/[D2] = kt$$

The elimination half-life can be obtained by solving the above differential equation.

$$t1/2e = 0.693/k$$

This equation helps to find the half-life of a drug, given its fixed rate constant **k**.

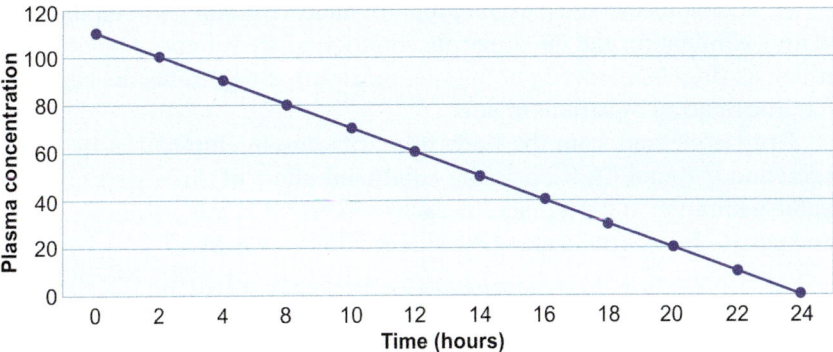

FIG. 2: Zero-order kinetics.

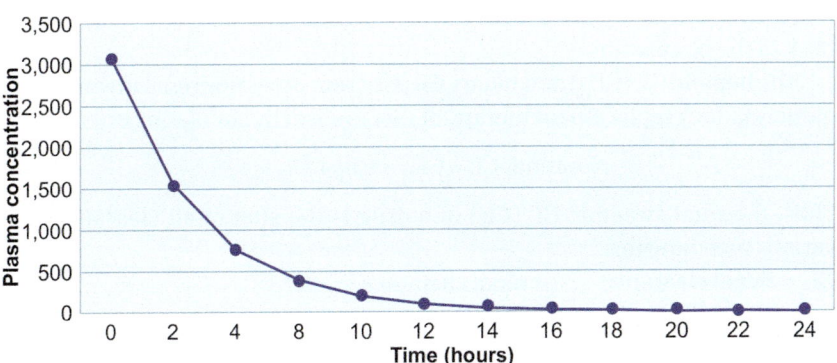

FIG. 3: First-order kinetics.

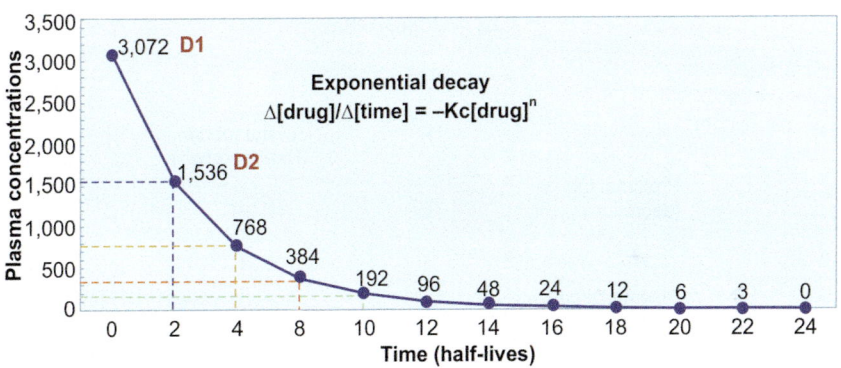

FIG. 4: Elimination half-life curve.

Alternatively, another half-life equation which is dependent on k, which is correlate with Vd and clearance (CL).[13]

$$t_{1/2e} = 0.693 \times Vd(L)/CL(L/h)$$

where,
Vd is the volume of distribution or precisely apparent volume of distribution of a drug and is defined as the theoretical volume needed to account for all of the drug in the body based on the serum concentration in a blood sample.[12]

CL is clearance defined as the proportionality constant between the rate of drug elimination and the drug concentration or the volume of blood from which all drug is removed per minute (mL/min). It represents the capacity for drug removal by various organs.[14,15]

Drug is cleared from the body primarily due to elimination by renal excretion.[14] Renal CL (CL_r) is the combined effect of three step process namely filtration at the glomerulus, active secretion in the proximal tubule, and passive reabsorption along the kidney tubules (**Fig. 5**).

$$CL_r = (Fu \times GFR) + CL_{secretion} - CL_{reabsorption}$$

where,

Fu represents the unbound free drug concentration in the plasma, $CL_{secretion}$ represents the actively secreted drug in the kidney tubules $CL_{reabsorption}$ represents part of the drug which is reabsorbed from the glomerular filtrate back to the circulation.

The hepatic CL (CL_H) and biliary CL (CL_B) are other nonrenal means of CL namely kidney replacement therapy or metabolism by circulating esterases.[16]

$$\text{Nonrenal CL} = CL_H + CL_B + CL_{others}$$

Thus, the total systemic CL (Cl_S) of a drug is the sum of all clearances by various mechanisms.

CL_S = Renal clearance + Nonrenal clearance
$CL_S = (CL_r) + (CL_H + CL_B + CL_{others})$
$CL_S = [(Fu*GFR) + CL_{secretion} - CL_{reabsorption}] + [CL_H + CL_B + CL_{others}]$

However, since, it is not feasible to determine CL from each organ CL_S is often obtained by measuring the AUC after a single dose.

$$CLs = Dose/AUC$$

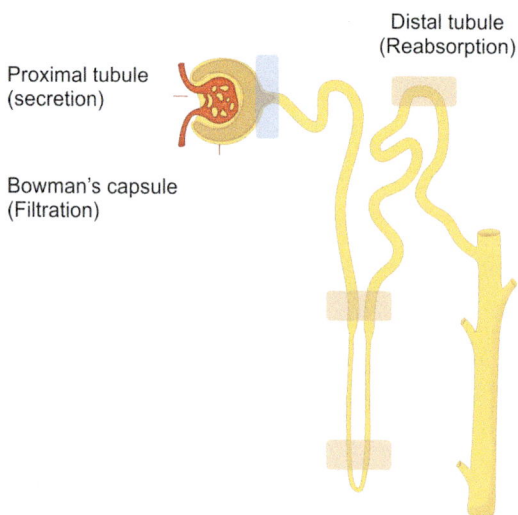

FIG. 5: Total renal clearance (CL_r).

It is an important means of dose adjustment in patients who have high or low CL relative to the usual value for the population; low CL leads to higher systemic exposure and vice-versa.[17]

The elimination rate constant (Kel) represents the fraction of drug eliminated per unit of time. Since, drug CL follows first order kinetics, a plot of log drug concentration versus time provides the elimination rate constant (Kel) as the slope (**Fig. 6**).[18]

Clearance is a parameter used to determine the rate at which drug must be administered to maintain the steady state plasma concentration which is a transition point between distribution and elimination.[15] It indicates completion of distribution of drug between the central and peripheral compartments and fluidity between them is nil. Vd can be calculated during steady-state (**Vss**) and is critical for obtaining the loading dose of a drug.[12]

$$\text{Loading dose (mg)} = [\text{Dp (mg/L)} \times \text{Vd (L)}]/F$$

Contrasting, the loading dose, which is reliant on Vd of the drug, the maintenance dose is dependent on CL.[12] Therefore, the maintenance dosing is calculated with the following equation:

$$\text{Maintenance dose rate (mg/hr)} = [\text{Dp (mg/L)} \times \text{CL (L/hr)}]/F$$

Dp represents the target plasma concentration of drug
F represents the bioavailability of drug (IV administration = 1)

On continual drug administration, the quantity of drug in the body at first will rise, however, later when the rate of elimination of the drug equals the amount administered per unit time, it will reach a steady-state (**Fig. 7**).

When the plasma concentration-time profile is identified subsequent to a single dose of a drug, the estimated profile following repeat administration of a fixed dose of drug given at regular intervals can be obtained by reproducing the single dose profile after each new dose (gray lines) and adding at each time the resultant concentrations related with each dose. The result (dashed line) is a typical sawtooth profile rising to a plateau.

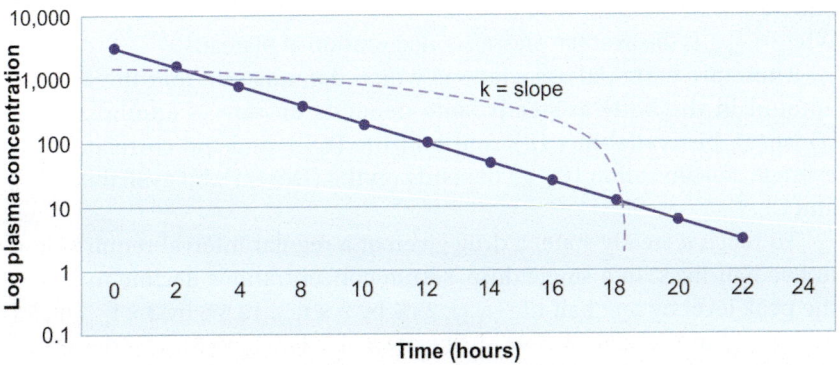

FIG. 6: First order rate constant (k) for elimination is obtained from a plot of log compound concentration versus time.

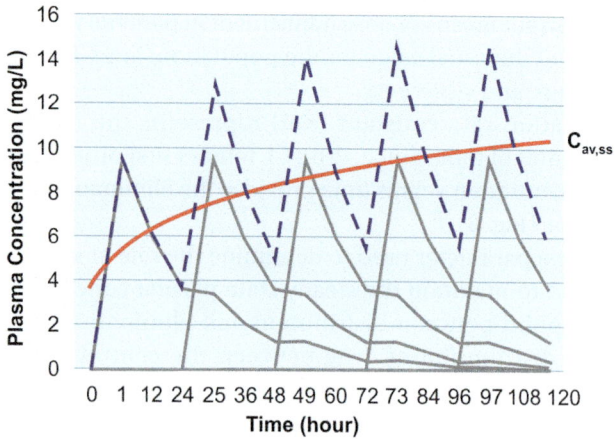

FIG. 7: Accumulation on approach to plateau.

The average amount in the body at plateau can be determined using the steady-state concept: Average rate of drug administered must be equal average rate of drug eliminated between doses.

$$\text{Average rate (in)} = F \cdot \text{Dose}/\tau$$

where,
F is the bioavailability of the drug
τ is the dosing interval

$$\text{Average rate (out)} = k \cdot A_{av,ss}$$

where,
$A_{av,ss}$ is the average amount of drug in the body over the dosing interval, τ, at plateau.
Equating at steady state,
Average rate (in) = Average rate (out)
Solving for $A_{av,ss}$ and replacing k with $0.693/t_{1/2}$:
Or
Solving for $C_{av,ss}$:
Equation 1:
Where $C_{av,ss}$ is the average plasma concentration at plateau.

These are essential associations which demonstrate that the average amount in the body at steady state depends on rate of administration (Dose/τ), bioavailability (F), and half-life ($t_{1/2}$), and the corresponding average concentration ($C_{av,ss}$) depends on the (Dose/τ), bioavailability (F), and CL.[19]

To reach a steady state, a drug given at a regular interval requires four to five half-lives. In a single dose, serum concentrations decline to 50% of the peak level by one half-life ($t_{1/2}$), 25% by $2 \times t_{1/2}$, 12.5% by $3 \times t_{1/2}$, 6.25% by $4 \times t_{1/2}$, and 3.125% by $5 \times t_{1/2}$. Therefore, by $4 \times t_{1/2}$ to $5 \times t_{1/2}$, the serum levels are decreased nearly by 94–97% of the peak level; the entire dose is thus eliminated from the body by $4 \times t_{1/2}$ to $5 \times t_{1/2}$.[20]

Drug accumulation does not occur indefinitely at a given dosing frequency because a steady state is eventually attained due to the concentration dependent process of elimination. Only when the process of elimination is impaired [for example chronic kidney disease (CKD)], the mean plasma levels of the drug specifically eliminated by the impaired pathway increase and may exceed the therapeutic window.

CHANGES IN PHARMACOKINETICS OF DRUGS IN CHRONIC KIDNEY DISEASE

Chronic kidney disease is a gamut of kidney dysfunction from mild kidney damage to kidney failure including end-stage renal disease (ESRD).[21] The National Kidney Foundation (NKF) defines CKD based on various findings including estimated glomerular filtration rate (*eGFR*) (**Table 1**). Albuminuria is a marker of kidney damage (increased glomerular permeability) (**Box 2** and **Table 2**).

In CKD, the GFR and organic anion transporting polypeptide (OATP), organic cation transporter (OCT)-mediated transport processes are affected leading to decreased CL and therefore, maintenance dose or frequency of

TABLE 1: Glomerular filtration rate (GFR) categories in chronic kidney disease (CKD).

GFR category	GFR (mL/min/1.73 m²)	Terms
G1	≥90	Normal or high
G2	60–89	Mildly decreased*
G3a	45–59	Mildly to moderately decreased
G3b	30–44	Morderately to severely decreased
G4	15–29	Severely decreased
G5	<15	Kidney failure

*Relative to young adult level.

Note: In the absence of evidence of kidney damage, neither GFR category G1 nor G2 fulfill the criteria for CKD.

Box 2: Chronic kidney disease (CKD) criteria (one of the following found for >3 months).

- Albuminuria [AER ≥ 30 mg/24 h; ACR ≥ 30 mg/g (≥3 mg/mmol)]
- Urine sediment abnormalities
- Electrolyte and other abnormalities due to tubular disorders
- Abnormalities detected by histology
- Structural abnormalities detected by imaging
- History of kidney transplantation

(ACR: albumin-to-creatinine ratio; AER: albumin excretion rate)

TABLE 2: Staging-based on albuminuria.

Category	AER (mg/24 h)	ACR (approximate equivalent)		Terms
		(mg/mmol)	(mg/g)	
A1	<30	<3	<30	Normal to mildly increased
A2	30–300	3–30	30–300	Moderately increased*
A3	>300	>30	>300	Severely Increased**

Notes:
*Relative to young adult level.
**Including nephrotic syndrome [albumin excretion usually >2200 mg/24 h. (ACR >2220 mg/g; >220 mg/mmol)]

(ACR: albumin-to-creatinine ratio; AER: albumin excretion rate; CKD: chronic kidney disease)

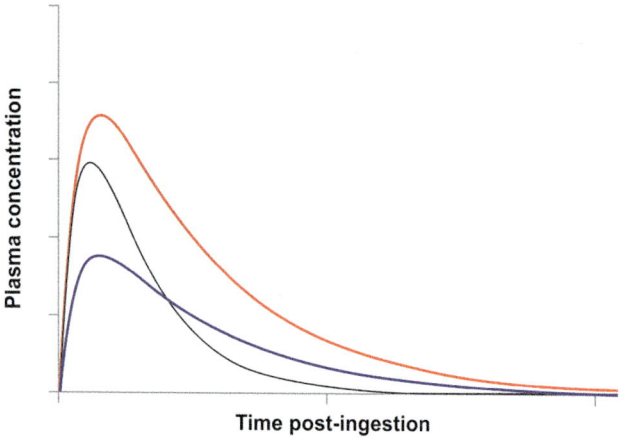

(CL: clearance; Vd: volume of distribution)

FIG. 8: Change in Vd or CL has different effects on time versus plasma concentration profile.

dosing should be reduced, e.g., methotrexate, atorvastatin, imatinib, and rosuvastatin. Decrease in the GFR, increases the active secretion. Hence, compared to only glomerulopathy, the dose reductions to a greater extent are required in tubulopathy which affects the active secretion. Additionally, the transporter efficiency for active secretion and reabsorption of drugs, both are dependent on factors like pH, alteration of which alters the drug CL.[10]

In CKD, a rise in Vd or a drop in CL leads to proportionate extension of $t_{1/2}$. If the CL drops to half, the AUC-time curve becomes twice, the $t_{1/2}$ will become twice its original duration of time (**Fig. 8**).

From the equations stated below, it is obvious that doubling the Vd results in halving of the peak plasma concentration unlike the AUC-time curve which remains unaltered.

$$\text{AUC} = \frac{\text{Dose}}{\text{Clearance}} \qquad C_{max} = \frac{\text{Dose} \times F}{VD}$$

As discussed previously, decline in kidney function may then result in drug accumulation and increase the risk of toxicity (**Figs. 9** and **10**), particularly in the case of treatment for a chronic disease.

Compared to nonend stage kidney disease (ESKD) patients, in ESKD patients, the $t_{1/2}$ of atenolol increases from 6 to 100 hours.

Though the effect of change in Vd or CL on the concentration-time profile is dissimilar, the action required is increasing the dosing interval to twice its original value (**Fig. 11**).

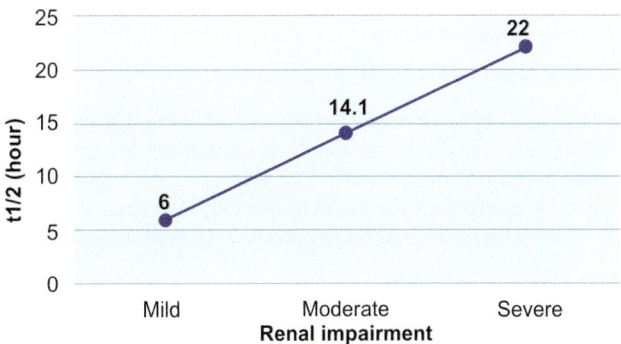

FIG. 9: Half-life of atenolol after administration of an administered a single 100 mg oral dose. In patients with normal renal function have a mean half-life of 6.0 ± 0.7 h. The presence of mild renal impairment (Group II) resulted in an increase to 14.1 ± 3.6 h and in the moderate to severe renal insufficiency patients (Group III) the mean half-life increased to 22.0 ± 4.5 h.

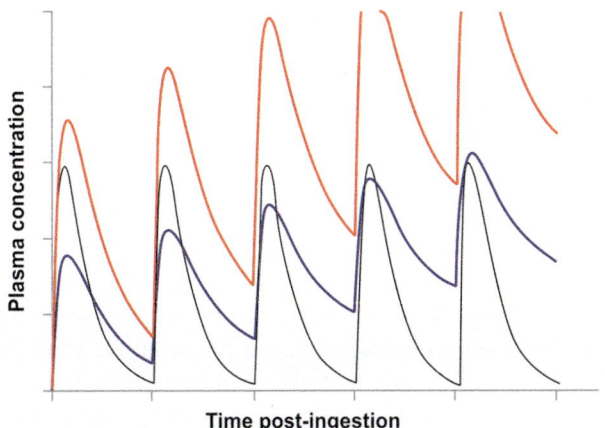

FIG. 10: In patients with transformed kinetics, constant dosing will lead to drug accumulation if the regimen is not modified. A decrease in clearance will lead to earlier onset of toxicity.

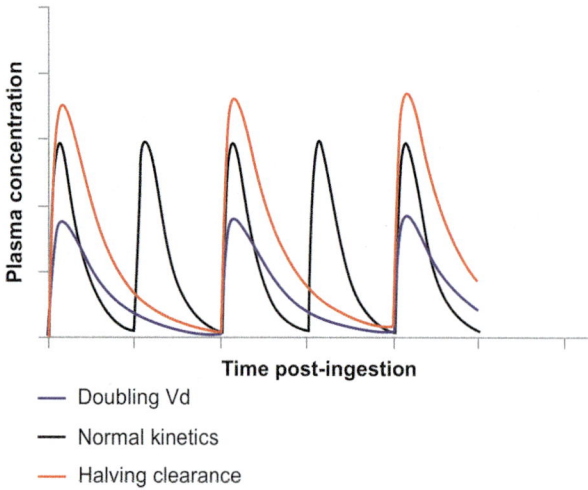

(CKD: chronic kidney disease; Vd: volume of distribution)

FIG. 11: In patients with transformed kinetics, lengthening the gap between doses will avoid the buildup of drug. The trough concentrations are comparable after the reduction in dosing rate, the maximum plasma concentration and average concentration are lesser when Vd is doubled. This may lead to suboptimal efficacy in CKD patients compared to otherwise normal subjects.

When the AUC prior to and post-kidney dysfunction is compared, the change in AUC is twice compared to initial value due to decrease in CL. The surge in the AUC and total drug exposure for a given dose increases the risk of adverse drug reactions.

Nevertheless, these changes do not occur alone, but simultaneously in patients with sepsis, kidney disease, and liver disease, hence, the representation is not as simple.

The association between various routes of CL has been shown in discussed previously in which the change in CL is related to the GFR (**Fig. 12**). However, the basis is a more generalized since, even in a patient with renal dysfunction, the nonrenal route of CL also may be affected due to the former which has not been considered.[10]

For instance, the nonrenal route, viz., the CL via drug disposition can also decline with deteriorating kidney function. Clinical evidence exists which shows substantial reductions in nonrenal CL ranging from 30 to 90% in patients with ESRD. CKD has been shown to significantly reduce the nonrenal CL and alter bioavailability of drugs mostly metabolized by the liver and intestine (**Fig. 13**).[22] Experimental studies in chronic renal failure models have explained these alterations in nonrenal CL as a consequence of reduced protein expression or downregulation of various cytochrome P 450 (CYP) enzymes (CYP2C6, CYP2C11, CYP3A2, and CYP) and thereby decreased metabolism; e.g., nimodipine CL was reduced by 87% due to decreased activity of CYP3A4 which is responsible for its dealkylation, similarly verapamil CL reduced by 54% due to decreased activity enzyme

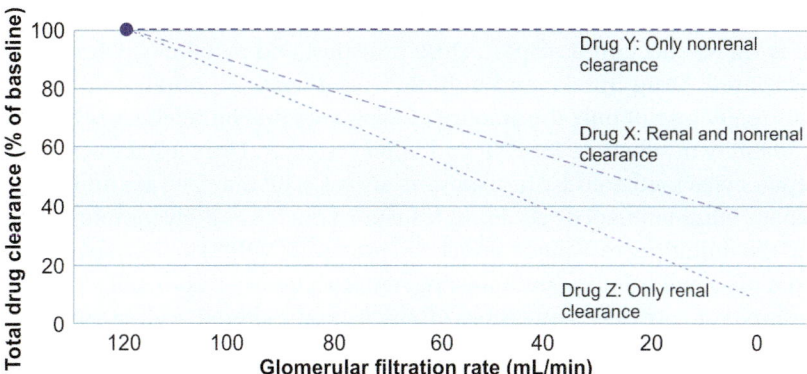

FIG. 12: Changes in total drug clearance with declining kidney function relates to the extent of drug clearance by the kidney. Drug Z is completely eliminated by renal route, hence, a drop in glomerular filtration rate (GFR) will lead to proportionate decrease in the total clearance; this will necessitate either reduction in dose or increasing the dosing interval to sustain the same mean plasma concentration. Drugs such as β-lactams, dabigatran, and atenolol are examples belonging to this group of solely renal clearance. Fluoroquinolones, rivaroxaban, and bisoprolol are drugs belonging to drug X-combined routes of clearance; lastly macrolides, metoprolol, and warfarin are examples belonging to drug Y which are cleared by nonrenal route only.[10]

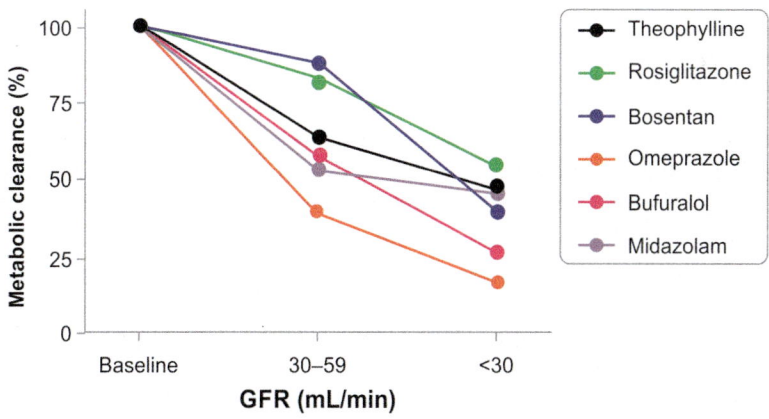

(GFR: glomerular filtration rate)

FIG. 13: Clearance via metabolism.

CYP3A4 causing demethylation.[10,23] Studies have also shown that the degree of inhibition of certain enzymes was not affected by dialysis but overturned entirely after renal transplantation.[24]

The effect of chronic renal failure (CRF) demonstrates as increase in bioavailability (F) for high extraction drugs (drugs with total CL_H highly dependent on hepatic blood flow).

Another way declining renal function affects nonrenal modes of drug CL is via its effect on transport. Drug transport and metabolism are closely associated. Drug uptake and outflow from intestinal, renal, and hepatic cells regulates not only the amount of drug available intracellularly but also availability of substrate for CYP and other enzymes. Drug uptake across the hepatocytes mediated by transporters such OATP may be rate limiting on hepatic elimination of drugs. Efflux transporters such as P-glycoprotein (Pgp) and the multidrug resistance associated protein 2 (MRP2) in the hepatocytes, renal proximal tubules, and intestinal enterocytes are responsible for CL of various types of drugs; expressions of which may be altered leading to changes in transport. In experimental models of chronic renal failure, an increase in protein, messenger ribonucleic acid (mRNA) expression of hepatic Pgp, hepatic MRP2 mRNA expression in kidney as well as liver was noted. Some in-vitro studies showed a decrease in OATP2 and renal OCT2 expression.

Likewise, expression and function of drug transporters in the intestine are also reduced in CRF) experimental models. Reduced intestinal Pgp and MRP2 protein expression and activity without change in mRNA have been found which suggests that protein degradation and not downregulation of transcription generally leads to decline in drug transporter function. Also, the increased levels of circulating uremic factors could inhibit transport function owing to their competition with the substrates, thus increasing bioavailability of drugs in CRF.[23] Several uremic toxins are known to directly inhibit the uptake of certain drugs by OATP in kidney as well as hepatocytes.[23]

ADJUSTING THE DOSING REGIMEN IN CHRONIC KIDNEY DISEASE: OPTIMAL APPROACH

Though there is clarity on the effects of CKD on the pharmacokinetic parameters of various drugs, the cut-off at which the dose adjustments should be begun in renal dysfunction is yet not clearly defined. It has been generally followed that a decline of <30% in any pharmacokinetic parameter does not need dose modifications. Further, the contribution of renal route of excretion should also be considered when recommending dose modifications. Occasionally, hepatically metabolised and eliminated drugs transform into potent metabolites for which renal elimination is the major route. In such cases, it is important to consider dose modifications to prevent drug accumulation. Renal excretion of morphine per se is merely 4% of its total elimination. Yet, in patients with renal dysfunction, morphine use leads to morphine intoxication. This is attributed to two major morphine metabolites, i.e., morphine-3-glucuronide and morphine-6-glucuronide, which are cleared via renal mechanisms but amass in patients with renal dysfunction. Similarly, mycophenolate metabolizes to mycophenolic acid glucuronide and accumulates but being inactive does not cause any signs of intoxication in these patients.[25,26] The former is up to 360 times more potent than the parent, and the latter is inactive. These can build-up in the patients with renal impairment and leads to gastrointestinal intolerance in severe CKD. Other examples include, meperidine metabolite normeperidine, which lowers the seizure threshold as it accumulates in uremic patients; benzodiazepine metabolites prolong sedation.[27] Several other general principles can be applied based on available data for the drug; accumulation of a negligibly toxic drug for a short treatment course can be exempted from dose modifications unlike a drug which is needed for a longer treatment duration since, this could lead to levels of toxic accumulation in patients with renal dysfunction.

Less toxic, short treatment course	Highly toxic, longer treatment course
Antibiotics	Metformin, digoxin, lithium, or colchicine

Thus, dose modifications would be necessary for particular drugs which are greatly affected by the deterioration of kidney function and increased risk of toxicity.[10]

OPTIMIZATION OF TREATMENT IN CHRONIC KIDNEY DISEASE

In patients with hepatic or renal impairment, the conventional approach is to initiate therapy with a lower dose and gradually increase it. This method is appropriate for chronic therapy in which target clinical effect can be achieved over a longer duration. Nevertheless, in acute conditions like infection or sepsis which necessitate prompt treatment with anti-infectives, this perspective may not be helpful.[28]

The desired plasma concentration to achieve clinical benefit without increasing risk of adverse effect is affected by many factors such as the patient perse, the disease condition and drug being prescribed for particular duration.[29] The outcomes of treatment can be determined based on the relevant parameter as per the disease condition, e.g., improvement in systolic and diastolic blood pressure, blood glucose levels, hemoglobin A1c (HbA1c), etc. Some outcomes may take a longer time to display a significant improvement, like anticancer drugs or immunosuppressants.[10]

Loading dose-reduced inappropriately may result in inappropriate plasma levels leading to inefficacy in patients with renal impairment. A loading dose equivalent to the typical maintenance dose for patients with normal renal function should be generally administered to patients with impaired renal function. Later, the dose and frequency should be personalized based on the desired plasma concentration.[30] Since, the objective of the loading dose is to attain a plasma concentration post first dose, changes in drug CL do not impact the loading dose administered. Hence, except CL, if no other pharmacokinetic parameters are altered, the loading dose does not need adjustment.

When quick onset of action is not necessary, the maintenance dose can be used right from the initial treatment to reach steady state concentrations. In renally impaired patients, if renal excretion decreases by ≥50%, the maintenance dose needs adjustment which can be either prolongation of interval or dose reduction or both. The extension of the interval should be proportionate to the extent of delay in drug excretion which in turn depends on the level of renal impairment. This option would be applicable for drugs with a wide therapeutic range and long half-life, however, it should be used cautiously since, it can lead to suboptimal concentration. The dose reduction method without the decrease in frequency, results in consistent plasma concentration of the drug. Decreases may be required for drugs mostly secreted in the proximal tubule in patients with kidney tubulointerstitial disease and for drugs that are mainly excreted via nonrenal pathways when GFR < 60 mL/min.[29] Though dose reduction method is more commonly used, it may be associated with increased risk of toxicity due to accumulation. Hence, in order to balance the risks and improve benefits a combination of these two methods is suggested.[29,30] This does not affect the steady state concentration (equation 1) but reduces the variation in the plasma concentrations. Further still, modifying either or both does not assure efficacy without safety concerns, therefore, therapeutic drug monitoring or biomarker of effect should be considered in CKD patients especially with drugs having a narrow therapeutic index, since, a small change in concentrations of such drugs can cause toxicity or loss of efficacy (**Fig. 14**).[29,30] On the contrary, large alterations in CL of drugs with a wide therapeutic index, may have only a negligible impact on response, and therefore, significant dose adjustments are not necessary, e.g., β-lactam antibiotics.[31]

Lastly, another important factor to be considered is the clinical correlation with plasma concentrations, since, these drugs may cause toxicity even within therapeutic range.[29]

Hence, in CKD patients maintaining drug concentration within therapeutic range are even more challenging when drugs with short half-life (e.g., heparin) are required to be administered. Patients with CKD are at high-risk of thrombosis. Therefore, anticoagulation with heparin is vital but since, heparin is predominantly eliminated by renal pathways, maintain its plasma concentration within therapeutic range is an arduous task. A slow first-order CL of heparin by renal excretion, leads to nonlinear pharmacokinetics with anticoagulation snowballing unreasonably at high

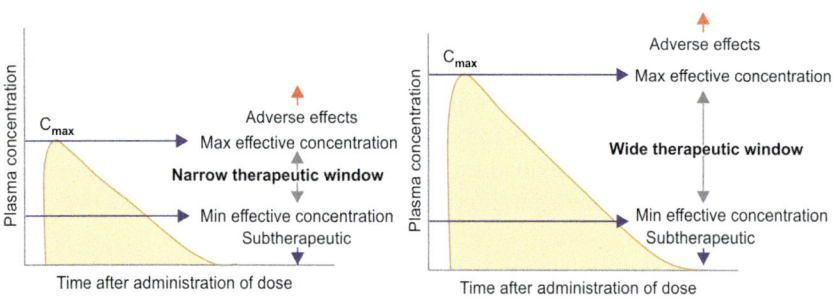

(Max: maximum; Min: minimum)

FIG 14: Therapeutic window.

therapeutic doses. This can lead to excessive anticoagulation in patients with moderate to severe renal dysfunction. Additionally, interpatient variability makes the anticoagulant response unpredictable. Therefore, conventional dosing of heparin is suggested in patients with severe renal impairment to prevent supratherapeutic anticoagulation.[32]

Renal pathway is an important excretion means for opioid drugs, via both tubular secretion and glomerular filtration. Significant increases in both the AUC-time curve (70%) and C_{max} (29%) have been demonstrated for dihydrocodeine in renal failure patients. Evidently, failure of renal excretion of the parent drug or its metabolites explains the disparity between CKD patients and normal subjects. In order to achieve plasma concentrations in CKD patients similar to normal subjects, the dose reduction in such cases is not necessary, merely extending the dosing interval is adequate. Yet validity of these data in other patients needs confirmation; hence, therapeutic monitoring should be considered.[33] Unlike dihydrocodeine, for repaglinide in patients with advanced CKD (**Fig. 4**) dose reduction as well as prolongation of dosing interval are necessary to match the AUC and plasma concentration with normal subjects because the increase in patients with CKD is relatively very high, 232% and 82%, respectively compared to dihydrocodeine 70% versus 29%.[34]

The conventional approach of adjusting the drug dose in proportion to the decrease in GFR is limited by several factors: the nonrenal processes affected by renal impairment, the contribution of intact tubules in drug elimination compared to glomerular filtration. In patients with comparable GFR, but difference in glomerular nephritis, proteinuria, hypoalbuminemia, but creatinine CL (CrCL) >90 mL/min, the CL of drugs can be decreased significantly owing to the impact on transporters and protein binding.[30] Joy et al., in his prospective in-vivo study found that there were significant pharmacokinetic differences between patients with glomerulonephritis and healthy subjects. Nevertheless, even though the kidney functions were affected to a variable degree across patient groups with glomerulonephritis, nonglomerular CKD, and ESRD patients there was no significant difference in-vivo metabolism and transporter functions.[35] But, studies have demonstrated differential effects depending on the drug in terms of effect on the pharmacokinetic parameters.

Consequently, it is not appropriate to oversimplify these findings of transformed pharmacokinetics to patients with different GFRs, kidney diseases, or other drugs. Yet, it can be stated that absorption may increase or decrease and is not adequately enumerated. The Vd is either unchanged or increased, the CYP-mediated CL is rather diminished, the renal excretion is either reduced or comparatively constant but CL_{NR} is not adequately determined or decreased.[30]

Given the variability in the pharmacokinetics of drugs, it is prudent to opt for therapeutic drug monitoring which though tedious takes into consideration the interindividual variability unlike population-based mean or median data. As mentioned previously, therapeutic drug monitoring

(TDM) is especially important in case of critically ill patients, for drug classes with narrow therapeutic index (e.g., warfarin and digoxin) and for drug classes (antimicrobials)[36] for which optimal plasma concentrations are critical determinants of clinical outcomes. The only limitation of TDM is the lack of quick turnaround time within clinically advantageous time span.[37] Only in cases which are not complicated, drug courses and dose intervals are shorter, TDM may not be necessary.[38]

LIMITATIONS OF ESTIMATED GLOMERULAR FILTRATION RATE

Though the measured GFR (mGFR) is the gold standard, due to its resource requirements and cost, eGFR is preferred to classify and monitor the severity of CKD. However, eGFR also has its own limitations. The true GFR could be nearly 50% or twice that of the estimated value which means that when the GFR is greater, this error would further rise.[39] For example, eGFR 30 mL/min may indicate an mGFR of 20–40 mL/min.

Also, automated eGFR do not give exactly the same results. For patients with a body surface area that deviates considerably from 1.73 m^2, the eGFR can be deindexed to give units of mL/min (**Box 1**).

Deindexed eGFR (mL/min): = eGFR (mL/min/1.73 m^2) × BSA ÷ 1.73

This value is used to decide the drug dosing. But, the eGFR is limited in patients with severe and morbid obesity since, these formulae were not corroborated in obese or severely obese population (BMI ≥ 35 kg/m^2).[40] More bias has been found with deindexed eGFR in the subgroup of patients with BMI ≥ 40 kg/m and males than females.[2] Thus, the mean actual GFR (mL/min) is about 10% higher than the automated eGFR, and >30% higher for those who are taller or heavier.[40] If drug's dose is reduced when a patient's GFR is <30 mL/min, the dose for the patient is usually higher if the deindexed eGFR is used to guide dosing. A study in obese population has suggested that regardless of the CKD stage, deindexation of eGFR leads to higher prejudice and misclassification and cannot be used as a proxy of mGFR.[41]

Some of the drugs dosing recommendation are stated in terms of eCrCl. The eCrCl is probably lower in patients with a lower body weight (<60 kg) and advanced age (>80 years). In obese patients (BMI > 30 kg/m^2), eCrCl based on actual body weight will overestimate GFR and vice-versa in underweight.

However, slight digressions in eGFR are not likely to be clinically meaningful and should not lead to an immediate dose adjustment (or cessation) but instead prompt ongoing monitoring of kidney function or TDM.[40]

CONCLUSION

'Relationship between drug concentration and time' and 'relationship between drug concentration and effect' are two important understanding before prescribing any medicine. While advising any therapeutics we need to be extremely cautious regarding these concepts. Constantly we need to evaluate risk versus benefit of given medicines while they reach both supra and sub therapeutic range. There are different formulas to calculate eGFR like Cockcroft–Gault formula, CKD-EPI, MDRD, etc. To offer best possible outcome we need to consider different PK parameters as well with host specific critical issues. Therapeutic drug monitoring could be one important strategy and should be utilized in patients who require. Clinical pharmacology principles could be immensely helpful to optimize therapy in CKD patients having multiple comorbidities.

REFERENCES

1. Turfus SC, Delgoda R, Picking D, Gurley BJ. Pharmacokinetics. In: Pharmacognosy (3rd edition). Jamaica: Elsevier; 2017.
2. Patel K, Kirkpatrick CM. Pharmacokinetic concepts revisited--basic and applied. Curr Pharm Biotechnol. 2011;12(12):1983-90.
3. Saghir SA, Ansari RA. Pharmacokinetics. In Reference Module in Biomedical Sciences. Amsterdam, The Netherland: Elsevier; 2018.
4. Benet LZ, Zia-Amirhosseini P. Basic principles of pharmacokinetics. Toxicol Pathol. 1995;23(2):115-23.
5. Sakai JB. Pharmacokinetics: The Absorption, Distribution, and Excretion of Drugs. Practical Pharmacology for the Pharmacy Technician. 2009:27-40.
6. Blowey DL. Drug Use and Dosage in Renal Failure. Comprehensive Pediatric Nephrology. 2008;991-1002.
7. Maddison JE, Page SW, Dyke TM. Clinical pharmacokinetics. In: Maddison JE, Page SW, Church DB (eds). Small Animal Clinical Pharmacology (2nd Edition). W.B. Saunders; 2008. pp. 27-40.
8. Davis JL. Pharmacologic Principles. In: Reed SM, Bayly WM, Sellon DC (eds). Equine Internal Medicine (4th Edition). W.B. Saunders; 2018. pp. 79-137.
9. Aldred EM, Buck C, Vall K. Pharmacology: A Handbook for Complementary Healthcare Professionals. Elsevier; 2009.
10. Lea-Henry TN, Carland JE, Stocker SL, Sevastos J, Roberts DM. Clinical Pharmacokinetics in Kidney Disease: Fundamental Principles. Clin J Am Soc Nephrol. 2018;13(7):1085-95.
11. Borowy CS, Ashurst JV. Physiology, Zero and First Order Kinetics. StatPearls. 2020.
12. Mansoor A, Mahabadi N. Volume of Distribution. StatPearls. 2020.
13. Hallare J, Gerriets V. Half Life. StatPearls. 2020.
14. Ward RM, Kern SE. Principles of Pharmacokinetics. In: Fetal and Neonatal Physiology (5th Edition). Elsevier; 2017.
15. Bardal SK, Martin DS. Pharmacokinetics. In: Applied Pharmacology. Elsevier; 2011.
16. Momper JD, Venkataramanan R, Nolin TD. Nonrenal drug clearance in CKD: Searching for the path less traveled. Adv Chronic Kidney Dis. 2010;17(5):384-91.
17. Collins JM. Pharmacokinetics, Pharmacodynamics, and Pharmacogenetics. In: The Molecular Basis of Cancer (3rd Edition). Elsevier; 2008.
18. Kerns EH, Di L. Pharmacokinetics. In: Drug-Like Properties: Concepts, Structure Design and Methods (2nd Edition). Elsevier; 2016.
19. Multiple-Dose Regimens. 2020. [online] Available from https://basicmedicalkey.com/multiple-dose-regimens/(Last accessed September, 2021).
20. Ito S. Pharmacokinetics 101. Paediatr Child Health. 2011;16(9):535-6.
21. Chronic Kidney Disease: Clinical Practice Recommendations for Primary Care Physicians and Healthcare Providers (6th edition). American Society of Nephrology.

22. Wan SH, Koda RT, Maronde RF. Pharmacokinetics, pharmacology of atenolol and effect of renal disease. Br J Clin Pharmacol. 1979;7(6):569-74.
23. Dreisbach AW, Lertora JJ. The effect of chronic renal failure on drug metabolism and transport. Expert Opin Drug Metab Toxicol. 2008;4(8):1065-74.
24. Dreisbach AW, Lertora JJ. The effect of chronic renal failure on hepatic drug metabolism and drug disposition. Semin Dial. 2003;16(1):45-50.
25. Michaud J, Dube P, Naud J, Leblond FA, Desbiens K, Bonnardeaux A, et al. Effects of serum from patients with chronic renal failure on rat hepatic cytochrome P450. Br J Pharmacol. 2005;144(8):1067-77.
26. Frances B, Gout R, Monsarrat B, Cros J, Zajac JM. Further evidence that morphine-6 beta-glucuronide is a more potent opioid agonist than morphine. J Pharmacol Exp Ther. 1992;262:25-31.
27. MacPhee IA, Spreafico S, Bewick M, Davis C, Eastwood JB, Johnston A, et al. Pharmacokinetics of mycophenolate mofetil in patients with end-stage renal failure. Kidney Int. 2000;57:1164-8.
28. Verbeeck RK. Pharmacokinetics and dosage adjustment in patients with hepatic dysfunction. Eur J Clin Pharmacol. 2008;64(12):1147-61.
29. Roberts DM, Sevastos J, Carland JE, Stocker SL, Lea-Henry TN. Clinical Pharmacokinetics in Kidney Disease: Application to Rational Design of Dosing Regimens. Clin J Am Soc Nephrol. 2018;13(8):1254-63.
30. Swan SK, Bennett WM. Drug dosing guidelines in patients with renal failure. West J Med. 1992;156(6):633-8.
31. Prescribing Drugs in Renal Disease. Pocket Companion to Brenner and Rector's The Kidney. 2011:665-700.
32. Doogue MP, Polasek TM. Drug dosing in renal disease. Clin Biochem Rev. 2011;32(2):69-73.
33. Hughes S, Szeki I, Nash MJ, Thachil J. Anticoagulation in chronic kidney disease patients-the practical aspects. Clin Kidney J. 2014;7(5):442-9.
34. Barnes JN, Williams AJ, Tomson MJ, Toseland PA, Goodwin FJ. Dihydrocodeine in renal failure: further evidence for an important role of the kidney in the handling of opioid drugs. Br Med J (Clin Res Ed). 1985;290(6470):740-2.
35. Marbury TC, Ruckle JL, Hatorp V, Andersen MP, Nielsen KK, Huang WC, et al. Pharmacokinetics of repaglinide in subjects with renal impairment. Clin Pharmacol Ther. 2000;67(1):7-15.
36. Joy MS, Frye RF, Nolin TD, Roberts BV, La MK, Wang J, et al. In vivo alterations in drug metabolism and transport pathways in patients with chronic kidney diseases. Pharmacotherapy. 2014;34(2):114-22.
37. Wong G, Sime FB, Lipman J, Roberts JA. How do we use therapeutic drug monitoring to improve outcomes from severe infections in critically ill patients? BMC Infect Dis. 2014;14:288.
38. Ates HC, Roberts JA, Lipman J, Cass AEG, Urban GA, Dincer C. On-Site Therapeutic Drug Monitoring. Trends Biotechnol. 2020;38(11):1262-77.
39. Begg EJ, Barclay ML, Kirkpatrick CJ. The therapeutic monitoring of antimicrobial agents. Br J Clin Pharmacol. 1999;47(1):23-30.
40. Stefani M, Singer RF, Roberts DM. How to adjust drug doses in chronic kidney disease. Aust Prescr. 2019;42(5):163-7.
41. Guebre-Egziabher F, Brunelle C, Thomas J, Pelletier CC, Normand G, Juillard L, et al. Estimated Glomerular Filtration Rate Bias in Participants with Severe Obesity Regardless of Deindexation. Obesity (Silver Spring). 2019;27(12):2011-7.

30. Protection of the Healthcare Workers in the Coronavirus Disease Pandemic

Khusrav Beji Bajan

INTRODUCTION

The coronavirus disease 2019 (COVID-19) pandemic has been devastating world over. Not only has it evolved into a dangerous always mutating threat, but also led to a crippling economy and millions to die. Waves after waves have surprised and shocked the entire healthcare systems globally. The bravest efforts to combat this menace have been from the frontline healthcare workers (HCWs).

In the first wave, without ammunition like vaccinations, poor supply of personal protective equipments (PPEs) and a lack of infrastructure, the frontliners-exhibited selflessness, bravery, and humanity to once again roll up their sleeves to combat this war.

It is imperative for the healthcare system to ensure safety of the frontline workers as they grapple 24×7, risking their and their families lives. We need to have guidelines and some protocols which would help enable HCWs safety.

GUIDELINES TO PROTECT THE PROTECTORS

- Appropriate use of PPE
    - Level of PPE to be divided as per the zone in the hospital
        - High risk zone [full PPE—hazardous materials (HAZMAT)]
            - Intensive care unit (ICU)/occupational therapy (OT)/emergency room (ER)/holding area/ambulance/scopy suites
        - Medium risk zone (N95 + surgical mask on top and goggles or face shield +/– surgical gown)
            - Outpatient department (OPD)/fever clinic/oncology/artificial kidney dialysis department (AKD)/imaging/ear, nose, and throat (ENT)/dental
        - Low risk zone (two surgical masks)
            - One other than above
- Appropriate donning and doffing procedures and dedicated areas
    - To have donn/doff buddies to guide
    - Videos/posters

- For any aerosol generating procedures (AGP) such as intubation, bronchoscopy, swab collection, and cardiopulmonary resuscitation (CPR).
  - Use extra gears in form of personal air purifying respirators (PAPRs) or honeywell shields over and above full PPE.
- Swab collection to be done only by qualified lab technician anywhere in the hospital and not to be done by doctors/interns/paramedics.
- Proper and appropriate accommodation to be provided to doctors keeping in mind social distancing in cafeterias, food halls, etc.
- Appropriate quarantine facilities for the doctors into hotels, etc., if similar facilities not available at their homes and to protect the family members from getting affected too.
- Working hours to be restricted to 6 hours in high risk zones. Also work:off ratio to be maintained at 7:3 days.
  - Minimum manpower to be utilized and rotation from high to medium to low risk zones done cyclically.
- Consider antibody testing at regular intervals for an insight into the immunity level.
- Appropriate environment to be created in the high risk zones.
  - Negative pressure:
    - \>12 to 15 air exchanges per hour or >145 L/sec/patient achieved
    - High efficiency particulate air (HEPA) filters deployed where appropriate
    - Ante room, if possible
      - To use engineering department skills to deal with heating, ventilation, and air conditioning (HVAC)
- Look after the mental health of the HCWs
  - Periodic consultations
  - Groups to discuss
  - Mentoring and "*hearing them out*" sessions
- Treatment of affected HCWs at top priority since, severity and mortality is five to tenfold higher amongst positive HCWs across all age groups.
  - Preferably a separate area in the same institute or any equivalent institute with proper hygiene and treatment facilities.
  - Provide additional leave for up to a month for the severe and prolonged cases.
  - Provide aggressive post-COVID syndrome care including physio and rehab.
- Adequate rest and appropriate nutrition including zinc, vitamin C, vitamin D, etc. (*only if evidence justifies its use*).
- Prioritize vaccination amongst all frontliners. Make efforts to allay vaccination hesitancy amongst the group.
- Have a task force to audit the breakthrough infections amongst the fully-vaccinated. Have genomics done for all such infections to understand the pattern of variants and vaccination efficacy.
- Have a specialized team to address the post-COVID syndrome and the quality-of-life goals amongst those who have been infected previously.

CONCLUSION

Frontline HCWs need a healthy and safe environment with access to facilities, infrastructure, drugs, and updated literature.

Government must provide adequate compensation in terms of remuneration and make periodic efforts toward maintaining the mental and physical health of the frontline HCWs holistically.

Utmost care must be exercised to provide PPEs, vaccinations (even booster doses when appropriate), and prompt and free treatment to all HCWs.

The entire healthcare system needs to unite to be able to avoid fatigue and burnout amongst fellow colleagues and to maintain a healthy work life balance.

SUGGESTED READINGS

1. Chen W, Huang Y. To protect health care workers better, to save more lives with covid-19. Anesth Analg. 2020;131(1):97-101.
2. The Lancet. COVID-19: Protecting health-care workers. Lancet. 2020;395(10228):922.
3. Udwadia ZF, Raju RS. How to protect the protectors: 10 lessons to learn for doctors fighting the Covid-19 coronavirus. Med J Armed Forces India. 2020;76(2):128-31.

31. The Immunology of Sepsis

Om Shrivastav

INTRODUCTION

Sepsis, the systemic inflammatory response to infection, is the major cause of death among critically ill patients. Both the pathogen and the host with respect to an inappropriate inflammatory response play role in immune mechanisms which contributes to sepsis. Also is the pathogenic role of immunity—cytokine storm and through immune paralysis. Apoptosis is a key mechanism in both of these also in multiorgan failure, which is a feature of severe sepsis. A number of polymorphisms are involved in susceptibility to sepsis, this includes cytokine genes, human leukocyte antigen (HLA) class II and caspase-12.

SEPSIS-ASSOCIATED HOST RESPONSE (BOX 1)

Sepsis and disruption of homeostatic functions go hand in hand and this has implications on metabolic, catabolic, and immune balance. This also impacts toward a state of persist inflammation that may last for weeks to months after infections are over, and is called chronic, critical illness since, a number of the functions disrupted may not return to normal for prolonged durations, much as the damage seen in noninfectious injuries. While these include a dysfunctional immune system, they may also represent altered mentation and impaired cognitive functions that may not return to normal for several months to years as part of the critical illness syndrome.

> **Box 1: Sepsis-associated host response.**
> - Key proinflammatory responses during sepsis:
>   - The activation of the complement system
>   - The coagulation system
>   - The vascular endothelium
>   - Neutrophils and platelets
> - Whereas, immune suppression is primarily caused by:
>   - The reprogramming of antigen-presenting cells
>   - The apoptosis
>   - Exhaustion of lymphocytes

The role of superantigens in chronic intensive care illness is unclear, however, the role of group A streptococcus is well defined.

Interaction between Pathogen and Host Immune Responses

Selection of both virulence and immune evasion strategies.

Immune evasion strategies:
- Camouflaging self from immune system
- Functional disruption of immune system
- Destroying elements of the immune system (e.g., microbial antigens presenting structures to initiate host response). As S counter strategy of host responses is important for a successful response to overcome cellular and immune dysfunction.

Effector T-cells have a recognized role in bacterial infections, however, the role in viral infections is still unclear.

Immune dysfunction may mimic a profound and prolonged immunodeficiency, especially in the number of viable CD4 counts, again reflective of viable T-cell population. This has been best described in the human immunodeficiency virus (HIV), but is also seen in cytomegalovirus (CMV) or other viral infections, often occurring as more than one infection at a point in time because the T-cell population has diminished. Prolonged T-cell dysfunction may also contribute to a number of malignancies, especially Kaposi's sarcoma.

ASSESSMENT OF HOST IMMUNE RESPONSES

While thorough intensive care management accompanied by nutritional support, antibiotic therapy, and prevention of secondary infections remain the cornerstones of treatment, uncontrolled infection, and therefore, sepsis still remains the largest cause of death. Recurrent nosocomial infections leading to mortality are largely reflective of multiple compartments of immune breakdown over prolonged periods of intensive care units (ICU) patients. This includes primarily the helper T-cells or CD4 counts, but also suppressor T-cells (CD8 cells), but also natural killer (NK) cells, compliments, and immunoglobulins. A major and often disregarded factor in immune dysfunction is the presence of multiple drugs that have a suppressive effect on the central nervous system, and therefore the brain, besides knocking out major components of the immune system.

The role of cellular markers and genomic evaluation of a critically ill patient cannot be overemphasized. Key elements, such as tumor necrosis factor-alpha (TNF-α), besides C-reactive protein and anti-pro-brain natriuretic peptide (BNP) are significantly contributory besides other markers in establishing the state of inflammation and impaired cell-mediated immunity (CMI).

There are other elements in the immune system that include chemokines and cytokines that should be measured, but unfortunately require referenced laboratories and are both time consuming and labor intensive. These may well become the markers of a broken down CMI that lends to mortality in sepsis in the very foreseeable future.

Along with granulocyte-macrophage colony stimulating factor (GM-CSF), flow-cytometric monocytic HLA receptor (mHLA-DR) is useful as a diagnostic biomarker for immunosuppression and as a surrogate outcome for intervention.

IMMUNE DYSFUNCTION IN SEPSIS

As a consequence of ongoing sepsis, homeostatic functions all across the board involving both innate and CMI are either severely impaired or completely depleted. This, therefore, leads to recurrent infections, poor response of agents requiring robust CMI, and coagulopathy. Not only the lifespan of combat inducing cells to pathogens is drastically decreased, the hematopoietic system which continuously has an accelerated production and delivery of protective elements of the immune system gradually shows slowing and ultimately paralysis of all productive elements in sepsis. Consequent to these features tissue regeneration and wound healing is also impaired.

Consequent to the features described above the host responses of specifically-directed measures such as systemic inflammatory response syndrome (SIRS) and compensatory anti-inflammatory response syndrome (CARS) become gradually impaired and then completely dysfunctional.

Chronic sustained infections and subsequent inflammatory responses increase morbidity, length of stay, requirement for additional therapy, not limited to antibiotics, and mortality. A feature that commences between 10th and 15th day in ICU patients is called persistent critical illness and this is defined of a patient needing to stay in ICU, independent of infections, but rather dictated by age, sex, and other comorbidities.

Critical illness is hallmarked by dysfunction of neutrophils, macrophages, monocytes, complement system, and immunoglobulins besides multipole components of the immune system.

The process of physiological aging undergoes a catastrophic insult as a consequence of the features described above. This is termed as immunosenescence.

T-cells which become dysfunctional, critically because of shortening of telomeres, is a process that is described as thymic involution. Hematopoietic cell dysfunction is a major feature of T-cell paralysis and dysfunctional T-cell population.

Conditions that mimic autoimmune diseases may also manifest that lead to a self-feeding cycle of requiring immunosuppression and worsening of sepsis. This is largely due to the inability of the immune system to make robust antigen presenting cells (APCs) which are the most important elements in consequent immune dysfunction.

Behavioral Pattern of Cytokines in Sepsis

Both protective and damaging elements are regulated by the cytokine system, and this intricate feature is constantly being played in milder or self-limiting infections. In sepsis, however, the proinflammatory cytokines supersede all protective measures and subsequently leads to a partially or irreversible process that dictates poor patient recovery.

T Cell

A number of infections which may be described as opportunistic that include bacterial, viral, fungal, protozoal, either singularly or in combination, will present themselves when functional T-cells fall by anywhere between 15–20% of a patient's pre-existing count. A ratio of CD4:CD8 cells that exceeds 0.3% is protective, and the chance of an opportunistic infection is <20%. Conversely, if this ratio is 0.1% or below, the chance of an opportunistic infection approaches 40–70%.

Gamma Delta T Cells

The TY-cell receptor plays an important role in pathogenesis involving the gut mucosa. Upon recognizing the lipid surface of pathogen, the gamma delta T cells ($\gamma\delta$ T cells), which are a subset of T cells, release several proinflammatory cytokines which includes, besides others, the interferons and IL-17.

Additionally, because of the decreased circulation of CD4 and APCs, besides neutrophils, the presence of CD8 cells leads to the cytotoxic function being enhanced and several disruptions of the cross-linking cell lineages that are protective in septicemia.

T Helper Cells (Th cells)

The activation of T cells is almost singularly dependent on the presentation of APC, by the B cell and the major histocompatibility complex-II (MHC-II) for the next stage of immunological response. The next stage of cascade activation of both adaptive and innate immunity follows this presentation of the APC to the CD4 cells. Upon activation, CD4 cells differentiate into one of several T-cell subsets including Th1, Th2, Th3, Th17, Th22, Th9, or T follicular helper (TFH).

The process of program cell death or apoptosis is the first major casualty of robust CD4 cell function due to sepsis. The other major mechanisms that influence Th1 function involve histone and chromatin that undergo both remodeling and methylation sepsis. In addition to these disruptions, the Th17 reduced function leads to increased bacterial infections and impaired clearing of fungal infections.

Regulatory T cells

A key feature of T-cells is the regulatory component that suppresses a number of responses especially odd autoimmune diseases that would otherwise manifest as clinically significant conditions. These are called T-regulatory cells or Tregs. In all states of inflammation, but especially sepsis, the Tregs have a deleterious effect on recovery and therefore, adverse outcomes in sepsis. This is largely due to the impact that the Tregs have an uncontrolled infections in ICU. This failure of auto regulation is significantly contributory to the presence of sepsis-induced prolonged inflammation and immune dysregulation.

Other Components

In assessing immune dysfunction in the earliest part of septicemia, the other components of immune responses are:
- B cells
- Natural killer cells, neutrophils, monocytes, and macrophages
- Complement studies and immunoglobulin quantification should also be considered, but interpreted carefully since, there occurs a transient reduction of responses.

B Cells

The role of B cells in sepsis is diverse, involves several phenotypes and has a major impact in sepsis immune biology. B-cell effectiveness reduces progressively in septic shock and two key predictors of survival from B-cell populations, CD5+ B1a-type cells are significantly depleted. These dysfunctions in turn have decisive down regulatory effect on cytokine production and reduced interferon signaling.

Innate response activator (IRA) B-cell population, which is phenotypically and functionally distinct from B1a cells and depends on pattern recognition receptors (PRRs), which produces GM-CSF. This impaired competence of B-cells leads to recurrent infections in the elderly, even after septic episodes have concluded. Concurrent with these dysfunctions, there also occurs depleted abilities of IRA B-cell generation, a hyper stimulatory GM-CSF, and IRA-regulated interleukin-3 (IL-3) production. All of these dysfunctions have a role in increasing mortality, recurrent infections, and poor immune response.

Natural Killer Cells

The cytotoxic function of NK cells is significantly impeded during sepsis. This subsegment identified by CD16 and CD56 markers is dysfunctional and has consequences on the interferon-γ (IFN-γ) expression as well. The combined effects of these impediments in function have, therefore, a role in the activation of viruses like CMV, commonly associated with septicemia.

Neutrophils

Neutrophils are a crucial component of the inherent innate systems of defense and have a major role in the control of infections before they become the reason for sepsis in ICUs. The impact that sepsis has a disruption of basic innate immunity functions and is diverse at multiple levels. The neutrophil production from the bone marrow during sepsis is such that immature neutrophil forms like band forms flood the circulation. This in turn has implications on fully functional complement system and anti-inflammatory cytokines. The impact on an already exhausted immune system is grievous since, the cell signaling, neutrophil immune senescence, and a fractured toll-like-receptor (TLR) activation and response impact on persistent infections and have a presence upon a weakened immune system, even after patients recover from sepsis. Neutrophils also elaborate neutrophil extracellular traps (NETs). This mechanism entails the release of antimicrobial proteins anchored to a chromatin network of activated neutrophils. The deoxyribonucleic acid (DNA) of the NETs has embedded in it multiple components that elaborate diverse pathways for antimicrobial control. Granule and cytoplasmic proteins, including neutrophil elastase (NE), myeloperoxidase (MPO), cathepsin G, proteinase 3 (PR3), gelatinase, LL-37, lactoferrin, and calprotectin as well as histones H1, H2A, H2B, H3, and H4.

Monocytes and Macrophages

The physical characteristics of the monocytes that enable it to be functional in sepsis are altered. The reduced capacity of blood monocytes of the patients with sepsis release proinflammatory cytokines after endotoxin [lipopolysaccharide (LPS)] challenge "endotoxin tolerance" which has been suggested to facilitate poor short-term and long-term sepsis outcomes. Various mononuclear cell signaling pathways are altered and contribute to endotoxin tolerance, reduced antigen presentation related to diminished HLA-DR cell surface expression. Persistent reductions in HLA-DR cell surface expression, monocytes from the patients with sepsis also demonstrate a reduced ability to secrete the proinflammatory cytokines TNF, IL-1, IL-6, and IL-12 after LPS challenge. The reduced monocyte capacity to secrete proinflammatory cytokines suggest that intracellular signaling has shifted toward the production of anti-inflammatory mediators which are associated with hospital acquired, ongoing, and secondary infections which ultimately increase sepsis-associated mortality. Reduced monocyte HLA-DR expression is a surrogate marker of monocyte "anergy", development of ongoing infections, and mortality.

KEY POINTS
- Sepsis-associated host response gets disrupted and can have long-term implications on immune balance.
- The interaction between pathogen and host immune response is a complex mechanism of immune evasion strategies on the part of the pathogen.
- T cells are disrupted very early in sepsis and they have implications on other immune responses.

- Host immune responses need to be measured in a serial manner to access the extent of suppression of the host immune system.
- The growing role of cellular markers and genomic evaluation is emphasized.
- Chronic-sustained infections have a deleterious effect on all components of the host immune system that persists even after the infection has been controlled.
- The role of T-cells subpopulations, like $\gamma\delta$ cells or T helper cells, are responsible for activation of MHC-II and determining the next stage of the inflammatory cascade in sepsis.
- Other components of the defense include also disruption of primarily neutrophils, monocytes, B cells, and NK cells, besides other components.

SUGGESTED READINGS

1. McBride MA, Owen AM, Stothers CL, Hernandez A, Luan L, Burelbach KR, et al. The metabolic basis of immune dysfunction following sepsis and Trauma. Front Immunol. 2020;11:1043.
2. Cao C, Ma T, Chai YF, Shou ST. The role of regulatory T cells in immune dysfunction during sepsis. World J Emerg Med. 2015;6(1):5-9.
3. Pons S, Arnaud M, Loiselle M, Arrii E, Azoulay E, Zafrani L. Immune consequences of endothelial cells activation and dysfunction during sepsis. Crit Care Clin. 2020;36(2):401-13.
4. Nascimento DC, Alves-Filho JC, Sônego F, Fukada SY, Pereira MS, Benjamim C, et al. Role of regulatory T cells in long term immune dysfunction associated with sepsis. Crit Care Med. 2010;38(8):1718-25.
5. Bermejo-Martin JF, Andaluz-Ojeda D, Almansa R, Gandía F, Gómez-Herreras JI, Gomez-Sanchez E, et al. Defining immunological dysfunction in sepsis: A requisite tool for precision medicine. J Infect. 2016;72(5):525-36.
6. Delano MJ, Ward PA. Immune systems role in sepsis progression, resolution and long-term outcomes. Immunol Rev. 2016;274(1):330-53.
7. Pool R, Gomez H, Kellum JA. Mechanisms of organ dysfunction in sepsis. Crit Care Clin. 2018;34(1):63-80.
8. Immunology and Infectious Diseases – Medscape.
9. Infectiousdiseasesclinicsuptodate.om

32. Coronavirus Disease and Cardiovascular System

Ajit Desai, Nikesh Jain

INTRODUCTION

The first case of coronavirus disease 2019 (COVID-19), caused by severe acute respiratory syndrome coronavirus 2 (SARS-CoV-2) virus was diagnosed on 12th December, 2019 in Wuhan, Hubei province of China. It spread rapidly throughout China and all parts of the world, and on 11th March, 2020 World Health Organization declared COVID-19 as "Pandemic". COVID-19 pandemic is still ongoing with emergence of different variants throughout the world.

Severe acute respiratory syndrome coronavirus 2 primarily affects respiratory system causing pneumonia. Severe COVID-19 triggers cytokine storm causing multiorgan damage with frequent cardiac involvement. In addition to cytokine storm, the hyperinflammatory state causes plaque rupture, thromboembolic phenomenon, endothelial dysfunction, microangiopathy contributing to cardiac damage. Cardiovascular manifestations increase COVID-19 morbidity and mortality. Patients with risk factors for cardiovascular disease (CVD) such as diabetes, hypertension (HTN), dyslipidemia, etc., and with pre-existing CVD are more vulnerable to develop cardiac complications. Even de novo cardiac complications occur frequently, irrespective of severity of COVID-19 infection.

There is a complex pathophysiology link between COVID-19 infection and cardiac manifestations. As there is no definitive treatment for COVID-19 infection, with most of world's population yet to be vaccinated, understanding detailed pathophysiology can help timely and appropriate management of patients.

In this review, we will discuss in detail about pathophysiological link between COVID-19 and cardiovascular manifestations, various cardiac manifestations and its management. Most recommendations are from nonrandomized studies and recommendations from various scientific bodies.

ETIOLOGY AND EPIDEMIOLOGY OF CORONAVIRUS DISEASE 2019 AND CARDIOVASCULAR INVOLVEMENT

Severe acute respiratory syndrome coronavirus 2 is a member of genus *Betacoronavirus* and is the seventh coronavirus known to infect humans.

Till date there have been approximately 22 crores cases in world with 3.31 crores cases in India causing approximately 46 lacs deaths in world with 4.41 lacs deaths in India till date.

Severe acute respiratory syndrome coronavirus 2 causes pneumonia and adult respiratory distress syndrome (ARDS), and in addition multiorgan involvement with special predilection for cardiovascular system.

Baseline Cardiovascular Disease and Coronavirus Disease 2019

There is strong correlation between pre-existing cardiovascular risk factors and severity of COVID-19 infection. Though it may vary widely from 4 to 40% depending on population studied, study period, and scale of study.

In early study from China, 32–46% of patients had underlying diseases, including hypertension (15–31%), CVD (14.5–15%), coronary artery disease (CAD) (4.2%), and diabetes (10–20%). Mortality rates were higher in patients with pre-existing risk factors—10.5% for CAD, 7.3% for diabetes, 6% for hypertension, as against crude mortality of 2.3%.

In a recent study from New York, USA—hypertension was present in 56.6% of patients, CAD in 11.1% of patients, congestive heart failure (HF) in 6.9%, obesity in 41.7% of patients, and diabetes in 33.8% of patients.

In a small study from India of 144 patients—diabetes was present in 11.1%, hypertension in 2.1%, and CAD in 0.7%.

Coronavirus Disease 2019 and Cardiovascular Manifestations

Severe acute respiratory syndrome coronavirus 2 directly or indirectly affects cardiovascular system, with heart frequently involved by multifactorial mechanism as will be discussed below. Impact will be greater in patients with pre-existing CVD and its risk factors. Rate of myocardial involvement ranged from 7 to 28%. In one study, patients with CVD had fatality rates of 22.7%. The extent of myocardial involvement ranged from asymptomatic elevations of cardiac biomarkers to severe manifestations such as myocardial infarction (MI), heart failure, stress cardiomyopathy, and out of hospital cardiac arrest.

Impact on Cardiovascular Care

After COVID-19 pandemic, there was significant decline in admission for acute coronary syndrome (ACS) and percutaneous coronary intervention (PCI) by 40–50%. This has been confirmed by three large studies from Northern California, Italy, and England. Rates of hospitalization were more pronounced for non-ST segment elevation myocardial infarction (NSTEMI). In spite of decline in admissions for ACS, mortality for STEMI was more compared to pre-COVID era, and rates out of hospital cardiac arrest was also found to be higher.

Possible explanations were:
- Patient's fear of contacting COVID infection and avoiding medical care unless emergent situation arises
- Redistribution of healthcare system—evaluation and management of stable coronary disease patients were not on priority, unless not relieved with medical therapy or getting unstable.
- Change in lifestyle during pandemic

PATHOPHYSIOLOGY: IN RELATION TO CARDIOVASCULAR SYSTEM

Coronaviruses are enveloped, single-stranded ribonucleic acid (RNA) viruses with surface projections that correspond to surface spike proteins. The natural reservoir of SARS-CoV-2 seems to be the chrysanthemum bat, with pangolins as likely intermediate host, but not confirmed but the intermediate host remains unclear. The transmissibility and infectivity of SARS-CoV-2 is greater than that of influenza or SARS-coronavirus. Transmission occurs primarily by a combination of spread by droplet, and direct and indirect contact, and may possibly be airborne as well. The viral incubation period is 2–14 days, (mostly 3–7 days). It is contagious during the latency period. SARS-CoV-2 can initially be detected 1–2 days prior to onset of upper respiratory tract symptoms.

The host receptor through which SARS-CoV-2 enters cells to trigger infection is angiotensin-converting enzyme 2 (ACE2). ACE2 is involved in SARS through its function as the coronavirus receptor. Binding of the SARS-CoV-2 spike protein to ACE2 facilitates virus entry into lung alveolar epithelial cells, where it is highly expressed, through processes involving cell surface associated transmembrane protein serine 2 (TMPRSS2). Within the host cell cytoplasm, the viral genome RNA is released and replicates leading to newly formed genomic RNA, which is processed into virion-containing vesicles that fuse with the cell membrane to release the virus. In addition to the lungs, ACE2 is highly expressed in human heart, vessels, and gastrointestinal tract.

Coronavirus 2019 is primarily a respiratory disease, but it can directly or indirectly involve cardiovascular system, especially with severe infection. Many patients also have pre-existing CVD, or its risk factors such as HTN, diabetes, obesity, dyslipidemia. In both scenarios, there is increased morbidity and mortality.

Cardiovascular manifestations are attributed to either direct viral injury or as a consequence of hyperimmune response to infection. In severe infection, there is hyperimmune response with increase in inflammatory markers such as interleukins (IL-2, 6, and 7), tumor necrosis alpha, granulocyte colony-stimulating factor, C-X-C motif chemokine 10 (CXCL10), chemokine (C-C motif) ligand 2, complement and macrophage activation, causing cytokine release syndrome (CRS). Higher viral load and severe infection have been attributed to higher levels of inflammatory markers. Disseminated intravascular coagulation has been in >70% of severe cases.

Autopsy studies have showed coronary thrombosis in microvasculature and endothelitis as major mechanism of myocardial involvement causing myocarditis, myocardial dysfunction, and HF. Myocarditis appears several days after initiation of fever. Mechanisms of SARS-CoV-2-induced myocardial injury may be related to upregulation of ACE2 in the heart and coronary vessels. Cardiac injury leads to activation of the innate immune response with release of proinflammatory cytokines, as well as to the activation of adaptive autoimmune type mechanisms through molecular mimicry.

Hyperinflammatory state predisposes to plaque rupture/erosion and type I MI, or decompensation of pre-existing CAD. Type II MI can be caused by demand–supply mismatch due to hypoxia, hemodynamic, and respiratory derangement. Severe hypoxia itself can have myocardial depressant effect. Patient can also manifest as stress cardiomyopathy due underlying infection and CRS. Right ventricular strain may be present due to pulmonary embolism (PE), severe hypoxia caused by pneumonia and, ARDS.

Myocardial involvement can still happen in mild-to-moderate cases, though majority may be subclinical. In a study of 100 recovered patients, cardiac MRI showed myocardial involvement in 78% of patients with ongoing inflammation in 60% of patients.

Relationship between Hypertension, Angiotensin-converting Enzyme 2, and Coronavirus Disease 2019

Though initial studies found higher prevalence of HTN and presence of severe disease in HTN patients, it was found most likely to be confounding due to age and associated comorbidities. Initial speculation about patients taking angiotensin-converting enzyme (ACE) inhibitors and angiotensin receptor blockers (ARBs) being more vulnerable to infection and severity was refuted in later studies. Instead in experimental models, it was postulated that ARBs may have a protective effect. Recent observational study of over 8,910 patients from 169 hospitals in Asia, Europe, and North America did not show a harmful association of ACEIs or ARBs with in-hospital mortality, while a Wuhan study demonstrated that in 1,128 hospitalized patients use of ACEI/ARB was associated with lower risk of COVID-19 infection or serious complication or deaths from COVID-19 infection. Guidelines from major CV Societies advocate that patients on or ARBs should not stop their treatment.

CARDIOVASCULAR MANIFESTATIONS IN CORONAVIRUS DISEASE 2019

Myocarditis

Myocardial injury is an important prognostic marker and is strongly associated with mortality. Myocardial injury can range from asymptomatic elevation in cardiac biomarkers like troponin and NT-pro BNP to severe involvement causing bi-ventricular dysfunction and HF. Acute cardiac injury was found in 8–12% of COVID-19 patients, and it was 13 times more common in severely ill patients. High levels of inflammatory markers, cardiac biomarkers, and CRS were associated with fulminant myocarditis and high mortality. In studies, high NT-pro BNP (27.5%) and troponin T (TnT) (10%) were also associated with high levels of inflammatory markers. Though most cases of myocarditis may improve with resolving COVID-19 infection and CRS, few may persistently manifest as dilated cardiomyopathy.

In severe cases, evaluation relies on serial monitoring of cardiac biomarkers and bedside two-dimensional (2D) echocardiography. 2D echocardiography may reveal varying grades of left ventricular (LV) dysfunction depending on severity. In fulminant myocarditis, there may be severe biventricular dysfunction resulting in cardiogenic shock. Cardiac MRI revealed biventricular myocardial interstitial edema along with late gadolinium enhancement. Extent of involvement depends on severity of involvement. In fulminant cases, autopsy studies have shown infiltration of interstitium with mononuclear inflammatory cells.

Acute Coronary Syndrome

Acute coronary syndrome can be due to plaque rupture, demand–supply mismatch, endothelial dysfunction, coronary artery spasm, hypercoagulability (thromboembolic environment) and decompensation of pre-existing CAD. Presentation of ACS in COVID-19 infection may be atypical, most may not complain of chest pain, and present with unexplained tachycardia, HF, or cardiogenic shock. Manifestations of ACS are similar to those without COVID-19 infection.

In an early study from China, up to 27.8% had elevated TnT levels during index hospitalization for COVID-19. In a case series by Bangalore et al. among 18 patients with STEMI, 5 underwent PCI. This study also showed high prevalence of nonobstructive CAD, variable presentation, and poorer prognosis even after revascularization. In another series from Italy of 28 patients with STEMI, 17 (60.7%) had critical disease and 11 (39.3%) had nonobstructive CAD. Delayed presentation with ACS was also a concern during pandemic as discussed earlier. Delayed presentation was frequently complicated by mechanical complications like cardiogenic shock with in-hospital mortality up to 42.9%

Acute coronary syndrome was not always present during active inflammatory stage; it may also present during early stage or even in those recovering from infection. There may be diagnostic dilemma, as myocarditis or stress cardiomyopathy can cause similar clinical and laboratory features as ACS.

Stress Cardiomyopathy

A study noted increased incidence of stress cardiomyopathy in pandemic, compared to prepandemic era. It is frequently complicated by HF, cardiogenic shock, arrhythmias, and hypertensive crisis. It frequently recovers after resolution of COVID-19 and inflammatory state. In a study of 12 cases of stress cardiomyopathy, the mean age was 70.8 years and commonly occurred in female patients. Study showed elevated troponin level in 11 patients, no significant CAD on invasive coronary angiography in two patients, CAD in artery supplying a different territory in one case, negative computed tomography coronary angiography in five cases, and no CAD on autopsy in one case; angiography was not done in three cases.

Heart Failure

Heart failure in COVID-19 can be due to myocarditis, ACS, tachyarrhythmia, acute right stress (cor pulmonale), and decompensation of chronic HF. Patients with HF complain of dyspnea, palpitations, and fatigue, and is difficult to differentiate it from symptoms of ARDS caused by COVID-19. Cardiac markers can guide in diagnosis of myocardial involvement. HF ranged from 4.1 to 23% in various studies and had poor prognosis. In a study from China, 23% of inpatients had HF. In retrospective studies HF was found in 49–52% of patients who died. On imaging, in addition to classical COVID features, additional features due to HF, were higher ratio of central and gradient distribution, ratio of expansion of small pulmonary veins was higher, and these features subsided with HF treatment.

Acute cor pulmonale due to PE or severe hypoxia secondary to ARDS has been described in COVID-19. Both scenarios are more common in severely ill patients.

Arrhythmias

Potential causes for various arrhythmias include—cardiovascular complications like myocarditis, ACS, hyperinflammatory state, hypoxia, metabolic abnormalities—acidosis, hypokalemia, drugs—hydroxychloroquine (HCQ), azithromycin, remdesivir, fever unmasking channelopathies like Brugada syndrome.

Atrial fibrillation followed by atrial flutter was the most common tachyarrhythmia notes, whereas sinus bradycardia was the most common bradyarrhythmia noted. Incidence of malignant arrhythmia was found to be 5.9% in an initial study from China. In a study from Hubei province, 7.3% reported with palpitations. In another study, 17% presented with arrhythmias in general cohort, while it was present in 44% of patients admitted to ICU, and 11% of patients had ventricular tachyarrhythmias (VT). In a study of 143 patients, nonsustained VT occurred in 15.4% and premature ventricular contractions in 28.8% of patients with sustained ventricular arrhythmias though uncommon occurred as ventricular fibrillation in 1.4% and ventricular tachycardia in 0.7%. Severe bradyarrhythmias occurred as complete atrioventricular (AV) block in 1.4% and sinus arrest in 0.7%, with most requiring permanent pacemaker implantation.

Prolonged QTc (>500 ms) was found in 6.1% patients at time of admission in a multicentre New York cohort. HCQ and azithromycin commonly used in treatment were found to be associated to be increased incidence of prolonged

QTc, especially when used as combination therapy (up to 20% and 33% in studies). There was no difference in mortality noted for patients receiving HCQ + azithromycin or azithromycin alone. No patients had Torsades de Pointes (TdP), although only 1 patient had TdP in one study.

Thromboembolism

Hyperinflammatory states and hypercoagulability predispose to thromboembolic states and remain a major challenge in critically ill patients. The risk of venous thromboembolism was found to be 31-40% in critically ill patients, while risk of PE was found to be up to 20-23% in two case series from Italy. Unexplained worsening of hypoxia or hemodynamic instability, and unexplained tachycardia should raise suspicion for diagnosis. D-dimer will be invariably raised in CRS, so bedside 2D echocardiography and CT pulmonary angiography if feasible should be done for diagnosis of PE. Treatment decision for thrombolysis can be done based on combination of 2D echocardiography feature and hemodynamic instability.

Disseminated intravascular coagulation (DIC) occurred in 71.4% of patients who died of COVID-19 infection. DIC patients showed high levels of inflammatory markers and D-dimer, high fibrinogen levels, low antithrombin levels, elevated protein C levels, and pulmonary microvascular thrombosis and occlusion with fibrin deposition.

Apart from PE, there have been many reports of other systemic venous and arterial thrombosis.

Multisystem Inflammatory Syndrome in Children

Children with COVID-19 are manifesting with an inflammatory syndrome sharing features similar to Kawasaki Disease. Children usually presented with fever, gastrointestinal symptoms, rash, and mucosal changes. They frequently developed vasculitis with coronary involvement causing dilatation and coronary thrombosis, and also myocarditis with ventricular dysfunction and cardiogenic shock in few patients.

EVALUATION AND MANAGEMENT OF CARDIAC MANIFESTATIONS IN COVID-19 INFECTION

Outpatients

Patients being managed as home-based care should be educated regarding cardiac symptoms. Cardiac biomarkers and electrocardiogram (ECG) should be advised if any symptom arises. D-dimer should be measured as a marker for hypercoagulability and anticoagulation advised if elevated.

Patients with pre-existing CV risk factors and pre-existing CVDs should be monitored more closely and preferably admitted as per risk profile of patients. CV risk factors such as HTN, diabetes, and dyslipidemia should be under control. HF medications optimized. Specific laboratory evaluation such as NT-pro BNP, ECG, 2D echocardiography, troponin, and sugars as clinically indicated.

Inpatients

Principles of evaluation and management include—optimizing pre-existing CV risk factors and CVDs, and diagnosing cardiac manifestations early with appropriate management. Laboratory investigations should be used judiciously and interpreted based on underlying clinical scenario.

Effect of Current Anticoronavirus Disease 2019 Therapies

- Current antiviral therapies remdesivir, favipiravir, and lopinavir-ritonavir have not shown to have benefit on mortality. Remdesivir has been shown to only shorten the duration of hospital stay, but no effect on mortality.
- Role of HCQ and azithromycin either alone or in combination is still controversial.
- Randomized Evaluation of COVID-19 Therapy (RECOVERY) study showed beneficial role of dexamethasone only in patients requiring oxygen or mechanical ventilation. No benefit in patients not requiring any respiratory support.
- Studies have also shown beneficial role of anticoagulation [antiplatelets, low-molecular-weight heparin (LMWH)] in moderate-to-severe disease, and showed effectiveness in improving from hypoxia and weaning from ventilator, as guided by autopsy studies.

Acute Myocardial Injury and Acute Myocarditis

- Routine screening and evaluation with cardiac biomarkers and 2D echocardiography for clinically suspected myocarditis is recommended.
- In critically ill patients, NT-pro BNP, troponin, and bedside 2D echocardiography remain mainstay of diagnosis. Treatment is usually supportive—management of HF, arrhythmias, and avoidance of cardiotoxic drugs.
- Cardiac MRI can be used for diagnosis in relatively stable and serially followed up for complete recovery.
- Endomyocardial biopsy—can be selected patients where possibility of alternative diagnosis like "giant" cell myocarditis is a possibility and specific immunotherapy can be given. Endomyocardial biopsy can be considered for patients with severe biventricular dysfunction, malignant arrhythmias and in young patients, where alternative diagnosis is more likely.
- *Mechanical circulatory support devices*: Depending on local resources and expertise, extracorporeal membrane oxygenation (ECMO) has been used in 1–25% of patients. ARDS requires veno-venous ECMO, and is switched veno-arterial ECMO if there is severe LV dysfunction. Ventricular assist devices may be used depending on local resource considerations during COVID-19 pandemic.

Acute Coronary Syndrome

- High index of suspicion should be there to diagnose ACS due to atypical presentation.

- For patients presenting with NSTEMI/STEMI, COVID status should be determined before planning any intervention.
- *For COVID-19 patients presenting as "unstable angina"/NSTEMI*: Patient should be stabilized with medical therapy with antiplatelets, statins, anticoagulation, nitrates, and intervention planned once recovered from COVID-19 infection.
- *ST segment elevation myocardial infarction (Flowchart 1)*: Irrespective of COVID-19 status, all STEMI patients should receive standard care as it carries high morbidity and mortality.
- Decision to revascularize with either thrombolysis or primary PCI should be guided as follows:
  - Patients with severe infection (ARDS and multiorgan involvement) decision to revascularize should be done on case-to-case basis, with risk/benefit ratio of therapy, team approach and discussion with family, and if therapy will alter prognosis significantly.
  - *Patients with mild-to-moderate infection*: Primary PCI remains the therapy of choice. Though fibrinolysis was initially preferred, many may still require intervention as rescue PCI or pharmacoinvasive strategy, and realizing that many may be at high bleeding risk.

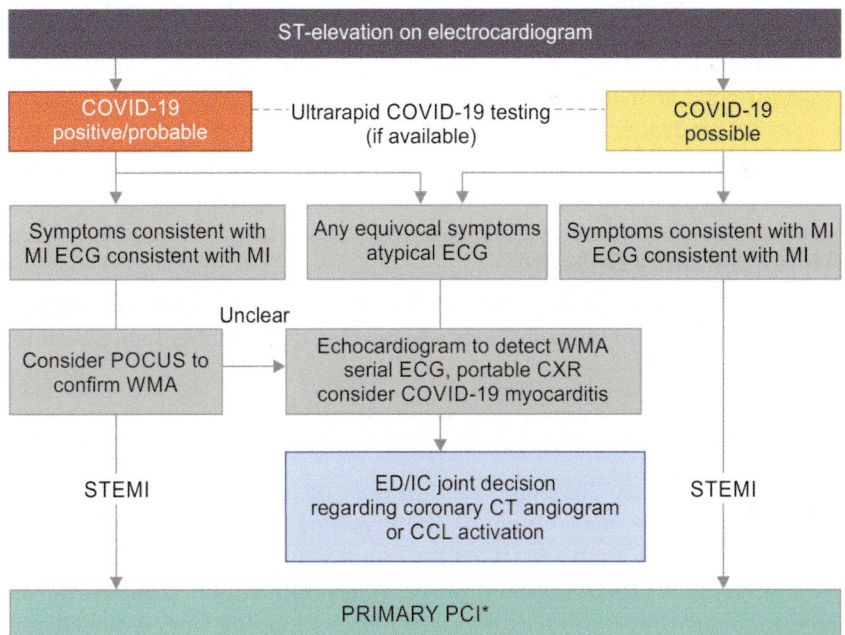

*Primary PCI should always be performed with the universal use of personal protection equipment (PPE) for aerosolized and droplet precautions for the entire CCL team.

(CCL: cardiac catheterization laboratory; COVID: coronavirus disease; ED: emergency department; IC: interventional cardiology; PCI: percutaneous coronary intervention; POCUS: point of care ultrasound; WMA: wall motion abnormalities)

FLOWCHART 1: Algorithm for decision making in patients presenting with ST segment elevation myocardial infarction (STEMI).

- Irrespective of COVID-19 status all catheterization laboratory staff should wear proper personal protection equipment.
- STEMI mimics like myocarditis and stress cardiomyopathy which are seen frequently should be ruled out before any treatment decision. ECG and 2D echocardiography feature suggestive of involvement of noncontiguous areas favor STEMI mimics.

Heart Failure
- Guideline directed medical therapy (GDMT) including ACE inhibitor/ARB should be continued for all chronic HF patients and doses optimized as per HF status during COVID-19 infection.
- Patients who develop de novo HF should be initiated on GDMT with ACEI/ARB, β-blockers and diuretics as per congestive state.
- Low threshold for intubation in acute HF to avoid respiratory distress and aerosolization with emergency intubation.
- Advanced cardiac support devices as discussed above.

Arrhythmias
- It should be managed medically as per standard guidelines.
- Do ECG at baseline and monitor serially after starting HCQ, azithromycin for QT prolongation.
- Cardioversion/Defibrillation is used for unstable atrial fibrillation or ventricular arrhythmias.
- Severe bradyarrhythmia like complete heart block (CHB) or sinus pause may require pacemaker if not resolved after acute state of infection. Temporary pacemaker is used for interim period as required.

Acute Pulmonary Embolism
- Indications for fibrinolysis remain the same as per standard guidelines.
- Catheter directed fibrinolysis should be done if patient has high bleeding risk.

CONCLUSION

Coronavirus disease 2019 involves not only respiratory system, but also has cardiovascular involvement. Pathophysiological relationship between COVID-19 and CV manifestations is complex. Patients with pre-existing CV risk factors or CVD are more prone to develop cardiac complications. Treatment of these CV complications is challenging and is based on guidelines for patients without COVID-19 infection.

SUGGESTED READINGS

1. World Health Organization. (2021). Report of the WHO-China Joint Mission on Coronavirus Disease 2019 (COVID-19). [online] Available from https://www.who.int/docs/default-source/coronaviruse/who-china-joint-mission-on-covid-19-final-report.pdf [Last accessed September, 2021].

2. Zhu N, Zhang D, Wang W, Li X, Yang B, Song J, et al. A novel coronavirus from patients with pneumonia in China, 2019. N Engl J Med. 2020;382:727-33.
3. Zhou P, Yang XL, Wang XG, Hu B, Zhang L, Zhang W, et al. A pneumonia outbreak associated with a new coronavirus of probable bat origin. Nature. 2020;579:270-3.
4. World Health Organization. (2021). WHO Coronavirus Disease (COVID-19) Dashboard. [online] Available from https://covid19.who.int/ [Last accessed September, 2021].
5. Wu Z, McGoogan JM. Characteristics of and Important Lessons From the Coronavirus Disease 2019 (COVID-19) Outbreak in China: Summary of a Report of 72 314 Cases From the Chinese Center for Disease Control and Prevention. JAMA. 2020;323:1239-42.
6. Liang W, Guan W, Chen R, Wang W, Li J, Xu K, et al. Cancer patients in SARS-CoV-2 infection: a nationwide analysis in China. Lancet Oncol. 2020;21:335-7.
7. Epidemiology Working Group for NCIP Epidemic Response, Chinese Center for Disease Control and Prevention. [The epidemiological characteristics of an outbreak of 2019 novel coronavirus diseases (COVID-19) in China]. Zhonghua Liu Xing Bing Xue Za Zhi. 2020;41:145-51.
8. Guan WJ, Ni ZY, Hu Y, Liang WH, Ou CQ, He JX, et al. Clinical Characteristics of Coronavirus Disease 2019 in China. N Engl J Med. 2020;382:1708-20.
9. Chow YW, Pietranico R, Mukerji A. Studies of oxygen binding energy to hemoglobin molecule. Biochem Biophys Res Commun. 1975;66:1424-31.
10. Richardson S, Hirsch JS, Narasimhan M, Crawford JM, McGinn T, Davidson KW, et al. Presenting characteristics, comorbidities, and outcomes among 5700 patients hospitalized with COVID-19 in the New York City area. JAMA. 2020;323:2052-9.
11. Mohan A, Tiwari P, Bhatnagar S, Patel A, Maurya A, Dar L, et al. Clinico-demographic profile & hospital outcomes of COVID-19 patients admitted at a tertiary care centre in North India. Indian J Med Res. 2020;152:61-9.
12. Bonow RO, Fonarow GC, O'Gara PT, Yancy CW. Association of Coronavirus Disease 2019 (COVID-19) with Myocardial Injury and Mortality. JAMA Cardiol. 2020;5:751-3.
13. Shi S, Qin M, Shen B, Cai Y, Liu T, Yang F, et al. Association of cardiac injury with mortality in hospitalized patients with COVID-19 in Wuhan, China. JAMA Cardiol. 2020;5:802-10.
14. Bangalore S, Sharma A, Slotwiner A, Yatskar L, Harari R, Shah B, et al. ST-segment elevation in patients with COVID-19—A case series. N Engl J Med. 2020;382:2478-80.
15. Puntmann VO, Carerj ML, Wieters I, Fahim M, Arendt C, Hoffmann J, et al. Outcomes of cardiovascular magnetic resonance in patients recently recovered from coronavirus disease 2019 (COVID-19). JAMA Cardiol. 2020;5:1265-73.
16. Garcia S, Albaghdadi MS, Meraj PM, Schmidt C, Garberich R, Jaffer FA, et al. Reduction in ST-Segment Elevation Cardiac Catheterization Laboratory Activations in the United States During COVID-19 Pandemic. J Am Coll Cardiol. 2020;75:2871-2.
17. De Filippo O, D'Ascenzo F, Angelini F, Bocchino PP, Conrotto F, Saglietto A, et al. Reduced Rate of Hospital Admissions for ACS during Covid-19 Outbreak in Northern Italy. N Engl J Med. 2020;383:88-9.
18. Solomon MD, McNulty EJ, Rana JS, Leong TK, Lee C, Sung SH, et al. The Covid-19 Pandemic and the Incidence of Acute Myocardial Infarction. N Engl J Med. 2020;383:691-3.
19. De Rosa S, Spaccarotella C, Basso C, Calabrò MP, Curcio A, Filardi PP, et al. Reduction of hospitalizations for myocardial infarction in Italy in the COVID-19 era. Eur Heart J. 2020;41:2083-8.

20. Mahfam MM, Spata E, Goldacre R, Curnow C, Bray M, Holings S, et al. COVID-19 pandemic and admission rates for and management of acute coronary syndromes in England. Lancet. 2020;396:381-9.
21. Xiang D, Xiang X, Zhang W, Yi S, Zhang J, Gu X, et al. Management and Outcomes of Patients With STEMI During the COVID-19 Pandemic in China. J Am Coll Cardiol. 2020;76:1318-24.
22. Mohammad MA, Koul S, Olivecrona GK, Götberg M, Tydén P, Rydberg E, et al. Incidence and outcome of myocardial infarction treated with percutaneous coronary intervention during COVID-19 pandemic. Heart. 2020;106:1812.
23. Li Q, Guan X, Wu P, Wang X, Zhou L, Tong Y, et al. Early transmission dynamics in Wuhan, China, of novel coronavirus-infected pneumonia. N Engl J Med. 2020;382:1199-207.
24. Huang C, Wang Y, Li X, Ren L, Zhao J, Hu Y, et al. Clinical features of patients infected with 2019 novel coronavirus in Wuhan, China. Lancet. 2020;395:497-506.
25. Liu PP, Blet A, Smyth D, Li H. The science underlying COVID-19: Implications for the cardiovascular system. Circulation. 2020;142:68-78.
26. Hoffmann M, Kleine-Weber H, Schroeder S, Krüger N, Herrler T, Erichsen S, et al. SARS-CoV-2 cell entry depends on ACE2 and TMPRSS2 and is blocked by a clinically proven protease inhibitor. Cell. 2020;181:271-80. e8.
27. Magro C, Mulvey JJ, Berlin D, Nuovo G, Salvatore S, Harp J, et al. Complement associated microvascular injury and thrombosis in the pathogenesis of severe COVID-19 infection: A report of five cases. Transl Res. 2020;220:1-3.
28. Tang N, Li D, Wang X, Sun Z. Abnormal coagulation parameters are associated with poor prognosis in patients with novel coronavirus pneumonia. J Thromb Haemost. 2020;18:844-7.
29. Mehra MR, Desai SS, Kuy S, Henry TD, Patel AN. Cardiovascular Disease, Drug Therapy, and Mortality in Covid-19. N Engl J Med. 2020.;382. e.102.
30. Bean DM, Kraljevic Z, Searle T, Bendayan R, Pickles A, Folarin A, et al. Treatment with ACE-inhibitors is associated with less severe disease with SARS-Covid-19 infection in a multi-site UK acute Hospital Trust. medRxiv. 2020.
31. de Abajo FJ, Rodríguez-Martín S, Lerma V, Mejía-Abril G, Aguilar M, García-Luque A, et al. Use of renin–angiotensin–aldosterone system inhibitors and risk of COVID-19 requiring admission to hospital: a case-population study. The Lancet. 2020;395(10238):1705-14.
32. Li J, Wang X, Chen J, Zhang H, Deng A. Association of Renin-Angiotensin System Inhibitors With Severity or Risk of Death in Patients With Hypertension Hospitalized for Coronavirus Disease 2019 (COVID-19) Infection in Wuhan, China. JAMA Cardiol. 2020;5(7):1-6.
33. Mancia G, Rea F, Ludergnani M, Apolone G, Corrao G. Renin-Angiotensin-Aldosterone System Blockers and the Risk of Covid-19. N Engl J Med. 2020;382(25):2431-40.
34. Reynolds HR, Adhikari S, Pulgarin C, Troxel AB, Iturrate E, Johnson SB, et al. Renin-Angiotensin-Aldosterone System Inhibitors and Risk of Covid-19. N Engl J Med. 2020;382(25):2441-8.
35. Zhang P, Zhu L, Cai J, Lei F, Qin JJ, Xie J, et al. Association of Inpatient Use of Angiotensin Converting Enzyme Inhibitors and Angiotensin II Receptor Blockers with Mortality Among Patients With Hypertension Hospitalized With COVID-19. Circ Res. 2020;126(12):1671-81.
36. Hu H, Ma F, Wei X, Fang Y. Coronavirus fulminant myocarditis saved with glucocorticoid and human immunoglobulin. Eur Heart J. 2020; ehaa190.
37. Inciardi RM, Lupi L, Zaccone G, Italia L, Raffo M, Tomasoni D, et al. Cardiac involvement in a patient with coronavirus disease 2019 (COVID-19). JAMA Cardiol. 2020;5:819-24.

38. Singh S, Desai R, Gandhi Z, Fong HK, Doreswamy S, Desai V, et al. Takotsubo Syndrome in Patients with COVID-19: a Systematic Review of Published Cases. SN Compr Clin Med. 2020;1-7.
39. Guo T, Fan Y, Chen M, Wu X, Zhang L, He T, et al. Cardiovascular implications of fatal outcomes of patients with coronavirus disease 2019 (COVID-19). JAMA Cardiol. 2020;5:811-8.
40. World Health Organization. (2020). The Cardiotoxicity of Antimalarials: World Health Organization Malaria Policy Advisory Committee Meeting. [online] Available from https://www. who.int/malaria/mpac/mpac-mar2017-erg-cardiotoxicityreport-session2.pdf. [Last accessed September, 2021].
41. Bessière F, Roccia H, Argaud L, Charrière R, Chevalier P, Argaud L, et al. Assessment of QT intervals in a case series of patients with coronavirus disease 2019 (COVID-19) infection treated with hydroxychloroquine alone or in combination with azithromycin in an intensive care unit. JAMA Cardiol. 2020;5:1067-9.
42. Mercuro NJ, Yen CF, Shim DJ, Maher TR, McCoy CM, Zimetbaum PJ, et al. Risk of QT interval prolongation associated with use of hydroxychloroquine with or without concomitant azithromycin among hospitalized patients testing positive for coronavirus disease 2019 (COVID-19). JAMA Cardiol. 2020;5:1036-41.
43. Grillet F, Behr J, Calame P, Aubry S, Delabrousse E. Acute pulmonary embolism associated with COVID-19 pneumonia detected with pulmonary CT angiography. Radiology. 2020;296:E186-8.
44. Poissy J, Goutay J, Caplan M, Parmentier E, Duburcq T, Lassalle F, et al. Pulmonary embolism in patients with COVID-19: Awareness of an increased prevalence. Circulation. 2020;142:184-6.
45. Cavalcanti AB, Zampieri FG, Rosa RG, Azevedo LCP, Veiga VC, Avezum A, et al. Hydroxychloroquine with or without Azithromycin in mild-to-moderate COVID-19. N Engl J Med. 2020;383:2041-52.
46. Wang Y, Zhang D, Du G, Du R, Zhao J, Jin Y, et al. Remdesivir in adults with severe COVID-19: A randomised, double-blind, placebo-controlled, multicentre trial. Lancet. 2020;395:1569-78.
47. RECOVERY Collaborative Group, Horby P, Lim WS, Emberson JR, Mafham M, Bell JL, et al. Dexamethasone in hospitalized patients with COVID-19: Preliminary report. N Engl J Med. 2021;384(8):693-704.
48. European Society of Cardiology. (2021). ESC guidance for the diagnosis and management of CV disease during the COVID-19 pandemic. [online] Available from https://www.escardio. org/Education/COVID-19-and-Cardiology/ESC-COVID-19- Guidance. [Last accessed September, 2021].
49. Mahmud E, Dauerman HL, Welt FG, Messenger JC, Rao SV, Grines C, et al. Management of acute myocardial infarction during the COVID-19 Pandemic: A Consensus Statement from the Society for Cardiovascular Angiography and Interventions (SCAI), the American College of Cardiology (ACC), and the American College of Emergency Physicians (ACEP). J Am Coll Cardiol. 2020;96:336-45.
50. Mahmud E, Dauerman HL, Welt FGP, Messenger JC, Rao SV, Grines C, et al. Management of Acute Myocardial Infarction During the COVID-19 Pandemic: A Position Statement From the Society for Cardiovascular Angiography and Interventions (SCAI), the American College of Cardiology (ACC), and the American College of Emergency Physicians (ACEP)). J Am Coll Cardiol. 2020;76(11):1375-84.

33. Nutrition in Diabetes: Relevance and Current Evidence

Shashank R Joshi

INTRODUCTION

A wide spectrum of patients, ranging from malnourished, lean, thin built with central obesity, normal weight with normal built, overweight, obese and morbidly obese, present at a diabetes clinic. The current endeavor in managing patients with diabetes is with transcultural approach which apart from medications includes lifestyle and culturally sensitive healthy eating patterns which are individualized.[1]

Structured medical nutrition therapy (MNT) remains one of the core component for effective and long-term diabetes care. An individualized MNT program is recommended for all people with type 1 diabetes mellitus (T1DM) or type 2 diabetes mellitus (T2DM) or gestational diabetes mellitus by majority of national and international organizations for diabetes and endocrinology. One of the important elements of MNT is to support weight loss in all overweight or obese patients with prediabetes and T2DM. The other common elements of MNT which remain common across the stages of diabetes include portion control, carbohydrate distribution, use of low glycemic index carbohydrates, and high fiber content.[2] Many of the patients are also having some or other kind of comorbidities and their nutrition needs also should be met. Some susceptible patient may require proper nutrition planning to prevent hypoglycemia episodes. Hydration maintenance should also be given proper attention, specifically in elderly patients, active patients, or athletes or in patients with chronic kidney disease or heart failure (**Fig. 1**).

GOALS OF NUTRITION THERAPY

- To promote and support healthful eating patterns, emphasizing a variety of nutrient-dense foods in appropriate portion sizes, to improve overall health and achieve and maintain body weight goals.
- Attain individualized glycemic, blood pressure, and lipid goals to delay or prevent the complications of diabetes.
- To address individual nutrition needs based on personal and cultural preferences, health literacy and numeracy, access to healthful foods, willingness and ability to make behavioral changes, and existing barriers to change.

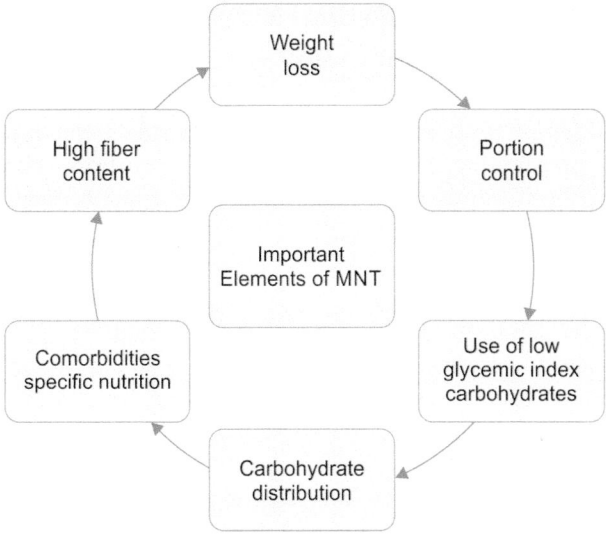

(MNT: medical nutrition therapy)

FIG. 1: Important elements of MNT.

- To maintain the pleasure of eating by providing nonjudgmental messages about food choices while limiting food choices only when indicated by scientific evidence.
- To provide an individual with diabetes the practical tools for developing healthy eating patterns rather than focusing on individual macronutrients, micronutrients, or single foods.

EFFECTIVENESS AND EVIDENCES

Medical nutrition therapy is found to reduce glycosylated hemoglobin (HbA1c) by 1–2% in patients with T2DM over 6 months and improvement in cholesterol parameters when incorporated with exercise.[3] In a multicentric randomized controlled trial (Look AHEAD study) conducted in the US with patients with T2DM, intensive lifestyle intervention compared to diabetes supports education showed a short-term as well as a long-term significant reduction in weight and glycemic parameters.[4] A similar randomized controlled study from Malaysia involving 230 patients with T2DM receiving either usual care or UC with structured lifestyle intervention based on a transcultural diabetes-specific nutrition formula (DSNF) showed a significant weight loss and reduction in HbA1c at 6 months.[5] Following such numerous studies, various national and international organizations have recommended proper MNT as first line recommendation for diabetes, prediabetes, and obesity.

Newer Evidences about Medical Nutrition Therapy, Incretin Axis, and Glycemic Control

There are direct and indirect effects of nutrients on glycogen-like peptide-1 (GLP-1) secretion from intestinal enteroendocrine L-cells. On a meal ingestion, enteroendocrine cells release GLP-1, an important incretin, that acts on both pancreatic β-cells to enhance insulin secretion and α-cells to suppress glucagon secretion.[6] Additionally, GLP-1 has favorable effects at pancreatic and extrapancreatic sites, viz. facilitating increased β-cell proliferation and reduced β-cell apoptosis in pancreas, reduced gluconeogenesis in liver, increased lipogenesis in adipose tissue, increased glucose uptake and storage in skeletal muscles, reducing gastric emptying, supporting neuroprotection, reducing appetite, supporting cardiac and renal protection, and improving endothelial function.[7] The secretion profile for GLP-1 is biphasic with an early peak approximately 30 minutes after nutrient ingestion and a second, more prolonged peak at 60–120 minutes.[8]

Diabetes-specific Nutrition Formulas—Beyond Just Protein Supplements

Many of times, just a simple diet plan prescribed to the patient may not fulfil all the disease specific requirements or adequate macronutrient proportion as recommended. That's where the need for DSNF comes in. DSNF, which contain resistant and complex carbohydrates, high fiber, high quality proteins, and high amount of monounsaturated fatty acids, are scientifically designed for people with diabetes that helps maintain blood glucose levels in normal range, helps reduce body weight when used as complete or partial meal replacement, and helps support improvement in lipid and lipoprotein profiles that reduce risks for developing vascular disease with its associated long-term complications. The resistant carbohydrates, "lente carbs" are not easily broken down by the pancreatic amylases leading to their slower absorption and thereby reduced glycemic response. Clinical research also suggests that resistant carbohydrates, dietary fiber, proteins, and unsaturated fatty acids have a positive impact on GLP-1 secretion.[9-11] In a crossover study which assessed GLP-1 response with DSNF compared to oat meal and no meal, it was found that DSNF improved glycemic control and elevated GLP-1 release compared to a healthful breakfast food (oat meal) or skipping breakfast.[12]

A systematic review and meta-analysis by Elia et al. involving of 23 clinical studies found that incorporating DSNF in the lifestyle regimen could significantly reduce the postprandial glucose, peak glucose as well as area under the cure (AUC) glucose.[13] A randomized controlled study by Tatti et al. in obese patients with T2DM established that use of DSNF with hypocaloric diet compared to only hypocaloric diet over 6 months could support a significantly greater weight loss, improvement in HbA1c, cholesterol, and blood pressure compared to baseline.[14] Similarly, DSNFs have been studied in several clinical trials conducted in >13 countries for several endpoints and

DSNFs have been found to enhance GLP-1 secretions, improve glycemic control, improve cholesterol parameters, improve blood pressure, reduce body weight, reduce insulin requirements, reduce healthcare costs, and lower the mortality rates.[5,12,15-18] In a real-world study conducted in India where DSNF was introduced to obese patients with T2DM along with dietary counseling, a clear reduction of AUC of ambulatory glucose profile (AGP) was seen overall at the end of 1 year and AUC reduced by 64% ($p < 0.0001$). There was also reduction of lipids and blood pressure but not statistically significant, except for triglyceride lowering (TG 69 mg% drop; $p < 0.003$).[19]

Based on the findings of various studies, the following clinical recommendation for DSNFs in patients with T2DM could be postulated based on patient body mass index (BMI):[20-22]

- Overweight and obese patients with BMI > 23 who are unable to eat a balanced diet (sick day/travel/unavailability of balanced food/missed meals)—replacement with DSNF are recommended to achieve target BMI and achieve calorie deficit of 250 kcal/day.
- Normal BMI patients (18-22.9) unable to eat a balanced diet (sick day/travel/unavailability of balanced food/missed meals)—replacements with DSNF are recommended.
- Underweight patients with BMI < 18, recommend good balanced diet, and supplement with DSNF to meet desired BMI as per physician's judgment.

As a conclusion to the above discussion, MNT remains one of the vital elements to successful diabetes care. The nutritional invention should be transculturally adopted and individualized in order to ensure better compliance for better clinical outcomes. In case of overweight and obese patients, MNT should also support weight loss. The individual nutrients in MNT should be considered in order to support portion control, carbohydrate distribution, use of low glycemic index carbohydrates, high fiber content, monounsaturated fatty acids, and good quality protein. The nutrients play a biochemically relevant role on GLP-1 secretion leading to clinically meaningful benefits for the patient. DSNFs could be relevant intervention along with MNT for better clinical outcomes in patients with diabetes.

REFERENCES

1. Handelsman Y, Mechanick JI, Blonde L, Grunberger G, Bloomgarden ZT, Bray GA, et al. American Association of Clinical Endocrinologists Medical Guidelines for Clinical Practice for developing a diabetes mellitus comprehensive care plan. Endocr Pract. 2011;17 Suppl 2:1-53.
2. Sievenpiper JL, Chan CB, Dworatzek PD, Freeze C, Williams SL. Erratum to "Nutrition Therapy": Canadian Journal of Diabetes 2018;42(S1):S64-S79. Can J Diabetes. 2019;43(2):153.
3. Pastors JG, Franz MJ, Warshaw H, Daly A, Arnold MS. How effective is medical nutrition therapy in diabetes care? J Am Diet Assoc. 2003;103(7):827-31.
4. Look AHEAD Research Group, Wadden TA, West DS, Delahanty L, Jakicic J, Rejeski J, et al. The Look AHEAD study: a description of the lifestyle intervention and the evidence supporting it. Obesity (Silver Spring). 2006;14(5):737-52.

5. Chee WSS, Gilcharan Singh HK, Hamdy O, Mechanick JI, Lee VKM, Barua A, et al. Structured lifestyle intervention based on a trans-cultural diabetes-specific nutrition algorithm (tDNA) in individuals with type 2 diabetes: a randomized controlled trial. BMJ Open Diabetes Res Care. 2017;5(1):e000384.
6. Kahn SE, Cooper ME, Del Prato S. Pathophysiology and treatment of type 2 diabetes: perspectives on the past, present, and future. Lancet. 2014;383(9922):1068-83.
7. João AL, Reis F, Fernandes R. The incretin system ABCs in obesity and diabetes - novel therapeutic strategies for weight loss and beyond. Obes Rev. 2016;17(7): 553-72.
8. Brubaker PL, Anini Y. Direct and indirect mechanisms regulating secretion of glucagon-like peptide-1 and glucagon-like peptide-2. Can J Physiol Pharmacol. 2003;81(11):1005-12.
9. Grysman A, Carlson T, Wolever TM. Effects of sucromalt on postprandial responses in human subjects. Eur J Clin Nutr. 2008;62(12):1364-71.
10. Bodnaruc AM, Prud'homme D, Blanchet R, Giroux I. Nutritional modulation of endogenous glucagon-like peptide-1 secretion: a review. Nutr Metab (Lond). 2016;13:92.
11. Psichas A, Sleeth ML, Murphy KG, Brooks L, Bewick GA, Hanyaloglu AC, et al. The short chain fatty acid propionate stimulates GLP-1 and PYY secretion via free fatty acid receptor 2 in rodents. Int J Obes (Lond). 2015;39(3):424-9.
12. Devitt AA, Oliver JS, Hegazi A, Mustad VA. Glycemia Targeted Specialized Nutrition (GTSN) improves postprandial glycemia and GLP-1 with similar appetitive responses compared to a healthful whole food breakfast in persons with type 2 diabetes: a randomized, controlled trial. J Diabetes Res Clin Metab. 2012;1(1):20.
13. Elia M, Ceriello A, Laube H, Sinclair AJ, Engfer M, Stratton RJ. Enteral nutritional support and use of diabetes-specific formulas for patients with diabetes: a systematic review and meta-analysis. Diabetes Care. 2005;28(9):2267-79.
14. Tatti P, di Mauro P, Neri M, Pipicelli G, Mussad VA. Effect of a low-calorie high nutritional value formula on weight loss in type 2 diabetes mellitus. Mediterr J Nutr Metab. 2010;3:65-9.
15. Alish CJ, Garvey WT, Maki KC, Sacks GS, Hustead DS, Hegazi RA, et al. A diabetes-specific enteral formula improves glycemic variability in patients with type 2 diabetes. Diabetes Technol Ther. 2010;12(6):419-25.
16. Sun J, Wang Y, Chen X, Chen Y, Feng Y, Zhang X, et al. An integrated intervention program to control diabetes in overweight Chinese women and men with type 2 diabetes. Asia Pac J Clin Nutr. 2008;17(3):514-24.
17. Han YY, Lai SR, Partridge JS, Wang MY, Sulo S, Tsao FW, et al. The clinical and economic impact of the use of diabetes-specific enteral formula on ICU patients with type 2 diabetes. Clin Nutr. 2017;36(6):1567-72.
18. Yu XY, Zhang H. Effects of a nutritional liquid supplement designed for diabetes mellitus on postprandial glucose and pregnancy outcomes in patients with gestational diabetes mellitus. Zhonghua Yi Xue Za Zhi. 2013;93(43):3450-3.
19. Joshi S, Vadgama J, Sound R, Mody P. Impact of Diabetes Specific Nutrition On Glycemic Variability In Obese Type 2 Diabetes Subjects. Endocrin Pract. 2018;24(S1):315.
20. Misra A, Chowbey P, Makkar BM, Vikram NK, Wasir JS, Chadha D, et al. Consensus statement for diagnosis of obesity, abdominal obesity and the metabolic syndrome for Asian Indians and recommendations for physical activity, medical and surgical management. J Assoc Physicians India. 2009;57:163-70.
21. Ditschuneit HH, Flechtner-Mors M, Johnson TD, Adler G. Metabolic and weight-loss effects of a long-term dietary intervention in obese patients. Am J Clin Nutr. 1999;69(2):198-204.
22. Look AHEAD Research Group, Wing RR. Long-term effects of a lifestyle intervention on weight and cardiovascular risk factors in individuals with type 2 diabetes mellitus: four-year results of the Look AHEAD trial. Arch Intern Med. 2010;170(17):1566-75.

Index

Page numbers followed by *b* refer to box, *f* refer to figure, *fc* refer to flowchart, and *t* refer to table.

A

Acidosis 230
Acromegaly 62
Acute coronary syndrome 78, 229, 232
Acute rheumatic fever 15, 19
   classification of 16
   clinical features of 16
   history of 15
   treatment of 19
Adipose tissue 240
Adiposity-based chronic disease 47, 49
Adrenal steroids 78
Adrenergic crisis 81
Adult treatment panel 117
Ageusia 150
Agitation 89
Airway
   eosinophilic inflammation of 176
   epithelial cell 174
   inflammation, pathway of 180*f*
Alanine
   aminotransferase 42
   transaminase 85
Albumin 129, 138
   excretion rate 203, 204
Albuminuria 203
   staging-based on 204*t*
Alcohol 43
Alcoholic liver disease 128
Allergic asthma, severe 177
Allergic eosinophilic asthma 176
Allergic rhinitis 37
Allogeneic hematopoietic stem cell transplant 113
Alprazolam 193
Ambulatory blood pressure monitoring 103
Ameliorates postural hypotension 191
Amiodarone 88
Amitriptyline 193
Amlodipine 28, 59
Amoxapine 193
Amphepramone 120
Amphetamines 82
Anaphylactoid reaction 29
Anemia 29
   refractory 110
Angina 78
Angioedema 29
Angiopoietin 130
Angiotensin 23
   receptor
      blockers 21, 23*f*, 23*t*, 25, 26, 29, 124, 158, 228
      neprilysin inhibitor 134
Angiotensin-converting enzyme 25, 115, 124, 158, 191, 227, 228
   inhibitor 21, 23*t*
      mechanism of action of 23*fc*
Anorexia 85, 89
Anosmia 150, 151
Anticholinergic burden 192, 193*t*
Anticoagulants 150
Antideoxyribonuclease B 17
Antidepressants, tricyclic 78, 88, 191
Antidiabetic medications, use of 159
Antidiuretic hormone 86, 91
   ectopic production of 88
Antigen detection test 17
Antihypertensive effects 27
Anti-immunoglobulin E therapy 177
Anti-interleukin-5 therapy 177
Antimicrobials 212
Antinuclear antibodies 142
Antipsychotic drug 88
Antithymocyte globulin 112
Antivirals 150
Aortic coarctation 78
Aortic dissection 78, 81
   acute 81
Aortic regurgitation 18
Aortic valve 18

Apnea 38
  hypopnea index 39
  obstructive 37
Apparent mineralocorticoid excess syndrome 56, 61
Appetite
  loss of 149
  reducing 240
  suppressants 78
Arginine vasopressin analogs 88
Arrhythmias 38, 230, 234
Arterial blood gas 87
Arterial hypertension 114
Aspartate aminotransferase 42
Aspartate transaminase 85, 129
Aspirin 123, 176
Asthma 65, 68, 71, 72f, 73, 174-176, 178t, 179t, 181t, 182
  acute 73, 88
  development of 68, 180f
  diagnosis of 174, 176
  exacerbation, management of 66fc
  severe 176, 177
  treatment of 67
Asthmatic patients, symptomatic 180
Ataxia 89
Atenolol 193
  half-life of 205f
Atherosclerotic cardiovascular disease 114
Atrial fibrillation 16, 47, 230
Atropine 193
Auscultation 16
Autoimmune
  diseases 220, 221
  hepatitis 43
Autonomic neuropathy 188
Autonomic regulation therapy 135
Azilsartan 28
Azithromycin 230, 231

B

B cells 222
Bacterial infections 142
Baroreceptor activation therapy 134, 134, 136
Basal glucose regulation 137
Basal insulin 138, 139
  long-acting 138
Beclomethasone dipropionate 69t, 193t
Benralizumab 177, 179, 181-183
Benzathine penicillin G 20
Benztropine 193
Beta-agonist
  long-acting 72
  short-acting 70
Betacoronavirus 225
Beta-lactam antibiotics 210
Bezafibrate infarction prevention trial 50
Bicarbonaturia 86
Bicytopenia 149
Biliary cirrhosis, primary 43
Bilirubin 42
Biochemical tests 59
Biopsy 144
Biotransformation 196
Bisphosphonate treatment 35
Black box warning 179
Blood 111
  eosinophil count 178
  investigations 149
Blood pressure 23, 98, 117, 190
  control 123
  elevated 115, 122, 128
  high 77
  lowering efficacy 27f
  systolic 48, 117
Blood urea nitrogen 79, 85
  increased 86
Bloom's taxonomy 11, 11b
Body mass index 117, 123, 129, 241
Bone
  metabolism 35
  mineral density 34
Bone marrow 111
  aspiration 144
Brain
  natriuretic peptide 39
  tumor 88
Bronchiectasis 88
Brugada syndrome 230
Budd–Chiari syndrome 43t
Budesonide 69
Bupropion hydrochloride 193
Burnout 1, 5
  prevention of 4
Burns 86

C

Calcium channel blockers 28, 59, 192
Calf tenderness 144
Canadian Cardiovascular Society 76

Cancer 93, 147
Candesartan 27
Captopril 193
Carbamazepine 88
Cardiac autonomic neuropathy 190
   prevelence of 188
Cardiac catheterization laboratory 233
Cardiac manifestations, management
   of 231
Cardiac metabolism 50
Cardiogenic shock 78
Cardiometabolic disorders 95, 96
Cardiovascular autonomic neuropathy,
   grading of 191
Cardiovascular care 226
Cardiovascular disease 47, 49, 50, 115,
   131, 156, 159, 172, 225, 226
   risk of 191
Cardiovascular disorders 97
Cardiovascular system 225, 227
Carditis
   acute 18
   chronic 18
Carotid intima-media thickness,
   higher 105
Cathepsin G 223
Central apnea 37
Central nervous system disorders 88
Cerebral infarction 44
Cerebral salt wasting 88
Cervical pillows 40
Challenges Facing Indian
   Healthcare 163
Chemoattractant receptor homologous
   molecule 175
Cheyne–Stokes respiration 89*t*
Chlorpheniramine 193
Chlorpromazine 193
Chlorthalidone 193
Cholangitis, primary sclerosing 43
Choledocholithiasis 45
Cholesterol 123
Cholesteryl ester transfer protein 123
Chorea 17, 19, 20
Ciclesonide 69
Cimetidine hydrochloride 193
Ciprofloxacin 88
Cleft palate 37
Clemastine 193
Clomipramine 193
Clonidine, abrupt cessation of 82
Clozapine 193
Cocaine 78, 82
Codeine 193
Colchicine 145, 193
Collagen vascular
   disease 142
   disorders 142
Coma 89
Confirmatory test 60
Congenital adrenal hyperplasia 56, 61
Congestive heart failure 23, 24
Conjunctivitis 150
Connective tissue disorders 37
Consumer health informatics 162
Convulsions 89
Copenhagen burnout inventory 1
Coronavirus disease 2019 (COVID-19)
      65, 148-151, 154-157, 159, 225, 226,
      228, 230, 233
   epidemiology of 148*f*, 152*t*, 225
   etiologies of 225
   exacerbation of 115
   infection 155, 225, 231
   novel 147
   pandemic 149, 215, 226
   prevalence of diabetes in 154
   severe 115, 118, 159, 225
   therapy 232
Coronary artery disease 24, 226
Coronary heart disease 47
Cortisol resistance, primary 56, 61
Cough 29, 149
C-reactive protein 19, 97, 142, 143, 149
   high-sensitivity 124
Creatine kinase 142
Creatinine 142
Culture bacteria 145
Cushing syndrome 56, 62, 78
Cyclic nucleotide-gated family 75
Cyclophosphamide 88
Cyclosporine 78
Cystic fibrosis 88
Cytokine 218, 221
   release syndrome 228
   storm 159
Cytomegalovirus 43, 219
Cytoplasmic proteins 223

D

Darifenacin 193
Daytime sleepiness 38
Decongestants 78

Delirium 149
Deoxycorticosterone-producing tumor 56, 61
Deoxyribonucleic acid 223
Depression 2
Desipramine 193
Diabetes mellitus 30, 93, 137, 147, 154, 155, 159, 172, 225
   complications of 157, 238
   prevention 124
   type 1 157, 188, 238
   type 2 21, 47, 50, 114, 123, 128, 159, 238
Diabetes, nutrition in 238
Diabetic autonomic neuropathy 188, 189, 194
   detection of 189
   signs of 190*b*
   symptoms of 190*b*
Diabetic ketoacidosis 149, 155
Diarrhea 86, 149, 151
Diastolic blood pressure 48, 77, 117
Diazepam 193
Dicyclomine 193
Diencephalic syndrome 78
Diethylpropion 120
Digital application programming interface 170
Digital health 162, 171
   advantages 164*f*
   types of 162
Digital outreach 162, 163, 173
Digoxin 193, 212
Dihexamers 139
Dipeptidyl peptidase-4 159, 160
Diphenhydramine 193
Dipyridamole 193
Direct renin inhibitor 23
Disopyramide phosphate 193
Disseminated intravascular coagulopathy 44
Diuretics 86, 90
Dizziness 78, 150
Domperidone 192
Down's syndrome 37
Doxepin 193
Drowsiness 89
Drugs, variety of 131
Dry cough 151
Dry powder inhaler 69, 71
Dual-energy X-ray absorptiometry 34
Duodenum carcinoma 88
Dupilumab 179-183
Dysautonomia 189
Dysglycemia-based chronic disease 47, 49
Dyslipidemia 114, 122, 225
   treatment of 191
Dysnatremias 84
Dyspnea 149

E

Ear-nose-throat 39
Echocardiography screening 17
Eclampsia 43, 78
Edema 86
Effector T-cells 219
E-health 162
   types of 162
E-healthcare network, comprehensive rural 166*f*
Electrocardiogram 34
Electroencephalogram 39
Electrolytes 142
Electronic health records 162
Elevated liver enzymes 43, 45
Embusartan 29
Emotional intelligence 4
Empirical therapy 145
Enalaprilat 81
Encephalitis 88, 150
Encompassing refractory anemia 110
Endocarditis 145
   peripheral signs of 145
Endocrine hypertension 56
Endogenous shyper 32
Endoscopic retrograde cholangiopancreatography 46
Endothelial damage 159
Endothelial nitric oxide synthase, reduced 50
Endurance exercise 88
Enteroendocrine cells 240
Enteropathy 29
Enuresis 38
Enzymes 206
Eosinophilia 177
   maturation of 174
Eosinophilic asthma 176
   diagnosis of 177
   late-onset 176
Eosinophilic phenotype 176
Eosinophils 174
   level of 176

Epilepsy 150
Episodic headache 57
E-prescribing 162
Epworth sleepiness scale 39
Erythema marginatum 16, 19
Erythrocyte sedimentation rate 19, 142, 143, 149
Erythropoietin 78, 112
  stimulating agents 112
Esmolol 81
Estimated glomerular filtration rate 98
  limitations of 212
Estrogens, high dose 78
Euvolemia 87
Euvolemic hyponatremia 87, 90
Ewing's sarcoma 88
Extracorporeal membrane oxygenation 232
Eyes 144

F

Factitious fever 142
Familial dysautonomia 78
Fasting glucose, elevated 115, 122
Fatigue 149
Fatty acids 241
Febuxostat 100
Fentanyl 193
Ferritin 142, 149
Fever 17, 19, 149, 151
Fibromuscular dysplasia 78
Fibrosis 129
Fimasartan 28, 29
Flapping tremors 89
Flash glucose monitoring techniques 139
Flavoxate 193
Flu pandemic 92
Fluid restriction 90
Fluorescence in situ hybridization 108, 109
Fluorodeoxyglucose 143, 144
Fluticasone
  furoate 69
  propionate 69
Fluvoxamine 193
Food and Drug Administration 65, 180
Formyl peptide receptor 2 175
Framingham heart study 114
Framingham risk score 123
Free fatty acids 118
Free thyroxine 32

French American British 109
Furosemide 193

G

Gallstone disease 43
  symptomatic 45
Gamma delta T cells 221
Gas infection, evidence of 17
Gaseous anesthetics 196
Gastrointestinal system 190
Gastrointestinal tract 196
Gastro-oesophageal reflux disease 38
Genetics 48
Genioglossus advancement 40
Genitourinary system 190
Gestational diabetes 114
Gestational hypertension 114
Global initiative asthma 65
Glomerular filtration rate 25, 203t
Glucocorticoids 19
Glucose-lowering drugs 159, 160f
Glucotoxicity 159
Glycated hemoglobin 118, 123
Glycemic control 240
Granulocyte colony stimulating factor 112
Guideline-directed medical therapy 135
Guillain–Barré syndrome 88, 150

H

Haloperidol 193
Hand grip test 191
Happy hypoxia 149
Head injury 88
Headache 38, 150
Health care information systems 163
Health infrastructure 163t
Healthcare 171
Hearing 216
Heart
  autonomic regulation of 134
  diseases 93
Heart failure 24, 30, 74, 230, 234
  unexplained right 38
Heart rate 74
  reduction 75
Hematopoietic stem cell transplantation 112
Hematuria 79
Hemoglobin 85, 139

Hemolysis 43, 45
Hemorrhage, subconjunctival 150
Heparin 210
Hepatic steatosis 129
Hepatitis
  B
    chronic 43
    immune globulin 45
  C, chronic 43
  E, acute 45
Herpes simplex hepatitis 43
Hiccup 89
Histocompatibility complex, major 175
Host immune responses 219
Human chorionic gonadotropin 121
Human immunodeficiency virus 109, 219
Human immunoglobulin 138
Human insulin 139
Human leukocyte antigen 15, 218
Hydralazine 81, 193
Hydrocephalus 88
Hydrochlorothiazide 28
Hydrocortisone 193
Hydrofluoroalkane 69, 71
Hydroxychloroquine 230
Hydroxylase deficiency 56, 61, 78
Hydroxysteroid dehydrogenase deficiency 56, 78
Hydroxyzine 193
Hyoid myotomy 40
Hyoscyamine 193
Hyperadrenergic state 82
Hyperaldosteronism, primary 59, 78
Hypercalcemia 62, 78
Hyperdeoxycorticosteronism 56, 61
Hyperemesis gravidarum 42, 43, 45
Hyperglycemia 157
Hyperglycemic hyperosmolar syndrome 155
Hyperinflammatory state 228, 230, 231
Hyperkalemia 29
Hyperlipidemia 114
Hypernatremia 84
Hyperparathyroidism 56
  primary 62
Hypertension 56, 57, 62, 79, 95, 103f, 147, 225, 228
  causes of 78
  endocrine causes of 56
  mendelian forms of 78
  postoperative 81
  secondary 56
  treatment of 191
  primary 21
Hypertensive crisis 229
Hypertensive emergency 77, 81, 82
Hypertensive encephalopathy 81
Hyperthyroidism 56, 62, 78
  symptomatic 35
  treatment 35t
Hypertonic hyponatremia 86
Hyperuricemia 95, 96, 97f
  cause of 96
  managing 98
Hypervolemia 86
Hypervolemic hyponatremia 90
Hypoglycemia 138, 139, 188
  severe 139
  symptoms of 139, 192
Hypokalemia 188, 230
Hyponatremia 84, 86, 87, 89, 90
  chronic 89
  management of 89
  signs of 89t
  symptoms of 87, 89t
Hypotension 28, 188
Hypothermia 89
Hypothyroidism 37, 38, 56, 62, 78
Hypovolemia 86
  signs of 86
Hypovolemic hyponatremia 90
Hypoxia 149, 228, 230
  severe 228

I

Ifosfamide 88
I-health 162
Imipramine 193
Immune
  dysfunction 220
  dysregulation 222
  function 157
  system 219
Immunoglobulins 219, 220
Impotence 38
Infection
  control measures 67
  mild-to-moderate 233
Infective endocarditis 16
Inflammation 50
  type 2 174

Inflammatory syndrome 231
Influenza
  A 92
  B 92
  seasons 93
  vaccination, importance of 92
Inhaled corticosteroid 66, 69-72, 179
  dose 69*t*, 71*t*
    high 68, 69
    low 68, 69
    medium 68, 69
  formoterol 67
Insulin 138
  degludec molecule 139
  detemir 138
  discovery of 137
  excess of 138
  glargine 137, 139
  receptor substrate 1 50
  resistance, effect of 50
  secretion 137
    impairment of 155
Intensive care unit 84, 159, 215, 219
Interferon 33, 157
Interleukin 97, 157
International Diabetes
    Federation 117
Interventional cardiology 233
Intracranial hemorrhage 78
Intracranial pressure, acute
    increased 78
Iridocyclitis 150
Ischemic heart disease 147, 188
Isosorbide preparations 193
Ivabradine, role of 75

J

Jaundice 42
  classification of 43*t*
Joint involvement 17

K

Kaplan–Meier curves 94*f*
Kaposi's sarcoma 219
Kidney 157, 196
  disease 147, 159, 205
    chronic 26, 97, 151, 196, 203, 203*b*,
        203*t*, 204, 206, 208
      treatment in 209
  injury, acute 149

L

Labetalol 81
Lactate dehydrogenase 142
Left ventricular
  ejection fraction 101
  end-systolic diameter 135
  failure 78
    acute 81
  hypertrophy 23, 30
  mass index 105
Legionella 88
Leukotriene receptor antagonists 69
Lineage dysplasia 110
Lipopolysaccharide 155
Lipoprotein
  cholesterol, high-density 115, 123
  high-density 48, 114, 117, 123, 124
Lipotoxicity 50
Lipotropic injections plan 121
Liver 144
  cirrhosis of 43
  disease 42-44, 46
    management of 45*t*
    pre-existing 46
  function tests 42
Long-chain 3-hydroxyacyl-coenzyme-A
    dehydrogenase 45
Loop diuretics 81
Loperamide 193
Losartan 27
Loss appetite 89
Low central venous pressure 86
Low dose inhaled corticosteroids 68, 69
Low molecular weight heparin 160
Low platelets syndrome 43, 45
Low-density lipoprotein 95, 123, 124
  cholesterol 118, 123
Lower glycemia 139
Lung 196
  abscesses 88
  carcinoma 88
  diseases 93
  function and symptom scores 181
  mucosa 176
Lymph nodes 144
Lymphoma 88

M

Macroglossia 38
Macrophages 222, 223

Marfan's syndrome 37
Masked hypertension 103, 105
  uncontrolled 104, 105
Maslach burnout inventory 1
Maslow's hierarchy 12
Mast cells, degranulation of 174
Meal ingestion 240
Mechanical circulatory support
  devices 232
Medical nutrition therapy 238, 239,
  239f, 240
Mediterranean fever 145
Memory, altered 38
Meningitis 88
Mepolizumab 69, 177, 179, 181-183
Mesothelioma 88
Metabolic abnormalities 230
Metabolic alkalosis 86
Metabolic complications, acute 155
Metabolic drivers 49
Metabolic dysregulation 128
Metabolic syndrome 95, 97, 114, 115,
  116t, 117, 122, 122t, 123, 123b, 130
  diagnosis of 123
  management of 119
  part of 128
  treatment of 120f
Metabolically healthy obese 49
Metabolic-associated fatty liver
  disease 128
Metabolism 197, 207f
Metoclopramide 192
Metoprolol 193
M-health 162, 163
  works 165
Microalbuminuria 191
  teatment of 191
Microbial antigens 219
Midodrine 192
Mineralocorticoid deficiency 86
Mineralocorticoid receptor 59
Mitochondrial modulation 51
Mitral regurgitation 18
Mitral stenosis 18
Mitral valve 18
  change, acute 18
Molecular weight of drug 197
Mometasone furoate 69
Monoamine oxidase inhibitor 78, 82
Monocyte 222, 223
  chemoattractant protein 97
Montelukast, risk of adverse effects
  of 71

Morphine 193
Mucosal changes 231
Multilineage dysplasia 110
Multiorgan dysfunction 148
Multiple endocrine neoplasia 57
Multisystem inflammatory
  syndrome 231
Muscarinic antagonist, long-acting 72
Muscle cramps 89
Myalgia 151
Myelodysplastic syndrome 108, 110,
  111t, 112, 112t, 113
  classification of 109
  diagnosis of 109f
  features of 109
  prognostication of 110
Myeloid leukemia, acute 108, 113
Myeloperoxidase 223
Myocardial glucose 130
Myocardial infarction 23, 24, 38, 81, 190
  acute 149
Myocardial injury 228
  acute 232
Myocardial oxygen demand 75
Myocarditis 228, 230
  acute 232
Myocardium 157
Myristic acid 138

N

Narcotics 88
Nasal dilators 40
Nasal oxygen, high-flow 147
National Rural Health Mission 169f
Natural killer cells 219, 222
Nausea 44, 78, 85, 89
Necroinflammation 129
Neoplasms 142
Neoplastic tumor 88
Nephropathy 30
Nervous system function 191
Neurofibromatosis 57
Neurovascular systems 188
Neutral protamine hagedorn 138
Neutrophils 222, 223
Nicardipine 59, 81
Nicotine 88
Nifedipine 59, 193
Nitric oxide 50, 97, 174
  synthase 95
Nitroglycerin 81
Nitroprusside 81

Nocturnal hypoglycemia 138, 139
Nonalcoholic fatty liver 129
　disease 95, 97, 114, 128-131
Nonalcoholic steatohepatitis 114
Noneosinophilic asthma, pathogenesis of 176
Noninfectious inflammatory diseases 141
Nonsteroidal anti-inflammatory drugs 19, 78, 143, 145
Noradrenergic drugs 120
N-terminal probrain natriuretic peptide 136
Numerous rheumatic diseases 141
Nutrition formula, diabetes-specific 239, 240
Nutrition therapy, goals of 238

O

Obesity 37, 38, 118, 147
　paradox 49
Obstructive pulmonary disease, chronic 71, 72, 93, 151, 176
Obstructive sleep apnea, risk factors 37
Olmesartan 21, 27, 28
Omalizumab 177, 179, 181
　treatment with 180
Ontarget trial 25
Ophthalmological manifestations 78
Oral appliances 40
Oral corticosteroids 66, 68, 70, 72
Oral ulcers 144
Orthostatic hypotension 191
Osmotic
　demyelination 84, 91
　diuretics 86
Osteoporosis 35
Osteotomy
　mandibular advancement 40
　maxillary advancement 40
Oxidative stress 159
Oxidized nonalcoholic steatohepatitis 129
Oxybutynin 193
Oxycarbamazepine 88
Oxytocin 88

P

Pancreatic carcinoma 88
Pancreaticobiliary disease 45
Pancytopenia 110, 149

Papilledema 150
Parasitic infections 142
Parasympathetic dysautonomia 192
Parasympathetic nervous system 74, 188
Paroxetine 193
Pathologic regurgitation 18
Percutaneous coronary intervention 226, 233
Permanent vision loss 44
Perphenazine 193
Personal air purifying respirators 216
Pharmacological therapy obesity 120
Phencyclidine 78, 82
Phenothiazines 191
Phenoxybenzamine 58
Phentermine 120
Phentolamine 81
Phenylpropanolamine 120
Pheochromocytoma 56, 57, 78, 82
Plasma aldosterone concentration 59
Plasma osmolality 87
Plasma renin state, high 82
Plasma-concentration profile 198f
Plasminogen activator inhibitor 129
Pneumonia 88, 156
Point of care ultrasound 233
Poisoning, lead 78
Polyarthralgia 19
Polycystic kidney disease 78
Polycystic ovarian syndrome 114
Polyneuritis 78
Porphyria, acute 78
　intermittent 88
Positional therapy 40
Positive airway pressure therapy 40
Positron emission tomography 144
Post-COVID
　fatigue syndrome 150
　syndrome 216
Postobstructive diuresis 86
Prazosin 191
Prediabetes 50
Predictable insulins 137
Prednisolone 193
Prednisone 193
Pre-eclampsia 43, 78
Pregnancy
　acute fatty liver of 43-45
　intrahepatic cholestasis of 43, 45
　jaundice in 42
Pressurized metered dose inhaler 67, 69, 71

Procyclidine 193
Promazine 193
Promethazine 193
Prophylaxis, secondary 20*t*
Propranolol 59
Proprotein convertase subtilisin/kexin type 9 123
Prostate cancer 88
Protamine 138
 zinc insulin 137, 138
Proteinuria 79
Pseudohyponatremia 86
Pulmonary arterial hypertension 59
Pulmonary capillary wedge 86
Pulmonary disorders 88
Pulmonary edema, acute 44, 81
Pulmonary embolism 78
 acute 234
Pulmonary function tests 174
Pulmonary hypertension 38
Pulmonary thromboembolism 150
Pupillomotor 190
Pyelonephritis 79
Pyrexia of unknown origin 141
Pyrilamine 193

Q

Quinidine 193

R

Ramipril 21, 25
Randomized controlled trials 67
Ranitidine 193
Rash 231
Reaction, rates of 197
Reactive oxygen species 157
Reflexes 89
Refractory cytopenia 110, 111
Refractory neutropenia 110
Refractory thrombocytopenia 110
Remdesivir 230
Renal blood flow 197
Renal disease 197
 progression of 25
Renal failure 44, 95
 acute 82
 chronic 207
Renal function 29
Renal impairment 209
Renal losses 86
 extra 86

Renal manifestations 79
Renal pathways 210
Renal tubular acidosis 86
Renal tumors 78
Renin-angiotensin-aldosterone system 22*f*, 60, 74, 97, 156, 157, 158*fc*, 191
Resistant hypertension 38
Reslizumab 177, 179-181, 183
 treatment 181
Respiratory depression 89
Respiratory distress syndrome, acute 149, 225
Respiratory disturbance index 39
Respiratory droplets 147
Respiratory failure 149
Respiratory system 190
Retinoic acid receptor 175
Rheumatic fever 20
 acute 19*t*
Rheumatic heart disease 15, 16*f*, 17, 18*b*, 19, 20
Rheumatic valvulitis 18
 acute 16
Rheumatoid factor 142

S

Salicylates 19
Saline infusion test 60
Saliva 196
Salt losing nephropathy 86
Salt restriction 90
Scopolamine 193
Seizures 89
Selective serotonin reuptake inhibitors 88
Sensorium, altered 89, 150
Sepsis 220, 221
 immunology of 218
Serologic tests 141
Serum
 creatinine, elevated 79
 osmolality 85
Severe acute respiratory syndrome 115, 150, 154, 226
Sexual dysfunction 114, 194
Sinoatrial node 75
Skin manifestations 17
Sleep apnea 37
 clinical score 39
 obstructive 37, 78
 syndrome 37
Sleep, poor quality of 38

Sleepiness, excessive day time 38
Small cell carcinoma 88
Solid tumors 141
Spinal cord section, acute 78
Spirometry 65
Spleen 144
Sputum eosinophil count 178
Stable angina 74
Steatosis, etiologies of 128
Steroids 150
    side effects of 145
Still's disease 145
Stomach carcinoma 88
Streptococcal infection 19
Streptococcal upper respiratory tract infection, group A 15
Stress cardiomyopathy 229
Stroke 16, 81, 88, 93, 150
Subarachnoid haemorrhage 88
Subclinical hyperthyroidism 32, 35
    causes of 33*fc*
    diagnosis of 33
Subcutaneous injection 138
Subcutaneous nodules 16, 19
Subdural hematoma 88
Subsequent inflammatory responses 220
Sudden cardiac death 24, 38
Sympathetic autonomic dysfunction 192
Sympathetic nervous system 74, 188
Sympathetic paraganglioma 56
Symptomatic cholecystitis 46
Syndrome of inappropriate antidiuretic hormone secretion 87, 91
    causes of 88*b*
Systemic inflammatory response syndrome 220
Systemic vasoconstriction 38

T

T helper cells 176, 221
Tachycardia 34, 57, 231
Target organ damage 105
Taste, loss of 151
T-cell 220, 221
    population 219
    regulatory 221
Tele diagnosis 171
Tele monitoring 171
Telehealth 162, 167
Telemedicine 162, 167
Telmisartan 25
Temporal arteries 144
    biopsy 144
Tender tooth 144
Tetradecanoic acid 138
Theophylline 193
Thermoregulatory causes 142
Thiazolidinediones 159, 160
Thromboembolism 231
Thymic stromal lymphopoietin 175, 180
Thymoma 88
Thyroid
    dysfunction 62
    function 87
    hormone 34
    stimulating hormone 32, 33, 35
Timolol maleate 193
Tiredness 38
Tissue
    peripheral 139
    sample 145
Tolterodine 193
Tonsils 37
Topiroxostat 100
Total cholesterol 48
Total renal clearance 200*f*
Toxic metabolites 155
Toxicity 205*f*
Transcend trial 25
Transformed kinetics 205*f*, 206*f*
Trazodone 193
Triamterene 193
Trifluoperazine 193
Triglycerides 117
    elevated 115
Trihexyphenidyl 193
Triiodothyronine 32
Tuberculosis 88, 142
Tubular necrosis, diuretic phase of acute 86
Tumor necrosis factor-alpha 118, 131, 219, 227
Typical telemedicine system 165, 165*f*

U

Unilineage dysplasia 110
Unstable angina 81, 233
Upper airway 39
    abnormalities 38
    obstruction 37
Urate lowering therapies 98, 98*f*
Urate transporter 1 96

Uric acid 95, 86
Uricases 101
Uricosurics 101
Urinary osmolality 87
Urinary pH 197
Urinary potassium 85
Urinary sodium 85, 87
Urine
  albumin 85
  osmolality 85, 86
  sodium 86
Uropathy, obstructive 78
Ursodeoxycholic acid 45
Uvulopalatopharyngoplasty 40

V

Vagal nerve stimulation 134
Vagus nerve 134
  stimulation 134
Valproate 88
Valsalva maneuver 190
Valsartan 27
Vaptans 90
Vinblastine 88
Vincristine 88
Viral hepatitis 43
  acute 45
Viral infections 142
Vitamin
  C 216
  D 216
Vomiting 44, 78, 85, 86, 89
von Hippel-Lindau disease 57

W

Waist circumference 115
Wall motion abnormalities 233
Warfarin 193, 212
Weakness 78
  and lethargy 89
Weight loss 119
White-coat hypertension 103
Wilson's disease 43

X

Xanthine oxidase 96
  inhibitors 98
  trials 99t

Z

Zero-order kinetics 199f
Zinc 216
ZOLL's LifeVest 171